Endocrine Hypertension

Guest Editor

LAWRENCE R. KRAKOFF, MD

ENDOCRINOLOGY AND METABOLISM CLINICS OF NORTH AMERICA

www.endo.theclinics.com

Consulting Editor
DEREK LEROITH, MD, PhD

June 2011 • Volume 40 • Number 2

SAUNDERS an imprint of ELSEVIER, Inc.

W.B. SAUNDERS COMPANY
A Division of Elsevier Inc.

1600 John F. Kennedy Boulevard ● Suite 1800 ● Philadelphia, Pennsylvania 19103-2899

http://www.theclinics.com

ENDOCRINOLOGY AND METABOLISM CLINICS OF NORTH AMERICA Volume 40, Number 2
June 2011 ISSN 0889-8529, ISBN-13: 978-1-4557-0441-5

Editor: Rachel Glover
Developmental Editor: Donald Mumford

Endocrinology and Metabolism Clinics of North America (ISSN 0889-8529) is published quarterly by Elsevier Inc., 360 Park Avenue South, New York, NY 10010-1710. Months of issue are March, June, September, and December. Periodicals postage paid at New York, NY and additional mailing offices. Subscription prices are USD 290.00 per year for US individuals, USD 503.00 per year for US institutions, USD 146.00 per year for US students and residents, USD 364.00 per year for Canadian individuals, USD 616.00 per year for Canadian institutions, USD 422.00 per year for international individuals, USD 616.00 per year for international institutions, and USD 216.00 per year for international and Canadian and foreign students/residents. To receive student/resident rate, orders must be accompanied by name of affiliated institution, date of term, and the signature of program/ residency coordinator on institution letterhead. Orders will be billed at individual rate until proof of status is received. Foreign air speed delivery is included in all *Clinics* subscription prices. All prices are subject to change without notice. **POSTMASTER:** Send address changes to *Endocrinology and Metabolism Clinics of North America*, Elsevier Health Sciences Division, Subscription Customer Service, 3251 Riverport Lane, Maryland Heights, MO 63043. **Customer Service: Telephone: 1-800-654-2452** (U.S. and Canada); **1-314-447-8871** (outside U.S. and Canada). **Fax: 1-314-447-8029. E-mail: journalscustomerservice-usa@elsevier.com** (for print support); **journalsonlinesupport-usa@elsevier.com** (for online support).

Reprints. For copies of 100 or more, of articles in this publication, please contact the Commercial Rights Department, Elsevier Inc., 360 Park Avenue South, New York, NY 10010-1710; phone: (+1) 212-633-3813; fax: (+1) 212-462-1935; e-mail: reprints@elsevier.com.

Endocrinology and Metabolism Clinics of North America is covered in *MEDLINE/PubMed (Index Medicus)*, *EMBASE/Excerpta Medica, Current Contents/Clinical Medicine, Current Contents/Life Sciences, Science Citation Index, ISI/BIOMED, BIOSIS*, and *Chemical Abstracts*.

Printed and bound by CPI Group (UK) Ltd, Croydon, CR0 4YY

Transferred to Digital Print 2011

Contributors

CONSULTING EDITOR

DEREK LEROITH, MD, PhD
Chief, Division of Endocrinology, Metabolism, and Bone Diseases, Department of
Medicine, Mount Sinai School of Medicine, New York, New York

GUEST EDITOR

LAWRENCE R. KRAKOFF, MD
Professor of Medicine; Director, Hypertension Program, Cardiovascular Institute, Mount
Sinai Medical Center, New York, New York

AUTHORS

RHONDA BENTLEY-LEWIS, MD, MBA, MMSc
Instructor in Medicine, Harvard Medical School, Diabetes Research Center and Diabetes
Unit, Massachusetts General Hospital, Boston, Massachusetts

ANGELA BOLDO, MD
Fellow, Division of Endocrinology, Dartmouth-Hitchcock Medical Center,
Lebanon, New Hampshire

ROBERT M. CAREY, MD, MACP
David A. Harrison III Distinguished Professor of Medicine; Dean, Emeritus, and
University Professor, Division of Endocrinology and Metabolism, Department of
Medicine, University of Virginia Health System, Charlottesville, Virginia

ROBERT G. DLUHY, MD
Professor of Medicine, Division of Endocrinology, Diabetes and Hypertension,
Harvard Medical School, Brigham and Women's Hospital, Boston, Massachusetts

ANDREA DUNAIF, MD
Charles F Kettering Professor of Endocrinology and Metabolism, Northwestern
University, Feinberg School of Medicine, Chicago, Illinois

RICHARD D. GORDON, MD, PhD, FRACP, FRCP
Professor of Medicine and Co-Director, Endocrine Hypertension Research Center,
University of Queensland School of Medicine, Princess Alexandra Hospital,
Woolloongabba; Greenslopes Private Hospital, Greenslopes, Brisbane, Australia

FLORENCIA HALPERIN, MD
Instructor in Medicine, Division of Endocrinology, Diabetes and Hypertension, Harvard
Medical School, Brigham and Women's Hospital, Boston, Massachusetts

VITALY KANTOROVICH, MD
Assistant Professor of Medicine, Division of Endocrinology and Metabolism,
University of Arkansas for Medical Sciences, Little Rock, Arkansas

LAWRENCE R. KRAKOFF, MD
Professor of Medicine; Director, Hypertension Program, Cardiovascular Institute, Mount Sinai Medical Center, New York, New York

MARIA I. NEW, MD
Professor of Pediatrics, Genetics and Genomics, Mount Sinai School of Medicine, New York, New York

LYNNETTE K. NIEMAN, MD
Senior Investigator, Program on Reproductive and Adult Endocrinology, *Eunice Kennedy Shriver* National Institute of Child Health and Human Development, National Institutes of Health, Bethesda, Maryland

SHARON L.H. ONG, BSc (Med), MBBS, FRACP
Consultant Nephrologist, Department of Nephrology, St George Hospital, Kogarah; Conjoint Lecturer, St George Hospital Clinical School, Faculty of Medicine, University of New South Wales, Sydney, New South Wales, Australia

KAREL PACAK, MD, PhD, DSc
Professor of Medicine, Section on Medical Neuroendocrinology, Program in Reproductive and Adult Endocrinology, *Eunice Kennedy Shriver* National Institute of Child Health and Human Development, National Institutes of Health, Bethesda, Maryland

ALAN A. PARSA, MD
Endocrine Fellow, Mount Sinai School of Medicine, New York, New York

EDUARDO PIMENTA, MD, FAHA
Clinical Research Fellow, Endocrine Hypertension Research Center, University of Queensland School of Medicine, Princess Alexandra Hospital, Woolloongabba; Greenslopes Private Hospital, Greenslopes, Brisbane, Australia

GIAN PAOLO ROSSI, MD, FACC, FAHA
Full Professor of Medicine and Chief Molecular Hypertension Laboratory, Dipartimento di Medicina Clinica e Sperimentale (DMCS) 'Gino Patrassi', Internal Medicine 4, University of Padua, University Hospital Padua, Padua, Italy

GARY L. SCHWARTZ, MD
Consultant, Division of Nephrology and Hypertension; Professor of Medicine, College of Medicine, Mayo Clinic, Rochester, Minnesota

ELLEN SEELY, MD
Professor of Medicine, Harvard Medical School; Director of Clinical Research, Division of Endocrinology, Diabetes, and Hypertension, Brigham and Women's Hospital, Boston, Massachusetts

SUSMEETA T. SHARMA, MBBS
Program on Reproductive and Adult Endocrinology, *Eunice Kennedy Shriver* National Institute of Child Health and Human Development, National Institutes of Health, Bethesda, Maryland

MICHAEL STOWASSER, MBBS, FRACP, PhD
Professor of Medicine and Co-Director, Endocrine Hypertension Research Center, University of Queensland School of Medicine, Princess Alexandra Hospital, Woolloongabba; Greenslopes Private Hospital, Greenslopes, Brisbane, Australia

ERIKA A. STROHMAYER, MD
Fellow, Division of Endocrinology and Diabetes and Bone Disease, Mount Sinai
School of Medicine, New York, New York

WILLIAM B. WHITE, MD
Professor of Medicine; Chief, Division of Hypertension and Clinical Pharmacology,
Pat and Jim Calhoun Cardiology Center, University of Connecticut School of Medicine,
Farmington, Connecticut

JUDITH A. WHITWORTH, AC, MBBS, DSc, MD, PhD, FRACP
Visiting Fellow, John Curtin School of Medical Research, Australian National University,
Acton, Canberra, Australian Capital Territory, Australia

SAMUEL M. ZUBER
Post-Baccalaureate Research Fellow, Section on Medical Neuroendocrinology,
Program in Reproductive and Adult Endocrinology, *Eunice Kennedy Shriver*
National Institute of Child Health and Human Development, National
Institutes of Health, Bethesda, Maryland

Contents

Multiple hormonal factors play a major role in the functional and structural abnormalities of hypertension (HT). At present, the kidneys and, in particular, renal Na$^+$ retention are thought to constitute a primary and sustaining mechanism in the development of HT. However, the precise renal and hormonal mechanisms leading to increased Na$^+$ reabsorption and HT remain unknown. Because the vast majority of HT is primary, this article focuses on the major endocrine systems, the RAS, aldosterone, and the SNS, that play a prominent role in the pathogenesis of HT.

Formal studies have not been performed to assess the cost-effectiveness of screening strategies for endocrine causes of hypertension. However, an understanding of the diagnostic accuracy of available screening tests and the clinical settings where disease identification will lead to improved health outcomes form the basis for a cost-effective strategy. Primary aldosteronism screening should be selective and restricted to settings where knowledge of the diagnosis has the greatest chance of improving health outcomes. Pheochromocytoma is rare; however, because it is a potentially fatal disease, screening strategies should err on the side of not missing the diagnosis, especially in high-risk clinical settings.

Pheochromocytoma is a tumor of the chromaffin cells in the adrenal medulla and sympathetic paraganglia, which synthesizes and secretes catecholamines. Norepinephrine, epinephrine, and dopamine all act on their target receptors, which causes a physiologic change in the body. High circulating levels of catecholamines can lead to severe hypertension and can have devastating effects on multiple body systems (eg, cardiovascular, cerebrovascular), and can lead to death if untreated. Although surgical treatment represents the only modality of ultimate cure, pharmacologic preoperative treatment remains the mainstay of successful outcome.

A few simple rules can allow physicians to successfully identify many patients with arterial hypertension caused by PA among the so-called essential hypertensive patients. The hyperaldosteronism and the hypoka-lemia can be cured with adrenalectomy in practically all of these patients. Moreover, in a substantial proportion of them, the blood pressure can be normalized or markedly lowered if a unilateral cause of PA is discovered. Hence, the screening for PA can be rewarding both for the patient and for the clinician, particularly in those cases where hypertension is severe and/or resistant to treatment, in which the removal of an APA can allow blood pressure to be brought under control despite withdrawal of, or a prominent reduction in, the number and doses of antihypertensive medications.

Glucocorticoid-remediable aldosteronism (GRA) is a hereditary form of primary hyperaldosteronism and the most common monogenic cause of hypertension. A chimeric gene duplication leads to ectopic aldosterone synthase activity in the cortisol-producing *zona fasciculata* of the adrenal cortex, under the regulation of adrenocorticotropin (ACTH). Hypertension typically develops in childhood, and may be refractory to standard thera-pies. Hypokalemia is uncommon in the absence of treatment with diuretics. The discovery of the genetic basis of the disorder has permitted the development of accurate diagnostic testing. Glucocorticoid suppres-sion of ACTH is the mainstay of treatment; alternative treatments include mineralocorticoid receptor antagonists.

Salt-sensitive forms of hypertension have received considerable renewed attention in recent years. This article focuses on 2 main forms of salt-sensitive hypertension (familial or genetic primary aldosteronism [PA] and Gordon syndrome) and the current state of knowledge regarding their genetic bases. The glucocorticoid-remediable form of familial PA (familial hyperaldosteronism type I) is dealt with only briefly because it is covered in depth elsewhere.

Low-renin hypertension occurs in children as a result of several genetic mutations that cause mineralocorticoid excess or excess stimulation of the mineralocorticoid receptor. This article discusses the genetic disorders that cause low-renin hypertension.

Diagnosis of Cushing's syndrome involves a step-wise approach and es-tablishing the cause can be challenging. Several pathogenic mechanisms have been proposed for glucocorticoid-induced hypertension, including a functional mineralocorticoid excess state, upregulation of the renin an-giotensin system, and deleterious effects of cortisol on the vasculature.

Surgical excision of the cause of excess glucocorticoids remains the optimal treatment. Antiglucocorticoid and antihypertensive agents and steroidogenesis inhibitors can be used as adjunctive treatment modalities in preparation for surgery and in cases where surgery is contraindicated or has not led to cure.

VISIT US ONLINE!
Access your subscription at:
www.theclinics.com

Foreword

Endocrine Hypertension

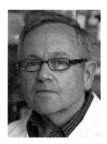

Derek LeRoith, MD, PhD
Consulting Editor

This issue on endocrine hypertension covers the basic mechanisms, clinical presentations, diagnostic criteria, and therapeutic modalities for a group of hypertensive disorders that, while they represent only a proportion of hypertensive conditions, are very important to consider since many are imminently treatable.

In an excellent introductory article Dr Carey provides an overview of hypertension including the general mechanisms involved. As he points out, 90% of hypertension in most communities is essential hypertension. The renin-angiotensin system (RAS) is obviously involved in these cases, together with aldosterone. On the other hand, there is ample evidence that activation of the sympathetic nervous system is also involved. As mentioned in the article, there are other causes of hypertension, most of which are endocrine in origin and are discussed in more detail in subsequent articles.

As discussed by Dr Schwartz in his article, almost 30% of adults in the United States are hypertensive, and it is clearly a major risk factor for many complications, leading to morbidity and mortality. The commonest form is essential hypertension and secondary causes include endocrine etiologies, especially of adrenal origin. The article describes the workup of hyperaldosteronism and pheochromocytomas, particularly from the important aspect of diagnostic criteria and accuracy, as well as cost-effectiveness.

Pheochromocytomas represent a reasonably rare cause for hypertension and the symptomatology is often similar to numerous other conditions. However, its importance lies in that fact that it should be considered a "high-risk" disorder. Thus the diagnostic workup, while important, is often not cost-effective, as discussed in the article by Drs Zuber, Kantorovich, and Pacak. Pheochromocytomas and the nonadrenal paragangliomas usually secrete norepinephrine and/or epinephrine, whereas the paragangliomas secrete dopamine. The classic diagnostic criteria are well described, as are the preoperative medical therapies; surgery remains the primary modality of treatment.

Endocrinol Metab Clin N Am 40 (2011) xiii–xv
doi:10.1016/j.ecl.2011.02.003
0889-8529/11/$ – see front matter © 2011 Elsevier Inc. All rights reserved.

endo.theclinics.com

Primary aldosteronism is still the classical form of hyperaldosteronism and hypertension commonly associated with hypokalemia. It is surgically curable as opposed to a number of less common, but related, causes of aldosterone-induced hypertension that are also treated by medical modalities and are described in more detail in other articles. Dr Rossi also reminds us that while Dr Conn made some fundamental discoveries on this condition, and the condition is often named after him, it was actually described two years prior in a more obscure journal.

The most common monogenic form of primary aldosteronism is glucocorticoid-remedial aldosteronism. The underlying cause is ectopic expression of aldosterone synthase due to a chimeric gene mutation. Nevertheless, aldosterone production is under the regulation of ACTH and therefore responds to glucocorticoid therapy. As discussed by Drs Halperin and Dluhy, the syndrome presents early in childhood and the genetic diagnosis makes it much easier to begin appropriate therapy in a timely fashion.

Drs Stowasser, Pimenta, and Gordon describe the less common syndromes that include familial or genetic primary aldosteronism (PA) and Gordon syndrome, both components of the "salt-sensitive" varieties of hypertension. Primary aldosteronism may be a component of MEN 1 or an autosomal-dominant familial form. Thus both genes that have been discovered are related to the various forms as well as genetic linkage studies that show association; however, the relationship between these genes and common causes of primary aldosteronism awaits further studies. Patients with Gordon syndrome, which is a unique clinical syndrome comprising hyperkalemia despite normal renal function, commonly demonstrate hypertension. Its pathophysiology has been studied and WNK kinases are apparently involved; the relationship of these kinases to PA is unclear.

Low renin hypertension of childhood has numerous etiologies, including 11b and 17a hydroxylase deficiencies, primary aldosteronism, dexamethasone suppressible hyperaldosteronism, and apparent aldosterone excess. As described in the article by Drs Parsa and New, many of the syndromes have classical presentation, diagnoses, and therapies, while variants of the syndromes are also seen.

Another treatable cause of hypertension is Cushing syndrome. As discussed by Drs Sharma and Nieman, 80% of all patients with Cushing syndrome develop hypertension due to the excess corticosteroids. The mechanisms include the excess glucocorticoids acting as a functional mineralocorticoid, stimulation of RAS, and other possible effects on the general vasculature. All of these potential mechanisms are well described in the article in addition to therapy that includes surgical removal of the tumor and certain medical therapies.

In a rather provocative article, Drs Ong and Whitworth discuss the latest evidence that glucocorticoids may not induce hypertension by the classically recognized mechanisms that include salt and water retention and sympathetic nervous system activation. The concept has been developed from studies in rodents where the authors show that glucocorticoid-induced hypertension may be the result of increased reactive oxygen species. On the other hand, glucocorticoid excess is associated with a reduction in prostacyclin synthesis. Whether these effects are relevant to the situation in humans is currently being studied.

Drs Strohmayer and Krakoff discuss the relationship between glucocorticoids (GC), hypertension, and cardiovascular disease. While GC may affect the cardiovascular system via its effect on blood pressure, it is well known to also induce insulin resistance and type 2 diabetes and its related hyperglycemia and hyperlipidemia, risk factors that are no less important.

It has been well established that oral contraceptives and hormone replacement therapy in postmenopausal women may induce hypertension. While the mechanisms involved include the renin-angiotensin system, there are apparently no obvious predisposing factors that have been discovered to date. On the other hand, as described by Drs Boldo and White, drospirenone, a progestin for postmenopausal replacement therapy, actually may induce weight loss and reduce blood pressure.

Polycystic ovarian syndrome has long been recognized as a disorder of insulin resistance with features of androgen excess. However, as discussed by Drs Bentley-Lewis, Seely, and Dunaif, hypertension is a previously unrecognized component of the syndrome. Whether the hypertension is the consequence of the excess weight or insulin resistance commonly associated with PCOS or due to other hormonal effects is as yet undefined. Nevertheless, therapy related to PCOS often reduces the blood pressure and, if inadequate, anti-hypertensive medication is warranted.

Dr Krakoff has collected a number of excellent contributions by authors that represent world experts in this area of endocrine hypertension. The issue represents an important up-to-date discussion on the various aspects of endocrine hypertension and to all the contributors we are indebted.

Derek LeRoith, MD, PhD
Division of Endocrinology, Metabolism and Bone Diseases
Department of Medicine
Mount Sinai School of Medicine
One Gustave L. Levy Place
Box 1055, Altran 4-36
New York, NY 10029, USA

E-mail address:
derek.leroith@mssm.edu

Preface

Endocrine Hypertension

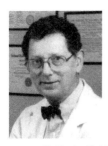

Lawrence R. Krakoff, MD
Guest Editor

Hypertension has emerged as a dominant cardiovascular risk factor and cause of cardiovascular disease in most of the world.[1] Effective reduction of high blood pressure, "control of hypertension," for prevention of future cardiovascular disease is now the main component of prevention for adult populations in both developed and developing nations.[2] The worldwide epidemic of hypertension has prompted public health initiatives and simplified approaches, such as the polypill therapy or attempts to reduce salt intake.[3,4] These are macrotherapies that are directed to large populations.

Among those with hypertension, a small fraction has rare identifiable disorders clearly identified with abnormal adrenal pathophysiology. The first or "big three" forms of adrenal hypertension to be described were: (1) pheochromocytoma, a tumor of adrenal chromaffin tissue; (2) Cushing's syndrome, due to excess production of cortisol, the human adrenal glucocorticoid; and (3) Conn's syndrome, an excess production of the mineralocorticoid, aldosterone, by an adrenal adenoma. Some were recognized long before the modern era of medical diagnosis, such as Cushing's syndrome or pheochromocytoma, because of unique clinical features. With the discovery of the various steroid hormones and their metabolic pathways, others have emerged during the past 60 years, such as primary aldosteronism and other disorders of mineralocorticoid secretion or adrenal steroid metabolism. Specific genetic diseases have recently become fully characterized and causative mutations verified. In some cases, unique and highly specific therapies have proven effective, such as the use of glucocorticoid therapy for glucocorticoid remediable aldosteronism, mineralocorticoid receptor antagonists for primary aldosteronism, or amiloride for Liddle's syndrome. Targeted alpha- and beta-receptor blockade or tyrosine hydroxylase inhibition has become available for the treatment of the catecholamine excess of pheochromocytoma. Research for the rare syndromes has thus been highly valuable for unraveling biochemical and genetic pathways and for developing specific targeted therapies. In this context, understanding of adrenal hypertension has provided the paradigm for personalized medicine.

Endocrinol Metab Clin N Am 40 (2011) xvii–xix
doi:10.1016/j.ecl.2011.04.001
0889-8529/11/$ – see front matter

Steroid hormones and catecholamines, the adrenal secretions, have also been actively studied for possible involvement in primary hypertension. Studies of adrenaline eventually led to characterization of noradrenaline as the sympathetic and central nervous system neurotransmitter. Altered metabolism or increased sensitivity to the catecholamines has been explored for a possible role in clinical hypertension and in various experimental models of hypertension. The high prevalence of low-renin essential hypertension prompted an extensive, if eventually futile, search for alternate mineralocorticoids. However, this search ultimately led to an unexpected form of genetic identifiable hypertension, gain of function mutations in the renal tubular Na epithelial channel.[5]

Another way to look at the significance of adrenal steroids and hypertension is by way of the transitions that occurred when steroids became recognized as effective drugs. The anti-inflammatory action of cortisol led to the development of synthetic glucocorticoids that, when used in supra-physiologic doses, were effective for many diseases ranging from arthritis syndromes and auto-immune diseases to neoplasia. While becoming highly valuable, glucocorticoid therapies reproduced the cardiovascular and metabolic disorders known to occur in naturally occurring Cushing's syndrome, hypertension, type 2 diabetes, dyslipidemias, and increased arteriosclerosis with a tradeoff of increased cardiovascular risk for the benefit of treatment of the primary disease. A more subtle tradeoff appeared when estrogen-progesterone analogues became used for birth control or hormone replacement after menopause. Hypertension and increased thrombotic events offset the value of these steroids, prompting abundant research to define the mechanisms accounting for the adverse effects of the "unnatural" uses of natural hormones and to develop safer analogues.

With widespread use of glucocorticoids or estrogen-progesterone-like drugs, the lessons of rare diseases or unusual metabolic pathways become the insights for understanding more widespread disorders. Improved and more accurate diagnostic testing for primary aldosteronism has led to the recognition that this disease is a major cause of resistant hypertension. Thus, the insights gained from basic research focused on the rare adrenal- and steroid-related forms of hypertension have led to important insights for the "population" diseases causing worldwide cardiovascular mortality.

The current literature dealing with adrenal hypertension and steroid-related hypertension in their various configurations is so abundant that a comprehensive compendium would be enormous and overly complex for application to address clinical issues. Yet to focus entirely on the solution of the clinical problems would omit awareness of current research that will provide future directions and also supplies the intellectual framework that has always made study of endocrine diseases so compelling. This issue is a collection of reviews by those in basic and clinical research who have devoted their efforts to advancing knowledge for "adrenal hypertension," including the rare diseases, the diseases of steroids as drugs, and a summary of adrenal mechanisms that might participate in primary hypertension.

Lawrence R. Krakoff, MD
Mount Sinai School of Medicine
One Gustave L. Levy Place, Box 1030
New York, NY 10029-6574, USA

E-mail address:
Lawrence.krakoff@mssm.edu

REFERENCES

1. Hypertension: uncontrolled and conquering the world. Lancet 2007;370:539.
2. Pereira M, Lunet N, Azevedo A, et al. Differences in prevalence, awareness, treatment and control of hypertension between developing and developed countries. J Hypertens 2009;27(5):963–75.
3. Combination Pharmacotherapy and Public Health Research Working Group. Combination pharmacotherapy for cardiovascular disease. Ann Intern Med 2005;143(8):593–9.
4. Yusuf S, Pais P, Afzal R, et al. Effects of a polypill (Polycap) on risk factors in middle-aged individuals without cardiovascular disease (TIPS): a phase II, double-blind, randomised trial. Lancet 2009;373(9672):1341–51.
5. Findling JW, Raff H, Hansson JH, et al. Liddle's syndrome: prospective genetic screening and suppressed aldosterone secretion in an extended kindred. J Clin Endocrinol Metab 1997;82:1071–4.

Overview of Endocrine Systems in Primary Hypertension

Robert M. Carey, MD, MACP

KEYWORDS

- Hypertension • Blood pressure • RAS • Aldosterone
- Sympathetic nervous system

Hypertension (HT) is the most prevalent cardiovascular disorder and a major public health problem in the United States as well as worldwide. The relationship between blood pressure (BP) and cardiovascular risk is continuous, consistent, and independent of other risk factors, and the higher the BP, the greater the chance of myocardial infarction, heart failure, stroke, end-stage renal disease, peripheral vascular disease, and mortality from all causes.[1] Approximately 90% of individuals with HT have primary (essential) HT, the root causes of which are still being explored. Of the causes of remediable HT (10%), the most prevalent conditions by far are primary aldosteronism (5%–10%) and renal vascular HT (1%–5%). Essentially, all of the specifically remediable causes of HT are endocrine disorders, which are described in detail later in this article.

Multiple endocrine systems have been demonstrated to play a role in primary HT, including renin-angiotensin system (RAS); mineralocorticoids and mineralocorticoid receptors (MRs); catecholamines and the sympathetic nervous system (SNS); the renal dopaminergic system; nitric oxide, endothelin, and cyclooxygenase metabolites; insulin and insulin resistance; the kinin system; vasopressin; and endogenous ouabain and cardiotonic steroids.

This article provides an overview of the endocrine mechanisms that most prominently contribute to the pathophysiology of primary HT: the RAS, mineralocorticoids, and the SNS.

THE RAS IN PRIMARY HT
Systemic RAS in HT

The RAS is a coordinated hormonal cascade of major significance in the control of BP and HT.[2] The RAS has become more complex with the discovery of several new

Division of Endocrinology and Metabolism, Department of Medicine, University of Virginia Health System, PO Box 801414, Charlottesville, VA 22908-1414, USA
E-mail address: rmc4c@virginia.edu

Endocrinol Metab Clin N Am 40 (2011) 265–277
doi:10.1016/j.ecl.2011.01.003
0889-8529/11/$ – see front matter © 2011 Elsevier Inc. All rights reserved.

endo.theclinics.com

components including functional angiotensin (Ang) type 2 (AT$_2$) receptors, the angiotensin-converting enzyme (ACE) 2–Ang (1-7)–*mas* receptor pathway and the (pro) renin receptor (**Fig. 1**).[3]

Although the RAS has been thoroughly studied, demonstration that the system is activated and participates in the pathophysiology of human HT has been elusive. In studies from the early 1970s, patients with primary HT were classified into 3 categories with respect to plasma renin activity (PRA): normal (60%), high (15%), and low (25%) PRA. Originally, it was thought that this classification would define the role of the RAS in primary HT.[4]

Low-renin hypertensive patients were considered to have volume expansion as the cause of HT, possibly related to excess production of a mineralocorticoid other than aldosterone.[5,6] Indeed, low-renin HT generally responded to diuretic therapy, including spironolactone, with normalization of BP.[7] However, many studies failed to demonstrate cryptic mineralocorticoid excess in low-renin primary HT,[8] and the pathophysiology of low-renin primary HT remains unknown at present.

Similarly, high-renin primary HT was thought to be associated with activation of the RAS, with clear involvement in the pathogenesis of the HT. In high-renin hypertensive patients, BP could be normalized by reducing the activity of the RAS with β-adrenergic antagonists, ACE inhibitors, or Ang receptor blockers.[5,7] Patients with HT and high levels of circulating renin were noted to have more severe HT and increased prevalence of ischemic heart disease, cardiovascular morbidity, and mortality as compared with patients with normal or low PRA.[9] Several later studies, however, demonstrated that this was not always the case,[10] and renin profiling to study the pathophysiologic mechanisms, diagnose HT, and design the treatment of HT was largely abandoned in the early 1990s.

Despite the disappointment that renin profiling has yielded, little consistent information concerning the pathogenesis of human primary HT, the RAS has been implicated in the pathophysiology of the nonmodulating hypertensive phenotype. Nonmodulation, a disorder of renal vascular and adrenal aldosterone secretory responsiveness to Ang II, occurs in approximately 40% of patients with primary HT. Nonmodulation is characterized by blunted aldosterone responses to Ang II during low Na$^+$ intake and reduced renal vasoconstriction to Ang II during high Na$^+$ intake.[11] Patients with nonmodulation have the inability to handle an Na$^+$ load, salt-sensitive HT, and normal

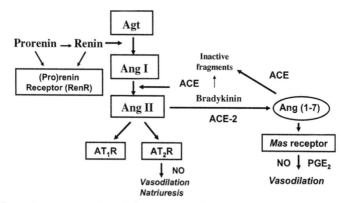

Fig. 1. Schematic representation of the RAS as understood in 2011. Agt, angiotensinogen; Ang, angiotensin; AT$_1$R, Ang type 1 receptor; AT$_2$R, Ang type 2 receptor; NO, nitric oxide; PGE$_2$, prostaglandin E$_2$.

to high circulating renin levels. A striking family history of HT and concordance of responses to Ang II in sibling pairs has suggested that nonmodulation is a genetic disorder, and angiotensinogen (Agt) gene polymorphisms were found in patients with nonmodulation.[11] In addition, the HT of patients with nonmodulation was completely abolished with ACE inhibition.[12] The nonmodulating phenotype has been confirmed by several independent research groups. However, not all studies have confirmed the existence of nonmodulation, and further work is required to determine whether the nonmodulating phenotype is a result of increased RAS activity alone or whether other mechanisms may play a role.

Although demonstration of the in vivo activation of the RAS in early or established HT has been difficult, there is no question that inhibition of the RAS has been efficacious in lowering BP in primary HT.[12,13] Multiple clinical trials have demonstrated that blocking the RAS with ACE inhibitors or Ang receptor blockers lowers BP and reduces cardiovascular morbidity and mortality.[14–20] RAS blockade not only lowers BP but also reduces target organ damage and BP variability, an independent risk factor for cardiovascular events and overall mortality.

The earliest pathophysiologic change demonstrable in primary HT is the process of vascular remodeling, a term used to characterize the functional, mechanical, and structural changes in small resistance arteries (100–300 μm) that engender reduction in lumen size and increased peripheral vascular resistance, a hemodynamic hallmark of HT.[21,22] However, even though vascular remodeling is already present in stage I HT, it is still unclear whether remodeling is a primary process or reflects early target organ damage resulting from increased BP. Small resistance artery remodeling in HT is characterized by an increased media to lumen ratio that derives from vascular smooth muscle (VSM) cell growth (hyperplasia and hypertrophy), apoptosis, elongation of cells, and altered composition of the extracellular matrix.[23,24] Ang II has been thought to play a substantial role in early vascular remodeling because it stimulates both VSM cell hyperplasia and hypertrophy.[21,22]

Besides the alterations in lumen size, typical of vascular remodeling, vascular injury in HT is characterized by inflammation.[21,22] Small arteries in HT have increased expression of surface adhesion molecules, inflammatory cell infiltration, cytokine production, chemokine exposure, and oxidative stress. Current evidence is quite convincing that vascular disease in HT is an inflammatory process and that chronic vascular inflammation may be the primary cause of HT.[22] Ang II is now recognized as a major inflammatory mediator in the vasculature, inducing its effects largely via oxidative stress.[23–25]

Ang II mediates many of its cellular actions by stimulating the formation of intracellular reactive oxygen species, including superoxide anion, hydrogen peroxide, hydroxyl free radial, and peroxynitrite.[26] Mediated by multiple redox-sensitive signaling pathways, reactive oxygen species are involved in virtually all stages of the vascular inflammatory process, including vascular cell permeability, leukocyte adhesion, transmigration, chemotaxis, cell growth, and fibrosis.

Ang II generally elicits enhanced vasoconstriction in human primary HT. The vasoconstrictor action of Ang II may be direct at the VSM cell or indirect via stimulation of the activity of the SNS. In addition, Ang II, via activation of the Ang type 1 (AT_1) receptor, is a major factor in eutropic inward remodeling observed at the earliest stages of HT. In patients with primary HT, AT_1 receptor blockade and β-adrenergic receptor blockade induced similar BP reduction, but only the former corrected resistance arterial structure.[27] Also, in spontaneously hypertensive rats (SHRs), both ACE inhibition and AT_1 receptor blockade normalize resistance artery structure. In summary, although it is clear that Ang II plays a major role in vascular remodeling, it is still unknown whether Ang II has a primary initiating role in HT or it simply mediates the vascular damage, even at an early stage, resulting from a primary increase in BP.

Tissue RAS in HT

The circulating RAS is only 1 component of the overall RAS, and tissue RAS that operates completely independently of the circulating RAS is present in the brain, kidney, heart, blood vessels, and adrenal gland. Although it is now probable that tissue RAS is activated even when the circulating RAS is normal or suppressed (eg, diabetic nephropathy), this concept has been difficult to establish in HT. In particular, it has been difficult to show the relative roles of the intrarenal RAS, as opposed to the systemic RAS, in the control of BP and HT in humans. This is an important issue because long-term regulation of BP involves the kidney, and the ability to sustain a hypertensive process chronically requires renal Na^+ retention.[28] Recent work, however, has helped clarify the tissue-specific sites, whereby the RAS regulates BP through a cross-transplantation approach in AT_1 (AT_{1A}) receptor–deficient mice.[29] Absence of AT_1 receptors exclusively in the kidney, with normal receptors elsewhere, was sufficient to lower BP by about 20 mm Hg. Thus, renal AT_1 receptors were demonstrated to have a unique and nonredundant role in the control of BP homeostasis. Because circulating aldosterone was unaffected in these experiments, BP is regulated by the direct action of AT_1 receptors on kidney cells, independent of mineralocorticoids. However, in addition to the renal AT_1 receptors, those outside the kidney made an equivalent, unique, and nonredundant contribution to BP control, that is, animals with a full complement of AT_1 receptors in the kidney, but without AT_1 receptors in extrarenal tissues, also had BP reductions of about 20 mm Hg. Together, this compelling evidence indicates that AT_1 receptors in either the vasculature or the central nervous system mediate the component of BP control that is independent of the kidney.

Ang peptides are synthesized in tissue sites.[30,31] Most, if not all, tissue Ang II is synthesized locally from tissue-derived Ang I. In addition, the beneficial actions of RAS blockers in treating HT are most likely due to interference with tissue Ang II rather than Ang II in the circulation.[32] Although it was originally thought that the renin required for local Ang I formation was locally synthesized, studies in nephrectomized animal models have proved that this is not always the case.[33] In many tissues, such as the heart and blood vessel wall, local Ang I synthesis depends on tissue uptake of kidney-derived renin.[34] In other tissues, such as the kidney, adrenal gland, and brain, renin is synthesized locally.

Intrarenal RAS in HT

The intrarenal RAS is considered to be the most important of the tissue RASs in the control of BP and HT. The intrarenal RAS was first recognized in the early 1970s, when it was demonstrated that intrarenal RAS inhibition markedly increased glomerular filtration rate and renal Na^+ and water excretion.[35,36] Since then, intrarenal RAS has increasingly been recognized as a crucial system in the regulation of Na^+ excretion and the long-term control of BP. Indeed, there is growing recognition that inappropriate activation of intrarenal RAS prevents the kidney from maintaining normal Na^+ balance at normal arterial pressures and is an important cause of HT.[37,38]

Several experimental models support the concept of an overactive intrarenal RAS in the development and maintenance of HT. These include 2-kidney, 1-clip Goldblatt HT; Ang II–infused HT; transgenic rat mRen2 HT with an extra renin gene; the remnant kidney model; and several mouse models overexpressing the renin or Agt gene. In many forms of HT, inappropriate activation of the intrarenal RAS limits the ability of the kidney to maintain Na^+ balance, when perfused at normal arterial pressure. In addition to Na^+ and fluid retention and progressive HT, other long-term consequences of an inappropriately activated intrarenal RAS include renal vascular, glomerular, and tubulointerstitial injury and fibrosis.[39]

Agt is the only known precursor of Ang II, and most of the intrarenal Agt messenger RNA and protein are localized to the proximal tubule cell, suggesting that intratubular Ang II is derived from locally formed Agt.[40] Both Agt and its metabolite Ang II from proximal tubule cells can be secreted directly into the tubule lumen.[40] A 2-week infusion of Ang II resulted in upregulation of intrarenal Agt messenger RNA and protein expression.[40] Therefore, a detrimental intrarenal positive feedback loop, whereby increased Ang II production stimulates its requisite precursor, may lead to markedly increased intrarenal Ang peptide levels in HT.

Renin is synthesized and secreted not only in the juxtaglomerular cells of the afferent arteriole but also by the renal connecting tubules, so that renin is probably secreted directly into the distal tubule fluid.[41] Because intact Agt can be detected in urine, it is possible that some of the proximally formed Agt is converted to Ang II in the distal nephron.[41,42] Indeed, Ang II infusion increased urinary Agt concentration in a time- and dose-dependent manner associated with increased renal Ang II levels.[42] Furthermore, collecting duct renin expression is upregulated by Ang II via the AT_1 receptor.[43] Therefore, several intrarenal mechanisms provide positive feedback control to enhance Ang II concentrations at both proximal and distal nephron sites, where Ang II has potent Na^+-retaining actions.

Studies have demonstrated that production of renin and Agt in the proximal tubule can increase BP independently of the circulating RAS.[44] Transgenic mice expressing human Agt selectively in the proximal tubule via the kidney androgen-regulated protein promoter, when bred with mice expressing human renin systemically, had a 20 mm Hg increase in BP despite having normal circulating Ang II. The increase in BP was managed with AT_1 receptor blockade, demonstrating Ang II–dependent HT. This finding constituted the first demonstration of systemic HT from isolated renal tissue activation of the RAS. Furthermore, isolated proximal tubule overexpression of both human renin and Agt increased BP, supporting the concept that intratubular RAS activation could induce HT. In these studies, it is unclear whether Ang I was first generated within the proximal tubule cell from intracellular cleavage of Agt by renin or whether the renin and Agt interaction occurred in the tubule lumen after secretion.

It now seems that the ability of Ang II to induce both HT and cardiac hypertrophy depends exclusively on the activation of AT_1 receptors within the kidney proximal tubule to increase Na^+ reabsorption.[45] Selective AT_1 receptor cross-transplantation studies demonstrate that animals with renal proximal tubule but not systemic AT_1 receptors were able to induce and sustain HT in response to systemic Ang II infusion. On the other hand, animals with systemic but not renal AT_1 receptors were unable to mount a hypertensive or cardiac hypertrophy response to Ang II. The ability of Ang II to induce HT was independent of aldosterone secretion. This represents strong evidence that renal proximal tubule AT_1 receptors are critical for the development of Ang II–induced HT. The importance of these receptors in human HT remains intriguing.

MINERALOCORTICOIDS IN PRIMARY HT

Aldosterone is a mineralocorticoid hormone synthesized and secreted by the adrenal zona glomerulosa in response to Ang II, K^+, and adrenocorticotropin (ACTH) that interacts with MRs in the renal cortical collecting duct, colon, and salivary and sweat glands to promote unidirectional Na^+ flux. Na^+ retention in response to aldosterone is accompanied by water retention such that inappropriately high aldosterone levels expand blood and extracellular fluid volumes, leading to HT. Nonepithelial sites of physiologic aldosterone action include the central nervous system, where it increases salt appetite, and the vascular wall, where it increases vascular contractility.[46]

The involvement of aldosterone in the pathophysiology of HT is clearly delineated in primary aldosteronism, in which there is a primary increase in aldosterone production by a unilateral adrenal aldosterone-producing adenoma (APA) or idiopathic bilateral adrenal hyperplasia. Patients with these disorders have Na^+ and water retention, hypokalemic alkalosis, and HT that, in the case of APA, is reversible with the removal of the adenoma. In the case of idiopathic adrenal hyperplasia causing primary aldosteronism, bilateral adrenalectomy does not cure the HT; other pathophysiologic factors must be involved in the HT of patients with this disorder. In recent years, there has been a revival of interest in the diagnosis of primary aldosteronism because this disorder is present in approximately 8% of hypertensive patients.[47] However, it has been much more difficult to demonstrate a role of aldosterone in primary HT. Although it is clear that MR antagonists, such as spironolactone, are effective in lowering BP of patients with resistant HT, these agents are only modestly effective in the early stages of HT. Interestingly, a four-corners analysis for the identification of genetic markers of BP did not identify plasma aldosterone as a familial correlate of HT.[48]

Experimentally, large doses of aldosterone that are associated with a 3-fold increase in plasma aldosterone levels and salt loading are required to induce arterial remodeling in humans. The major action of aldosterone on arteries is stimulation of collagen turnover and induction of fibrosis and perivascular inflammation. These changes are not characteristic of the eutrophic inward remodeling in small resistance arteries in primary HT. In uninephrectomized rats on a low Na^+ diet, large doses of aldosterone, which result in marked elevation of plasma aldosterone levels, do not induce perivascular fibrosis in the myocardium.[49]

Recently, several new concepts have emerged regarding the role of aldosterone and MRs that may be of major importance in HT: (1) extra-adrenal synthesis of aldosterone, (2) aldosterone induction of vascular and cardiac inflammation and fibrosis, (3) aldosterone induction of progressive cerebral and renal damage and cardiovascular disease, and (4) the action of gluococorticoid hormones at MRs.

The classic site of aldosterone biosynthesis is the adrenocortical zona glomerulosa. Recent research indicates, however, that the necessary chemical machinery (eg, aldosterone synthase) may be expressed in nonadrenal tissues, such as blood vessels, brain, heart, and kidney. In each of these nonadrenal tissues, local aldosterone production occurs, albeit in small quantities, because of aldosterone synthase expression in the tissue and aldosterone may serve as a paracrine substance to inflict tissue damage. On the other hand, nonadrenal tissue can take up aldosterone from circulating plasma; this action is easily demonstrated in the heart.[50] Irrespective of its origin, either via local synthesis or uptake from plasma, aldosterone can be detected in heart homogenate at 17-fold the concentration in plasma; its level is markedly increased after 3 hours of perfusion by Ang II or ACTH and is sensitive to dietary Na^+ and K^+. Recent work has demonstrated that the heart does not produce aldosterone in any appreciable quantity.[51] However, the possibility for vascular and/or renal aldosterone synthesis still remains.

Aldosterone induces fibrosis in the heart, as increased concentrations of the steroid (in combination with high Na^+ intake) induce myocardial interstitial fibrosis.[52] The fibrotic reaction induced by aldosterone is independent of elevated BP, and increased plasma aldosterone levels are not requisite for the steroid to mediate fibrosis. Selective MR blockade abrogates the cardiac effects of administered aldosterone.[53] In rats on a high Na^+ diet infused with Ang II and the nitric oxide synthase inhibitor N-nitro-L-arginine-methyl-ester (L-NAME), administration of the MR antagonist eplerenone or adrenalectomy abolished coronary vascular injury without lowering BP.[54] The protective effect of adrenalectomy was abolished by aldosterone replacement. Thus, in a high Na^+ environment aldosterone induces coronary damage through BP-independent mechanisms. In uninephrectomized rats receiving a high Na^+ diet and exogenous aldosterone, severe HT occurred after 2 weeks. The coronary vasculature was markedly inflamed with medial fibrinoid necrosis and perivascular inflammation associated with increased medial expression of vascular adhesion molecule 1, cyclooxygenase 2, osteopontin, and monocyte chemoattractant protein 1. MR blockade with eplerenone reduced BP and vascular inflammation to control levels. The fact that aldosterone itself is not toxic to tissues but requires a high Na^+ environment to induce these changes represents an intriguing unsolved problem.[46,55]

Aldosterone also has the capacity to induce progressive renal and cerebral vascular damage.[56,57] In the stroke-prone hypertensive rat, aldosterone seems to be a primary mediator of vascular inflammation in the brain and kidneys. MR antagonist administration or adrenalectomy afforded the same degree of tissue protection as did ACE inhibitors. Thus, Ang II per se is not sufficient to induce vascular and glomerular damage but aldosterone plays a key role in the pathology. Aldosterone causes microvascular damage, vascular inflammation, oxidative stress, and endothelial dysfunction, and MR antagonists are effective in preventing these changes.[58]

Aldosterone acts by binding to the MR, which was first characterized in classic Na^+-transporting epithelial cells and subsequently in a large number of nonepithelial cells, such as cardiomyocytes and VSM cells. Glucocorticoids bind to MR with equal affinity to aldosterone, but cortisol circulates at concentrations 1000-fold higher than aldosterone. In the epithelia, the blood vessels, and certain brain areas, however, MRs are protected against activation by glucocorticoids by expression of the enzyme 11β-hydroxysteroid dehydrogenase type 2, which converts cortisol to MR-inactive cortisone and the cofactor NAD to NADH. In epithelial tissues, such as the renal distal tubule, MRs can be activated by cortisol. However, glucocorticoids can occupy both the epithelial and nonepithelial MRs without activating the receptor, but in so doing, they may exclude aldosterone. The exact role of glucocorticoid activation of MRs in HT is the subject of intense investigation at present.[59]

The role of aldosterone in the pathophysiology of primary HT is still being investigated. However, the relationship of baseline plasma aldosterone concentrations to BP and to the incidence of HT has recently been evaluated in the Framingham study.[60] A 16% increase in the risk of increased BP and a 17% increase in the risk of HT were observed for each quartile increase in plasma aldosterone, with a 1.6-fold increased risk in the highest quartile. Thus, increased circulating aldosterone concentrations within the physiologic range predispose to HT.

THE SNS IN PRIMARY HT

Available evidence indicates that primary HT is commonly neurogenic, with documentation of high norepinephrine (NE) spillover.[61] The evidence that primary HT is neurogenic, that is, related to increased SNS activity, is summarized as follows: (1) the early stages of HT frequently are characterized by a hyperdynamic circulation, with increased heart rate and cardiac output triggered by enhanced sympathetic cardiovascular drive and attenuated parasympathetic nerve activity; (2) plasma NE concentrations are significantly elevated in patients with primary HT when compared with age-matched controls; (3) based on the administration of radiolabeled

NE, the rate of NE spillover from adrenergic neurons in the heart and kidneys is increased in young subjects with early HT; (4) hypertensive patients display lower ^{123}I-metaiodobenzylguanidine cardiac uptake and greater tracer washout compared with normotensive subjects, suggesting that cardiac sympathetic drive is enhanced in primary HT; (5) postganglionic sympathetic nerve traffic to skeletal muscle is characterized by an increased noradrenergic outflow in primary HT. Noradrenergic overactivity is proportional to the severity of the HT, absent in most forms of secondary HT, and potentiated in subjects with obesity and congestive heart failure; (6) microneurography and radiotracer dilution methodology to measure regional sympathetic activity demonstrate increased muscle sympathetic nerve activity and elevated systemic, cardiac, and renal NE spillover in patients with primary HT when compared with nonhypertensive normal control subjects. Thus, increased rates of sympathetic nerve firing and reduced neuronal NE reuptake contribute to sympathetic activation in HT.

Aging in humans is associated not only with increased BP but also with marked and sustained increases in SNS activity to several peripheral tissues.[62] Net whole-body SNS activity, as estimated by measuring NE spillover, was greater in older versus younger healthy adults. Increased net SNS activity is manifested in selected tissues, including heart, gastrointestinal tract, and skeletal muscles and is not present on a whole-body basis or in other regions. The critical mechanisms of increased SNS activity in aging have been identified. Increases in total and abdominal obesity and circulating adipose-sensitive signals, such as leptin, and increased subcortical suprabulbar brain noradrenergic activity play an important role.[63] This chronic activation of the peripheral SNS is thought to be a primary response of the central nervous system to stimulate thermogenesis to prevent increased fat storage in light of the increased obesity of aging. However, the increase in SNS activity is not only ineffective in achieving augmented thermogenesis but also associated with several adverse cardiovascular consequences. Indeed, HT commonly associated with obesity may be a secondary cardiovascular consequence of SNS overactivation, which was "intended" to stimulate thermogenesis and increase energy expenditure.[64]

The kidneys have long been considered predominant in the regulation of arterial BP because of their great capacity to return altered BP to its original level by increasing or decreasing Na^+ and water excretion. Activation of the sympathetic nerves to the kidneys increases tubule Na^+ reabsorption, renin release, and renal vascular resistance. These actions contribute to long-term pressure elevations by shifting the pressure-natriuresis curve to the right. In SHRs, renal sympathetic innervation is enhanced, and neonatal sympathectomy is accompanied by a decrease in arterial pressure.[65] Also, kidneys of SHRs have renal NE contents that are 1.5 to 3.0 times higher than those of age- and gender-matched control nonhypertensive rats.[66] However, treatment of rats with nerve growth factor resulting in noradrenergic innervation of the kidneys was not sufficient to increase BP. Nevertheless, when kidneys from neonatally sympathectonized SHRs are transplanted into untreated SHR recipients, there is a reduction in long-term arterial pressure and Na^+ sensitivity of the BP.[66] These findings suggest that neonatal sympathetic innervation in SHRs induces changes in renal function that govern the development and maintenance of HT.

Sympathetic nerve activity is increased in adult SHRs compared with Wistar Kyoto rats.[67] SHRs have elevated NE concentrations and tyrosine hydroxylase activities in skeletal muscles and white adipose tissue, increased excitability of superior cervical ganglion cells, and increased plasma NE levels. Also, obese Zucker rats have increased sympathetic activity compared with lean Zucker controls.[68] Humans with primary HT also have widespread increased SNS activity, as evidenced by cardiac NE spillover and muscle sympathetic nerve activity.[69] In heart and skeletal muscles, increased NE spillover of hypertensive subjects seems to be because of the decreased neuronal NE reuptake.

The increased SNS activity found in experimental and clinical (human) HT almost invariably involves the kidneys. Thus, renal sympathetic nerve activity is higher in SHRs than in normotensive controls as well as in obese Zucker versus lean Zucker rats and Wistar fatty versus Wistar lean rats. In patients with primary HT and obesity-related HT, renal NE spillover is elevated approximately 50% compared with lean normotensive controls.[70] NE spillover is also increased in the kidneys of hypertensive, but not normotensive, humans.[71]

SUMMARY

HT, the most prevalent cardiovascular disorder, is a major health problem throughout the world. Because the vast majority of HT is primary, this article has focused on the major endocrine systems, the RAS and the SNS, that play a prominent role in the pathogenesis of HT. In contrast to the defined remediable causes of HT discussed elsewhere in this issue, the cause of primary HT remains unknown. Clearly, multiple hormonal factors play a major role in the functional and structural abnormalities of HT. At present, the kidneys and, in particular, renal Na^+ retention are thought to constitute a primary and sustaining mechanism in the development of HT. However, the precise renal and hormonal mechanisms leading to increased Na^+ reabsorption and HT remain unknown. The role of cardiovascular hormones such as Ang II and aldosterone on target organ damage and their role in the induction of vascular inflammation have been appreciated. Although the understanding of the mechanisms of the remediable forms of HT, virtually all of which are endocrine, has markedly advanced, so far, these mechanisms have not clarified the underlying defects of primary HT.

Endocrinology has contributed greatly to the knowledge of the basis of HT and will certainly be at the forefront of new discoveries affecting this important condition.

REFERENCES

1. Chobanian AV, Bakris GL, Black HR, et al. Seventh report of the Joint National Committee on prevention, detection, evaluation, and treatment of high blood pressure. Hypertension 2003;42:1206–52.
2. Peach MJ. Renin-angiotensin system: biochemistry and mechanisms of action. Physiol Rev 1977;57:313–70.
3. Carey RM, Siragy HM. Newly recognized components of the renin-angiotensin system: potential roles in cardiovascular regulation. Endocr Rev 2003;24:261–71.
4. Brunner HR, Laragh JH, Baer L, et al. Essential hypertension: renin and aldosterone, heart attack and stroke. N Engl J Med 1972;286:441–9.
5. Laragh JH, Letcher RL, Pickering TG. Renin profiling for diagnosis and treatment of hypertension. JAMA 1979;241:151–6.
6. Sennett JA, Brown RD, Island DP, et al. Evidence for a new mineralocorticoid in patients with low-renin essential hypertension. Circ Res 1975;36:2–9.
7. Brunner HR, Sealey JE, Laragh JH. Renin subgroups in essential hypertension. Further analysis of their pathophysiological and epidemiological characteristics. Circ Res 1973;32(Suppl 1):99–105.
8. Tan SY, Mulrow PJ. Low renin essential hypertension: failure to demonstrate excess 11-deoxycorticosterone production. J Clin Endocrinol Metab 1979;49:790–3.
9. Alderman MH, Madhavan S, Ooi WL, et al. Association of the renin-sodium profile with the risk of myocardial infarction in patients with hypertension. N Engl J Med 1991;324:1098–104.

10. Meade TW, Cooper JA, Peart WS. Plasma renin activity and ischemic heart disease. N Engl J Med 1993;329:616–9.
11. Hollenberg NH, Williams GH. Abnormal renal function, sodium-volume homeostasis and renin system behavior in normal-renin essential hypertension: the evaluation of the non-modulator concept. In: Laragh JH, Brenner BM, editors. Hypertension: pathophysiology, diagnosis and management. 2nd edition. New York: Raven Press; 1995. p. 1837–56.
12. Unger T. The role of the renin-angiotensin system in the development of cardiovascular disease. Am J Cardiol 2002;89:3A–9A [discussion: 10A].
13. Dzau V. The cardiovascular continuum and renin-angiotensin-aldosterone system blockade. J Hypertens Suppl 2005;23:S9–17.
14. Sica DA. Combination angiotensin-converting enzyme inhibitor and angiotensin receptor blocker therapy: its role in clinical practice. J Clin Hypertens (Greenwich) 2003;5:414–20.
15. Julius S, Kjeldsen SE, Weber M, et al. Outcomes in hypertensive patients at high cardiovascular risk treated with regimens based on valsartan or amlodipine: the VALUE randomised trial. Lancet 2004;363:2022–31.
16. Dahlof B, Devereux RB, Kjeldsen SE, et al. Cardiovascular morbidity and mortality in the Losartan Intervention For Endpoint reduction in hypertension study (LIFE): a randomised trial against atenolol. Lancet 2002;359:995–1003.
17. Yusuf S, Teo KK, Pogue J, et al, Ontarget Investiagtors. Telmisartan, ramipril, or both in patients at high risk for vascular events. N Engl J Med 2008;358:1547–59.
18. ALLHAT Officers and Coordinators for the ALLHAT Collaborative Research Group. Major outcomes in high-risk hypertensive patients randomized to angiotensin-converting enzyme inhibitor or calcium channel blocker vs diuretic: the Antihypertensive and Lipid-Lowering Treatment to Prevent Heart Attack Trial (ALLHAT). JAMA 2002;288:2981–97.
19. Hansson L, Lindholm LH, Niskanen L, et al. Effect of angiotensin-converting-enzyme inhibition compared with conventional therapy on cardiovascular morbidity and mortality in hypertension: the Captopril Prevention Project (CAPPP) randomised trial. Lancet 1999;353:611–6.
20. Weber M. The telmisartan programme of research tO show Telmisartan End-organ proteCTION (PROTECTION) programme. J Hypertens Suppl 2003;21:S37–46.
21. Touyz RM. The role of angiotensin II in regulating vascular structural and functional changes in hypertension. Curr Hypertens Rep 2003;5:155–64.
22. Touyz RM. Molecular and cellular mechanisms in vascular injury in hypertension: role of angiotensin II. Curr Opin Nephrol Hypertens 2005;14:125–31.
23. Berk BC. Vascular smooth muscle growth: autocrine growth mechanisms. Physiol Rev 2001;81:999–1030.
24. Suzuki Y, Ruiz-Ortega M, Lorenzo O, et al. Inflammation and angiotensin II. Int J Biochem Cell Biol 2003;35:881–900.
25. Dandona P, Kumar V, Aljada A, et al. Angiotensin II receptor blocker valsartan suppresses reactive oxygen species generation in leukocytes, nuclear factor-kappa B, in mononuclear cells of normal subjects: evidence of an antiinflammatory action. J Clin Endocrinol Metab 2003;88:4496–501.
26. Taniyama Y, Griendling KK. Reactive oxygen species in the vasculature: molecular and cellular mechanisms. Hypertension 2003;42:1075–81.
27. Hall JE, Brands MW, Henegar JR. Angiotensin II and long-term arterial pressure regulation: the overriding dominance of the kidney. J Am Soc Nephrol 1999;10(Suppl 12):S258–65.

28. Schiffrin EL, Park JB, Intengan HD, et al. Correction of arterial structure and endo-thelial dysfunction in human essential hypertension by the angiotensin receptor antagonist losartan. Circulation 2000;101:1653–9.
29. Crowley SD, Gurley SB, Oliverio MI, et al. Distinct roles for the kidney and systemic tissues in blood pressure regulation by the renin-angiotensin system. J Clin Invest 2005;115:1092–9.
30. van Kats JP, Danser AH, van Meegen JR, et al. Angiotensin production by the heart: a quantitative study in pigs with the use of radiolabeled angiotensin infu-sions. Circulation 1998;98:73–81.
31. van Kats JP, Schalekamp MA, Verdouw PD, et al. Intrarenal angiotensin II: inter-stitial and cellular levels and site of production. Kidney Int 2001;60:2311–7.
32. van Kats JP, Duncker DJ, Haitsma DB, et al. Angiotensin-converting enzyme inhi-bition and angiotensin II type 1 receptor blockade prevent cardiac remodeling in pigs after myocardial infarction: role of tissue angiotensin II. Circulation 2000;102: 1556–63.
33. Chai W, Danser AH. Is angiotensin II made inside or outside of the cell? Curr Hy-pertens Rep 2005;7:124–7.
34. Re RN. Tissue renin angiotensin systems. Med Clin North Am 2004;88:19–38.
35. Kimbrough HM Jr, Vaughan ED Jr, Carey RM, et al. Effect of intrarenal angiotensin II blockade on renal function in conscious dogs. Circ Res 1977;40:174–8.
36. Levens NR, Freedlender AE, Peach MJ, et al. Control of renal function by intrare-nal angiotensin II. Endocrinology 1983;112:43–9.
37. Navar LG, Harrison-Bernard LM, Nishiyama A, et al. Regulation of intrarenal angiotensin II in hypertension. Hypertension 2002;39:316–22.
38. Navar LG, Kobori H, Prieto-Carrasquero M. Intrarenal angiotensin II and hyper-tension. Curr Hypertens Rep 2003;5:135–43.
39. Rüster C, Wolf G. Renin-angiotensin-aldosterone system and progression of renal disease. J Am Soc Nephrol 2006;17(11):2985–91.
40. Kobori H, Harrison-Bernard LM, Navar LG. Enhancement of angiotensinogen expression in angiotensin II-dependent hypertension. Hypertension 2001;37: 1329–35.
41. Rohrwasser A, Morgan T, Dillon HF, et al. Elements of a paracrine tubular renin-angiotensin system along the entire nephron. Hypertension 1999;34: 1265–74.
42. Kobori H, Nishiyama A, Harrison-Bernard LM, et al. Urinary angiotensinogen as an indicator of intrarenal angiotensin status in hypertension. Hypertension 2003;41:42–9.
43. Prieto-Carrasquero MC, Kobori H, Ozawa Y, et al. AT1 receptor-mediated enhancement of collecting duct renin in angiotensin II-dependent hypertensive rats. Am J Physiol Renal Physiol 2005;289:F632–7.
44. Lavoie JL, Lake-Bruse KD, Sigmund CJ. Increased blood pressure in transgenic mice expressing both human renin and angiotensinogen in the renal proximal tubule. Am J Physiol Renal Physiol 2004;286:F965–71.
45. Crowley SD, Gurley SB, Herrera MJ, et al. Angiotensin II causes hypertension and cardiac hypertrophy through its receptors in the kidney. Proc Natl Acad Sci U S A 2006;103:17985–90.
46. Rossi G, Boscaro M, Ronconi V, et al. Aldosterone as a cardiovascular risk factor. Trends Endocrinol Metab 2005;16:104–7.
47. Funder JW, Carey RM, Fardella C, et al. Case detection, diagnosis and treat-ment of patients with primary aldosteronism. A Clinical Practice Guideline of The Endocrine Society. J Clin Endocrinol Metab 2008;93:3266–81.

48. Watt GC, Harrap SB, Foy CJ, et al. Abnormalities of glucocorticoid metabolism and the renin-angiotensin system: a four-corners approach to the identification of genetic determinants of blood pressure. J Hypertens 1992;10:473–82.
49. Funder JW. Minireview: aldosterone and the cardiovascular system: genomic and nongenomic effects. Endocrinology 2006;147:5564–7.
50. Gomez-Sanchez EP, Ahmad N, Romero DG, et al. Origin of aldosterone in the rat heart. Endocrinology 2004;145:4796–802.
51. Funder JW. Cardiac synthesis of aldosterone: going, going, gone...? Endocrinology 2004;145:4793–5.
52. Brilla CG, Weber KT. Reactive and reparative myocardial fibrosis in arterial hypertension in the rat. Cardiovasc Res 1992;26:671–7.
53. Brilla CG, Matsubara LS, Weber KT. Anti-aldosterone treatment and the prevention of myocardial fibrosis in primary and secondary hyperaldosteronism. J Mol Cell Cardiol 1993;25:563–75.
54. Rocha R, Stier CT Jr, Kifor I, et al. Aldosterone: a mediator of myocardial necrosis and renal arteriopathy. Endocrinology 2000;141:3871–8.
55. Dluhy RG, Williams GH. Aldosterone–villain or bystander? N Engl J Med 2004; 351:8–10.
56. Rocha R, Chander PN, Zuckerman A, et al. Role of aldosterone in renal vascular injury in stroke-prone hypertensive rats. Hypertension 1999;33:232–7.
57. Rocha R, Chander PN, Khanna K, et al. Mineralocorticoid blockade reduces vascular injury in stroke-prone hypertensive rats. Hypertension 1998;31:451–8.
58. Joffe HV, Adler GK. Effect of aldosterone and mineralocorticoid receptor blockade on vascular inflammation. Heart Fail Rev 2005;10:31–7.
59. Gordon RD, Laragh JH, Funder JW. Low renin hypertensive states: perspectives, unsolved problems, future research. Trends Endocrinol Metab 2005;16:108–13.
60. Vasan RS, Evans JC, Larson MG, et al. Serum aldosterone and the incidence of hypertension in nonhypertensive persons. N Engl J Med 2004;351:33–41.
61. Esler M, Jennings G, Lambert G, et al. Overflow of catecholamine neurotransmitters to the circulation: source, fate, and functions. Physiol Rev 1990;70:963–85.
62. Seals DR, Dinenno FA. Collateral damage: cardiovascular consequences of chronic sympathetic activation with human aging. Am J Physiol Heart Circ Physiol 2004;287:H1895–905.
63. Esler M, Hastings J, Lambert G, et al. The influence of aging on the human sympathetic nervous system and brain norepinephrine turnover. Am J Physiol Regul Integr Comp Physiol 2002;282:R909–16.
64. Landsberg L. Insulin-mediated sympathetic stimulation: role in the pathogenesis of obesity-related hypertension (or, how insulin affects blood pressure, and why). J Hypertens 2001;19:523–8.
65. Caplea A, Seachrist D, Daneshvar H, et al. Noradrenergic content and turnover rate in kidney and heart shows gender and strain differences. J Appl Physiol 2002;92:567–71.
66. Grisk O, Rose HJ, Lorenz G, et al. Sympathetic-renal interaction in chronic arterial pressure control. Am J Physiol Regul Integr Comp Physiol 2002;283:R441–50.
67. Grisk O, Rettig R. Interactions between the sympathetic nervous system and the kidneys in arterial hypertension. Cardiovasc Res 2004;61:238–46.
68. Cabassi A, Vinci S, Cantoni AM, et al. Sympathetic activation in adipose tissue and skeletal muscle of hypertensive rats. Hypertension 2002;39:656–61.
69. Rumantir MS, Kaye DM, Jennings GL, et al. Phenotypic evidence of faulty neuronal norepinephrine reuptake in essential hypertension. Hypertension 2000;36:824–9.

70. Rumantir MS, Vaz M, Jennings GL, et al. Neural mechanisms in human obesity-related hypertension. J Hypertens 1999;17:1125–33.
71. Esler M, Jennings G, Korner P, et al. Assessment of human sympathetic nervous system activity from measurements of norepinephrine turnover. Hypertension 1988;11:3–20.

Screening for Adrenal-Endocrine Hypertension: Overview of Accuracy and Cost-effectiveness

Gary L. Schwartz, MD

KEYWORDS

- Screening • Secondary hypertension • Adrenal
- Diagnostic accuracy

Hypertension is a highly prevalent disorder afflicting 29% of adults in the United States.[1] It is a major risk factor for cardiovascular disease morbidity and mortality including myocardial infarction, congestive heart failure, stroke, renal disease, and dementia.[2–5] Multiple treatment trials have clearly shown the effectiveness of blood pressure control in preventing cardiovascular disease events.[6,7] Although control rates are improving, approximately 50% of adults with hypertension remain uncontrolled.[1] Most adults with increased blood pressure have primary or essential hypertension for which the cause is unknown. Generally, lifelong treatment is required. The proportion of patients with secondary or identifiable causes of hypertension is uncertain. Older studies suggest that secondary forms account for less than 10% of hypertension.[8] However, with the development of newer screening and diagnostic procedures, the frequency of some secondary forms of hypertension may be higher than previously believed.[9] Detection of secondary hypertension is important because, depending on the cause, it may be possible to cure the hypertension or tailor therapy to achieve control with fewer medications, reducing cost and side effects. In the case of endocrine causes of hypertension, identification is also important because undetected disorders can be fatal and confer adverse effects beyond those caused by increased blood pressure.

This article focuses on issues of accuracy and cost-effectiveness of screening strategies for 2 important endocrine causes of hypertension: primary aldosteronism,

This work was supported in part by US Public Health Service grants R01-HL53330, MO1-RR00039, GCRC grant MO1-RR00585, and funds from the Mayo Foundation.
The author has nothing to disclose.
Division of Nephrology and Hypertension, College of Medicine, Mayo Clinic, West 19, Mayo Building, 200 First Street SW, Rochester, MN 55905, USA
E-mail address: schwartz.gary@mayo.edu

a common secondary cause of hypertension; and pheochromocytoma, a rare secondary cause of hypertension. Cost-effectiveness of screening involves an understanding of the clinical contexts where the likelihood of these disorders is high enough to justify testing and where the potential adverse clinical consequences of missing the diagnosis justify the expense and risks associated with screening. It also requires an understanding of the diagnostic accuracy of current screening tests and strategies and the effect of positive and negative results on the probability of disease to limit further diagnostic investigations to those most likely to have one of these disorders.

BASICS OF COST-EFFECTIVENESS OF HEALTH INTERVENTIONS

Formal cost-effectiveness analysis is an analytical tool that assesses the costs and effects of an intervention designed to prevent, diagnose, or treat a disease compared with an alternative strategy designed to achieve the same goals.[10,11] A ratio is constructed in which the numerator is the net expenditure of health care resources (a monetary measure) and the denominator is the net improvement in health (a nonmonetary measure). In the context of the present discussion, for each of the endocrine causes of hypertension, the immediate costs are those associated with performing the relevant screening test(s) and any subsequent tests required to confirm the diagnosis and, where necessary, to identify subtypes of disease as well as costs related to any disease-specific interventions. Additional costs considered are those caused by patient time expended (lost wages), caregiving (paid or unpaid), travel expenses, and economic costs to employers. The most common measure of net improvement in health used in the denominator is quality-adjusted life years (QALYs) gained. The final value of the cost-effectiveness ratio represents the marginal effects in both the numerator and the denominator of the intervention compared with the alternative strategy, which, in the context of this discussion, represents the costs related to management of the blood pressure in the setting of an unrecognized endocrine cause and the estimated effect of missing the diagnosis on QALYs. No formal cost-effectiveness analyses have been performed for screening for the endocrine causes of hypertension considered here. The marginal effects on cost and health improvement arising from screening for endocrine causes of hypertension can only be discussed in general terms in this article.

PRINCIPLES UNDERLYING ACCURACY OF DIAGNOSTIC TESTING

Use of a screening test to evaluate for the presence of a disease requires an understanding of the mathematical relationships between test characteristics (ie, sensitivity and specificity) as well as some estimate of the likelihood that the disease is present (pretest probability) in various clinical contexts.[12] The relationship of a screening test result and the presence or absence of a disease is shown in **Fig. 1**. In this scheme, the screening test results are interpreted as either being positive or negative using a defined cut-point value (which is the case for most screening tests for endocrine hypertension). Sensitivity is defined as the proportion of people with the disease who have a positive test result. Specificity is the proportion of people without the disease who have a negative test result. As discussed in more detail later, sensitivity and specificity have not been clearly determined for many of the screening tests used to evaluate for endocrine hypertension. In part, this is because of the lack of an established gold standard used across studies to define the presence of the disease. Different gold standards for diagnosis yield different estimates of sensitivity and specificity. In addition, negative results of screening tests are less well studied than positive results in the medical literature because of a reluctance to perform confirmation

		DISEASE	
		Present	Absent
TEST	Positive	**True Positive** (a)	*False Positive* (b)
	Negative	*False Negative* (c)	**True Negative** (d)

Sensitivity = a/a+c   Specificity = d/b+d

Positive predictive value = a/a+b   Negative predictive value = c/c+d

Positive Liklihood ratio = $\frac{a/a+c}{b/b+d}$ Negative likelihood ratio = $\frac{c/a+c}{d/b+d}$

Fig. 1. Diagnostic test characteristics and definitions.

testing in persons with a negative screening test result. Thus, the false-negative rates for screening tests are often underestimated.

The ideal screening test would be characterized by having both a high sensitivity and specificity; however, for most screening tests, a trade-off between sensitivity and specificity is required when test results have a range of potential values; this is certainly the case for endocrine hypertension screening tests, which measure laboratory values that vary across a continuum (plasma renin activity [PRA]; serum aldosterone concentration; plasma or urine catecholamines or their metabolites; plasma, urine, or salivary cortisol). In these circumstances, the location of a cut-point that distinguishes normal from abnormal is arbitrary. Receiver-operator characteristic (ROC) curves are used to obtain the cut-point value that optimizes sensitivity and specificity for a given screening test (**Fig. 2**).

Test characteristics of sensitivity and specificity are important considerations when choosing a specific test to screen for a given disease. For example, the most sensitive test available should be used to screen for a dangerous but treatable disease such as pheochromocytoma. Highly sensitive screening tests are also useful when the probability of disease is low and the purpose of the test is to discover a disease, because a highly sensitive test is rarely negative in the presence of disease (few false-negative results). A highly sensitive test is most helpful when negative because it rules out the disease. In contrast, a highly specific test is best suited to confirm a diagnosis that is suggested by other data, because a highly specific test is rarely positive in the absence of disease (few false-positives). A highly specific test is most helpful when the result is positive because it rules in the disease.

Sensitivity and specificity of diagnostic tests are often determined using samples of persons with known disease (cases) and persons known not to have the disease (controls). With these extremes, the test may perform well. However, sensitivity/specificity may change when the test is applied to patients in clinical practice where the

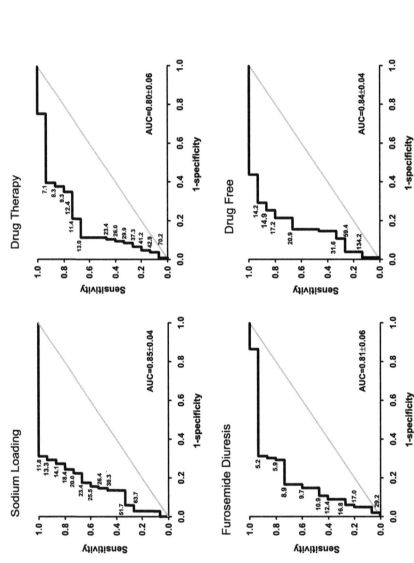

Fig. 2. ROC curves for the aldosterone/PRA ratio determined under 4 clinical conditions: drug therapy, concurrent antihypertensive drug therapy; drug free, after a minimum 2-week antihypertensive drug-free interval; sodium loading, after 4 days of high sodium diet; furosemide diuresis, after acute furosemide diuresis. Optimum cut-point in bold for each ROC curve is expressed using conventional units of ng/mL/h for PRA and ng/dL for aldosterone. (*From* Schwartz GL, Turner ST. Screening for primary aldosteronism in essential hypertension: diagnostic accuracy of the ratio of plasma aldosterone concentration to plasma renin activity. Clin Chem 2005;51(2):390; with permission.)

severity of disease may differ from the extremes used in case-control studies or when patients without the disease differ from the controls by frequently having other conditions that cause a false-positive result.

The predictive value of a test is defined as the probability of the disease given the test results (posttest probability, see **Fig. 2**). Positive predictive value is the probability of having the disease in a patient with a positive test result, whereas negative predictive value is the probability of not having the disease in a patient with a negative test result. Predictive value is determined from the sensitivity and specificity of the test and an estimate of the prevalence of the disease in the population being tested (pretest probability). For endocrine hypertension, there is variable information available regarding prevalence of disease in various clinical contexts, which influences the ability to estimate the predictive value of screening tests in all circumstances. The importance of pretest probability in test interpretation is illustrated by a positive result, even for a test with high specificity, likely being a false-positive if the pretest probability of disease is low. Similarly, a negative result, even for a test with high sensitivity, is likely to be a false-negative if the pretest probability of disease is high.

An alternative way of describing the performance of a diagnostic test is the use of likelihood ratios. The likelihood ratio for a particular value of a diagnostic test is defined as the probability of the test result in the presence of disease divided by the probability of the result in the absence of disease. It expresses how many times more or less likely a test result is present in persons with the disease compared with those without the disease. A major advantage of using likelihood ratios is that it is possible to summarize the information contained in a test result for any value of the test across the entire range of possible values rather than limiting interpretation at a single cutoff point. The potential value of using likelihood ratios across values of screening test results rather than a single cut-point are discussed later.

Because screening tests for endocrine hypertension are imperfect and characterized by intermediate sensitivities and specificities, the use of multiple tests is sometimes suggested as a screening strategy. Generally, multiple tests are performed in 2 ways. They can be performed in parallel (all at the same time), in which case a positive result from any single test is interpreted as evidence for disease, or they can be performed serially (consecutively) with subsequent tests performed based on positive results of a previous test. When performed serially, all tests must be positive to make the diagnosis.

In general, multiple tests performed in parallel increase the sensitivity and, therefore, the negative predictive value for a given pretest probability (prevalence) beyond that of any of the single tests at the expense of a lower specificity and positive predictive value. Parallel testing is useful when a sensitive screening strategy is desired but only 2 or more insensitive tests are available. This strategy misses fewer persons with the disease but increases the number without the disease who may undergo additional tests or interventions.

In general, multiple tests performed serially increases the specificity and, therefore, the positive predictive value for a given pretest probability (prevalence) beyond that of any of the single tests at the expense of a lower sensitivity and negative predictive value. Serial testing is useful when none of the available individual tests are highly specific. This strategy makes it more certain that a positive result represents disease, but at an increased risk that some with disease will be missed. When using 2 tests in series, use of the test with the higher specificity (and usually lower sensitivity) first is more cost-effective because it usually leads to the same number of cases identified with fewer patients subjected to both tests.

PRIMARY ALDOSTERONISM

Primary aldosteronism (PA) is the syndrome resulting from the autonomous overproduction of aldosterone. In general, it is caused by a unilateral aldosterone-producing adenoma (APA) or bilateral adrenal hyperplasia (idiopathic PA [IPA]). Other rare variants also occur. Morbidity arises from both increased blood pressure and non–blood pressure effects of aldosterone acting through the mineralocorticoid receptor inducing vascular injury and fibrosis in the heart and kidneys.[13–15] Thus, at the same level of blood pressure, patients with PA have higher morbidity and mortality than those with essential hypertension.[16] However, it is not certain whether, in the conditions of blood pressure control, morbidity or mortality outcomes differ between these groups. Distinction between the 2 major subtypes is important because removal of an APA may lead to cure of hypertension with attendant reduction in health risks and improvement in quality of life, whereas patients with idiopathic hyperaldosteronism (IHA) require lifelong treatment with antihypertensive drugs. However, targeted therapy using a mineralocorticoid receptor blocker may lead to improved blood pressure control with the need for fewer medications in some patients.

Screening for PA: Considerations Related to Cost-effectiveness

Although anecdotal clinical experience suggests detection of PA to be associated with improved blood pressure control and patient satisfaction, there are no data from clinical trials that directly link screening for PA to reduced morbidity, mortality, or improvements in quality of life. Given this limitation of evidence, screening should be restricted to patient subgroups for which the alternative treatment strategy, assuming a diagnosis of essential hypertension, could be reasonably considered to be inferior. Moreover, given the limitations of the currently recommended screening test (reviewed later), a decision regarding the relative harm of missing the diagnosis versus the potential costs and harms related to subjecting patients with false-positive screening results to further diagnostic studies also needs to be considered.

Screening for PA: Pretest Probability of Disease in Hypertensive Subsets

Current clinical guidelines from the Endocrine Society advise clinicians to limit screening for PA to patient subgroups with a high prevalence of the disease (pretest probability).[17] This is reasonable because screening restricted to hypertensive subgroups with a moderate prevalence of disease limits the number of false-positive screening results.

Estimates of the prevalence of PA vary across studies related in part to whether primary or referral populations are assessed (referral bias) and to variation in the reference standard used to confirm the diagnosis (verification bias).[18] However, PA seems to be the most common potentially curable secondary form of hypertension. In a study by Schwartz and Turner[19] using a community-based sample of adults with presumed essential hypertension (no referral bias) in which all participants (regardless of screening test results) underwent confirmatory testing for PA with dietary sodium loading, the prevalence was 13% (95% confidence interval 7%–20%). In a study by Mosso and colleagues,[20] assessing patients from primary care clinics (no referral bias) who underwent confirmatory testing with a fludrocortisone suppression test only if screening test results were positive, the prevalence of PA increased with the severity of hypertension (mild hypertension 2%, moderate hypertension 8%, severe hypertension 13%). Multiple studies have shown a high prevalence of PA, ranging from 17% to 23%, in patients referred with hypertension that is resistant or difficult to control.[21–24] The Primary Aldosteronism Prevalence in Hypertensives (PAPY) study screened 1125 newly diagnosed hypertensive adults for PA.[9] Screen-positive patients had the diagnosis confirmed with captopril suppression testing or with application of a validated logistic function. In this study, PA subtype (APA vs IHA) was determined in all diagnosed patients. The overall prevalence of PA was 11.2%, with 43% caused by APA and 57% caused by IHA. Thus, in the overall sample less than 5% of patients had an APA, which is the potentially curable form of PA.

Table 1 includes a complete listing of subgroups of the hypertensive population suggested for PA screening by the Endocrine Society,[17] with estimates of the prevalence of PA associated with each subgroup.[17,25] This list includes subsets with a moderate pretest probability of disease, and other subsets for which the pretest probability is presumed to be increased but remains uncertain. This uncertainty impairs determination of the predictive value of the screening test. In addition, this list includes subsets for which the pretest probability may be low, such as persons with hypertension and an adrenal incidentaloma. Motivation for screening such patients is derived from the possibility of finding surgically curable disease. This motivation must be tempered by the clinical context. The cost-effectiveness of screening a person with an adrenal mass but without hypokalemia and with easily controlled hypertension may not be justifiable, especially given that only 33% of patients with APA are cured with surgical removal of the tumor.[26] Also, if the pretest probability of disease is low (1%–2%), a higher rate of false-positive screening results will follow and, in the context of a known adrenal mass, the likelihood of performing further invasive diagnostic studies with their associated costs and risks will be high.

The other subsets recommended for screening (see Table 1) are those in which the alternative treatment strategy (assuming a diagnosis of essential hypertension) is often

Table 1
Hypertensive subsets considered for PA screening

Hypertensive Subset	Prevalence; Pretest Probability (%)
Moderate/severe hypertension (BP >160/100 mm Hg)	8–13
Resistant hypertension Defined by BP ≥140/90 mm Hg despite full doses of 3 complimentary antihypertensive drugs including a diuretic appropriate for level of renal function	17–23
Hypertension with unprovoked hypokalemia associated with renal potassium wasting[27]	50
Hypertension and an adrenal incidentaloma	1–10 (1–2 in the absence of severe hypertension or hypokalemia)
Hypertension and diuretic associated hypokalemia (especially if treatment resistant or in the presence of concomitant use of potassium-sparing diuretics or renin-angiotensin system blocking drugs)	Uncertain
Hypertensive first degree relatives of persons with PA	Uncertain
Hypertension and family history of early onset Hypertension or stroke (especially cerebral hemorrhage at a young age (<40 y)	Uncertain

Abbreviation: BP, blood pressure.
Data from Funder JW, Carey RM, Fardella C, et al. Case detection, diagnosis, and treatment of patients with primary aldosteronism: an Endocrine Society clinical practice guideline. J Clin Endocrinol Metab 2008;93:3268.

unsuccessful or is associated with the need for intensive treatment, with its associated high costs and negative effects on quality of life. In these settings, screening has a higher likelihood of being cost-effective. Screening of all persons for PA at the time of the diagnosis of hypertension cannot be supported by current knowledge.

Screening for PA: Plasma Aldosterone/Renin Ratio

The recommended screening test of choice for PA is the aldosterone/renin ratio (ARR), which represents the ratio of values of simultaneously measured plasma aldosterone concentration divided by PRA.[17] The rationale for the ARR as a screening test is based on the assumption that the usual dependency of aldosterone on renin is lost in PA and aldosterone becomes disproportionately increased relative to the concomitant renin. Moreover, as aldosterone causes extracellular volume expansion, renin becomes secondarily suppressed, resulting in a further increase in the ratio value. A single cut-point value of the ratio is used to distinguish positive from negative results. Values of the ratio differ by methods and units used to report measures of renin and aldosterone. Most often, plasma aldosterone is expressed in conventional units of ng/dL and PRA in conventional units of ng/mL/h. Sometimes PRA and plasma aldosterone concentration are expressed in Systeme International (SI) units and, more recently, direct renin concentration (DRC) is measured in some laboratories and expressed as mU/L. Conventional units of PRA are converted to SI units of ng/L/s, by multiplying by 0.2778; conventional units of aldosterone are converted to SI units of pmol/L by multiplying by 27.74. In some laboratories, the ratio is calculated using aldosterone expressed in SI units and PRA expressed in conventional units. Dividing such ratio values by 27.4 gives the corresponding value determined by using conventional units for both PRA and aldosterone. A PRA of 1 ng/mL/h is equivalent to a DRC of 8.2 mU/L. In this article, values of the ratio using conventional units for both PRA and aldosterone are used.

DIAGNOSTIC ACCURACY OF THE ARR

Few studies have determined the test characteristics of the ARR (sensitivity, specificity, predictive value, and likelihood ratios) at different cut-point values. In 2002, Montori and Young[27] reviewed 16 prospective studies (>3000 participants) of the ARR as a screening test for PA. They observed that none of these studies evaluated the ARR and reference standard independently of each other; only 2 studies evaluated screen-negative patients with the reference standard, and only 16.7% of the participants had both the ARR and the reference standard performed. Moreover, the origin of the study samples (primary care vs referral clinics), the conditions of measurement (on or off antihypertensive drug therapy), the details of measurement (time of day, body position), and the specific laboratory methods of measuring PRA and aldosterone varied among studies. They concluded that there were no published valid estimates of the test characteristics of the ARR when used to screen for PA in patients with presumed essential hypertension. Schwartz and Turner[19] conducted a study to determine the diagnostic accuracy of the ARR and to assess the effects of antihypertensive drug therapy with hydrochlorothiazide and variations in dietary sodium balance on test characteristics. This study overcame most of the deficiencies noted in the review by Montori and Young.[27] Referral bias was avoided by using a community-based sample of adults with presumed essential hypertension. All participants were subjected to confirmatory testing for PA regardless of the ARR results. The reference standard used for diagnosis of PA was 24-hour urine aldosterone excretion greater than or equal to 12 μg following 4 days of dietary sodium loading with greater than 200 mEq sodium in the 24-hour urine collection. Study personnel were blinded to the results of the screening test and reference standard until the time of data analysis. The overall prevalence of biochemical PA in the study sample was 13%. ROC curves were constructed for the ARR in each of the 4 clinical conditions studied, and the optimum cutoff values for the ARR were determined (see **Fig. 2**). **Table 2** summarizes the optimum cut-points of the ARR and their associated test characteristics in each of the clinical conditions assessed. This study showed that the optimum cutoff value of the ARR varied with clinical conditions, ranging from 8.9 when assessed in conditions of acute sodium diuresis to 14.9 with usual sodium intake and off antihypertensive drugs. Depending on the clinical conditions of testing, sensitivity varied from 73% to 93% and specificity varied from 71% to 84%. Predictive value of a positive test was poor (≤41%), suggesting that the diagnosis should not be based on the ARR alone. However, the predictive value of a negative test was high (≥95%) in all clinical conditions assessed. The study showed that the ARR had only fair diagnostic accuracy in screening for PA.

The modest sensitivities observed in the study by Schwartz and Turner[19] was expected because it is known that the ARR can vary greatly in individuals with known PA. In one study of repeated determinations of the ratio in random and standardized conditions in 71 patients with confirmed PA caused by aldosterone-producing adenomas, normal ARR values were observed in 31% of patients on at least 1 occasion, and in only 37% of patients were the ARRs increased on all occasions of measurement.[28] These observations support the recommendation of Gordon[29] to obtain repeated measures of the ARR. This is a form of parallel testing that, as previously noted, increases sensitivity (fewer false-negatives) at the expense of lower specificity (more false-positives). The cost-effectiveness of such a strategy has not been formally assessed.

The modest specificities observed in the study by Schwartz and Turner[19] was also expected, given the known high frequency of low PRA among patients with essential hypertension.[29] In a previous study, Schwartz and colleagues[30] measured

	Drug Therapy	Drug Free	Sodium Loading	Acute Diuresis
Optimum cut-point[a]	12.4	14.9	13.3	8.9
Sensitivity (%)	73	87	93	73
Specificity (%)	74	75	71	84
Likelihood ratio				
Positive test	2.8	3.4	3.2	4.4
Negative test	0.36	0.18	0.10	0.32
Predictive value (%)				
Positive test	29	33	32	41
Negative test	95	97	99	96

Table 2
Test characteristics of the ARR to screen for PA

Abbreviations: Drug therapy, concurrent antihypertensive drug therapy; drug free, after a minimum 2-week antihypertensive drug-free interval; sodium loading, after 4 days of high sodium diet; acute diuresis, after acute furosemide diuresis.

[a] Optimum cut-point expressed using conventional units of ng/mL/h for PRA and ng/dL for aldosterone.

Data from Schwartz GL, Turner ST. Screening for primary aldosteronism in essential hypertension: diagnostic accuracy of the ratio of plasma aldosterone concentration to plasma renin activity. Clin Chem 2005;51:390.

aldosterone and PRA in a large sample of 505 black and white adults with presumed essential hypertension 4 weeks off antihypertensive drug therapy. Using a cut-point value of 20, they determined the sensitivity, specificity, and predictive value of the ARR to identify combinations of PRA and aldosterone compatible with PA (low PRA defined as a value within the lowest quartile of the sample distribution and increased aldosterone for level of PRA defined as a value in the highest quartile predicted by linear regression on renin). Overall, the sensitivity of an increased ARR to identify combinations of PRA and aldosterone compatible with PA was 66% (80% in blacks vs 56% in whites). Overall specificity was 67% (46% in blacks and 84% in whites). Positive predictive value was only 34% (49% in whites and 27% in blacks). In 36% of instances, an increased ARR was solely a measure of low PRA without increased aldosterone for renin. The renin dependency of the ARR was also noted in a study by Montori and colleagues,[31] who measured PRA and aldosterone in a sample of 497 black and white adults with presumed essential hypertension in several conditions (in the supine position and in the seated position after 30 minutes of ambulation having been off antihypertensive drugs for 4 weeks and in the seated position after 30 minutes of ambulation following 4 weeks of treatment with hydrochlorothiazide). They observed that variation in the ARR was strongly and inversely dependent on variation in PRA and predominately an indicator of low PRA rather than an indicator of renin-independent aldosterone levels suitable to assess for PA. To improve the specificity of the ARR, some have advocated the addition of a minimum threshold value of aldo-sterone as part of the screening criteria.[32] This represents a serial test strategy. As previously noted, such a strategy increases specificity (fewer false-positives) but at the expense of further reductions in sensitivity (more false-negatives).

A practical problem facing clinicians in clinical practice is to decide which cut-point value of the ARR to use for a positive result. Suggested cut-point values for the ARR range from 15 to 100.[17,19] The most commonly used cut-point values for a positive ARR are 20 to 30.[17] The use of a single cut-point value to determine whether the test is considered positive or negative excludes useful information available from any single value obtained during screening. Reporting of likelihood ratios associated with ranges of values of the ARR could be used by the clinician to determine the impact of any measured value of the ARR on the probability of PA. As can be seen by inspection of the ROC curves (see **Fig. 2**), high values of the ARR have high spec-ificity for PA. In certain clinical settings (eg, hypertension with spontaneous hypoka-lemia associated with renal potassium wasting), a high value of the ARR by itself could be considered diagnostic for PA without the need for further confirmatory testing.

PHEOCHROMOCYTOMA

A pheochromocytoma is defined as a tumor arising from catecholamine-producing chromaffin cells in the adrenal medulla (intra-adrenal paraganglioma) or in extra-adrenal sympathetic and parasympathetic paraganglia (extra-adrenal paragan-glioma). As detailed later, pheochromocytomas are a rare cause of hypertension. Motivation for screening and case detection is the recognition that pheochromocy-toma can be fatal if unrecognized.

Screening for Pheochromocytoma: Considerations Related to Cost-effectiveness

Although a formal assessment of the cost-effectiveness of pheochromocytoma screening has not been performed, there are several issues that can be expected to influence this calculation. The first issue is the knowledge that pheochromocytoma can be a fatal disorder. Therefore, the potential health benefit (denominator) in the cost-effectiveness ratio is high. The second issue is the recognition that pheochromocytoma is rare in the population but clinical presentations raising the possibility of pheochromocytoma are common. In one reported series, only 1 of 300 patients evaluated for pheochromocytoma had the disorder.[33] A third issue relates to the diagnostic characteristics of the multiple available screening tests and how to use these most efficiently for case detection. A fourth issue relates to interpretation and clinical decision making for marginally increased screening test results. Further testing involving expensive imaging modalities can add significantly to the cost of case detection.

An analysis by Sawka and colleagues[34] illustrates how these issues can affect the cost of case detection. In this report, costs associated with 3 strategies of screening for pheochromocytoma (assuming diagnostic imaging for positive biochemical test results) in a population in which disease prevalence was 0.5% ranged from $60,000.00 to $116,000.00. Although these costs seem high, they may be reasonable when expressed as cost per life saved. However, given these cost estimates, it is obligatory that clinicians strive to identify the most effective and cost-efficient strategy for case identification.

Screening for Pheochromocytoma: Pretest Probability of Disease

Patients considered for pheochromocytoma screening include those with resistant hypertension, hyperadrenergic spells, a family history of pheochromocytoma, a hypertensive response to anesthesia, early onset hypertension (<20 years old), hypertension and unexplained cardiomyopathy, an incidental adrenal mass identified on imaging tests, and those with genetic disorders known to be associated with pheochromocytoma. Estimates of the prevalence of pheochromocytoma in some of these clinical subsets are summarized in **Table 3**.[35] For most patients encountered in clinical practice, the clinical indications for screening are often resistant hypertension or hyperadrenergic spells. The prevalence estimates of pheochromocytoma in such settings are low. As noted earlier, in settings where the prevalence of disease is low, a positive screening test result, even for a test with high specificity, is likely to be a false-positive. Therefore, clinical decision making is important when confronted with positive results from screening, especially if the results are only marginally positive. Considering test results in a binary fashion (positive or negative) is less informative than considerations related to the continuous nature of the results of screening tests for pheochromocytoma.

Table 3 Patient subsets and prevalence of pheochromocytoma	
Patient Subset	**Prevalence; Pretest Probability (%)**
Unselected hypertension population	0.2
Hypertension and suggestive symptoms	0.5
Adrenal incidentaloma	4
Hereditary forms of pheochromocytoma	
Multiple endocrine neoplasia type II	30–50
von Hippel-Lindau disease	15–20
Neurofibromatosis type I	1–5
Familial paraganglioma syndrome	20

Screening Tests for Pheochromocytoma

Diagnosis of pheochromocytoma requires biochemical evidence of excessive cate-cholamine production by the tumor. A variety of screening tests are available and consist of measurements of catecholamines (epinephrine, norepinephrine) or their metabolites (metanephrine, normetanephrine, or vanillylmandelic acid) in the blood or urine. The metabolites of epinephrine and norepinephrine can be reported as total metanephrines (metanephrine plus normetanephrine) or separately (fractionated metanephrines).

Most of the metabolism of catecholamines occurs within the cells that produce them, rather than after release into the circulation.[36] Within catecholamine-producing cells, vesicular stores of catecholamines are in a highly dynamic state of equilibrium with catecholamines in the cytoplasm. Active transport from cytoplasm to storage vesicles is countered by ongoing passive leakage of catecholamines from these vesicles. The small fractions of catecholamines that escape vesicular sequestration are subsequently metabolized by catechol O-methyl transferase and the metabolites are released into the circulation. This process accounts for most of the measured catecholamine metabolites in the plasma and urine. Within a catechol-amine-producing tumor, this process is occurring continuously and independently of catecholamine release, which often occurs only intermittently. This process provides a rationale for the observed higher diagnostic sensitivity of measures of plasma or urine catecholamine metabolites (metanephrines) than measures of plasma or urine catecholamines.[37,38] Among the catecholamine metabolites, vanillylmandelic acid has been shown to have poor diagnostic sensitivity and, thus, measurement of the fractionated catecholamine metabolites (metanephrine and normetanephrine in the plasma or urine) are the preferred screening tests for pheochromocytoma.[37–39]

Both plasma and urinary metanephrines are often measured by high pressure liquid chromatography with electrochemical detection. More recently, methods using gas chromatography with mass spectrometry or liquid chromatography with tandem mass spectrometry are being used. These newer methods of analysis are preferred because they are less susceptible to medication interference and nonspecific binding and, thus, are associated with higher diagnostic accuracy.[40]

Plasma metanephrines circulate freely in the plasma and are sulfated as they pass through the gastrointestinal circulation. The sulfated conjugates are excreted in the urine. Reported plasma metanephrines are usually measured in their free form, whereas reported urine metanephrines are measured after being deconjugated. Whether this results in differences in diagnostic performance between the tests is uncertain; however, plasma concentrations of free metanephrines are independent of renal function, which is not the case for urinary metanephrines. Thus, the plasma test is preferred in the presence of chronic kidney disease if glomerular filtration rate is less than 30 mL/min.[41]

DIAGNOSTIC ACCURACY OF PLASMA FREE AND URINARY FRACTIONATED METANEPHRINES

Several studies have assessed the test characteristics (sensitivity, specificity) of plasma free and urinary fractionated metanephrines (metanephrine and normeta-nephrine). Differences in results across studies can be influenced by several factors, including the analytical method used for determination of results, the sample studied (proportion of patients with sporadic vs hereditary pheochromocytoma, inclusion of patients with renal dysfunction), and the upper value of the reference range used to distinguish a positive from a negative test result. Test characteristics from more recent studies are summarized in **Table 4**.[38,40,42,43] In these studies, both sensitivity and specificity were slightly higher for plasma free metanephrines than for urinary fractionated metanephrines (for sensitivity, 96%–100% vs 86%–97%; for specificity, 89%–98% vs 86%–95%). However, these differences are small and the characteristics of these tests are similar. Plasma free metanephrines avoid the inconvenience of a 24-hour urine collection (especially in children) and the concerns associated with a possible incomplete collection. Also, plasma free metanephrines are not influenced by renal dysfunction.

As noted earlier, consideration of the continuous distribution of values for these tests in clinical decision making, rather than a binary positive or negative interpretation, is important. For example, values of plasma metanephrines that are greater than fourfold more than the reference range are associated with a virtual certainty of disease.[44] Values that are marginally more than the reference range must be interpreted carefully. Consideration of causes for false-positive results of either plasma or urine fractionated metanephrines should be made. These causes include concomitant use of drugs, especially phenoxybenzamine, tricyclic antidepressants, buspirone, and drugs containing catecholamines, such as decongestants and weight loss aids. Other settings associated with false-positive results include sudden discontinuation of drugs such as clonidine, benzodiazepines, or ethanol and severe, untreated sleep apnea. For plasma free metanephrines, performance of the test in the supine, rather than sitting, position may result in resolution of borderline elevations.[39] Diets rich in biogenic amines (ie, fruits and nuts) can cause up to a twofold increase in deconjugated normetanephrine levels (measured in the urine) but have no effect on plasma free metanephrines.[45] Repeating the test after consideration of these issues would be appropriate. For marginally increased plasma metanephrine or normetanephrine, values of the metanephrine/epinephrine ratio less than 4.2 and the normetanephrine/norepinephrine ratio less than 0.52 are consistent with a false-positive increase. The response of normetanephrine to oral clonidine can help distinguish false-positive from true-positive results.[44] Measurement of plasma chromogranin A or urine fractionated metanephrines in patients with marginally increased plasma metanephrines may improve diagnostic specificity.[46]

Screening for Pheochromocytoma: Multiple Testing Strategies

It is common in practice to order multiple screening tests in patients who are considered to be at high risk for pheochromocytoma. As noted previously, tests can be ordered in parallel or serially. Multiple tests ordered in parallel (all at the same time) increase the sensitivity of screening at the expense of lower specificity. This strategy is most often used when individual screening tests lack sensitivity, but this is not the

Table 4
Test characteristics of plasma free and urinary fractionated metanephrines[a]

Study	Plasma Free Metanephrines		Urinary Metanephrines	
	Sensitivity (%)	Specificity (%)	Sensitivity (%)	Specificity (%)
Perry et al[42]	—	—	97.1	91.1
Hickman et al[38]	100	97.6	85.7	95.1
Grouzmann et al[43]	96	89	95	86
Peaston et al[40]	100	96	—	—

[a] Tests characteristics based on a positive test defined as either metanephrine or normetanephrine more than the reference range, and a negative test defined as both metanephrine and normetanephrine within the reference range.

case for the recommended screening tests for pheochromocytoma and, thus, this practice is generally discouraged. In most patients encountered in clinical practice, the pretest probability of disease is low, and a parallel screening strategy most often leads to additional invasive testing in patients with false-positive results. However, in patients in whom the pretest probability is high (see **Table 3**), parallel testing may be justified.

As discussed earlier, several serial testing strategies have been suggested for further evaluation of marginally increased plasma or urine fractionated metanephrines to improve specificity and reduce the number of false-positive patients undergoing further invasive diagnostic tests.[44,46] In general, serial testing is useful when none of the available screening tests is highly specific. As noted in **Table 4**, both plasma and urine fractionated metanephrines have similar, but only moderate, specificity for pheochromocytoma. In general, serial testing increases specificity at the expense of lower sensitivity, and this must be kept in mind when using such strategies for identification of a potentially fatal disorder.

SUMMARY

Formal studies have not been performed to assess the cost-effectiveness of screening strategies for endocrine causes of hypertension. However, an understanding of the diagnostic accuracy of available screening tests and the clinical settings where disease identification will lead to improved health outcomes form the basis for a cost-effective strategy. PA may be common, but screening should be selective and restricted to those settings where knowledge of the diagnosis has the greatest chance of improving health outcomes. Pheochromocytoma is very rare; however, because it is a potentially fatal disease, screening strategies should err on the side of not missing the diagnosis, especially in high-risk clinical settings.

REFERENCES

1. Egan BM, Zhao Y, Axon RN. US trends in prevalence, awareness, treatment, and control of hypertension, 1988–2008. JAMA 2010;303:2043–50.
2. Kannel WB. Blood pressure as a cardiovascular risk factor. JAMA 1996;275: 1571–6.
3. Gorelick PB. Stroke prevention therapy beyond antithrombotics: unifying mechanisms in ischemic stroke pathogenesis and implications for therapy: an invited review. Stroke 2002;33:862–75.
4. Tozawa M, Iseki K, Iseki C, et al. Blood pressure predicts risk of developing end-stage renal disease in men and women. Hypertension 2003;41:1341–5.
5. Birns J, Kalra L. Cognitive function and hypertension. J Hum Hypertens 2009;23: 86–96.
6. Staessen JA, Wang JG, Thijs L. Cardiovascular protection and blood pressure reduction: a meta-analysis. Lancet 2001;358:1305–15.
7. Law MR. Use of blood pressure lowering drugs in the prevention of cardiovascular disease: meta-analysis of 147 randomised trials in the context of expectations from prospective epidemiological studies. BMJ 2009;338:b1665. DOI: 10.1136/bmj.b1665.
8. Sinclair AM, Isles CG, Brown I, et al. Secondary hypertension in a blood pressure clinic. Arch Intern Med 1987;147:1289–93.
9. Rossi GP, Bernini G, Caliumi C, et al. A prospective study of the prevalence of primary aldosteronism in 1,125 hypertensive patients. J Am Coll Cardiol 2006; 48:2293–300.

10. Mandelblatt JS, Fryback DG, Weinstein MC, et al. Assessing the effectiveness of health interventions for cost-effectiveness analysis. J Gen Intern Med 1997;12: 551–8.

11. Weinstein MC, Siegel JE, Gold MR, et al, for the Panel on Cost-Effectiveness in Health and Medicine. Recommendations of the Panel on Cost-effectiveness in Health and Medicine. JAMA 1996;276:1253–8.

12. Fletcher RH, Fletcher SW, Wagner EH. Diagnosis. In: Collins N, Eckhart C, Chalew GN, editors. Clinical epidemiology, the essentials. 2nd edition. Baltimore (MD): Williams & Wilkins; 1988. p. 42–75.

13. Holaj R, Zelinka T, Wichterle D, et al. Increased intima-media thickness of the common carotid artery in primary aldosteronism in comparison with essential hypertension. J Hypertens 2007;25:1451–7.

14. Diez J. Effects of aldosterone on the heart: beyond systemic hemodynamics? Hypertension 2008;52:462–4.

15. Reincke M, Rump LC, Quinkler M, et al. Risk factors associated with low glomerular filtration rate in primary aldosteronism. J Clin Endocrinol Metab 2009;94:869–75.

16. Milliez P, Girerd X, Plouin PF, et al. Evidence for an increased rate of cardiovas-cular events in patients with primary aldosteronism. J Am Coll Cardiol 2005;45: 1243–8.

17. Funder JW, Carey RM, Fardella C, et al. Case detection, diagnosis, and treatment of patients with primary aldosteronism: an Endocrine Society clinical practice guideline. J Clin Endocrinol Metab 2008;93:3266–81.

18. Kaplan NM. Is there an unrecognized epidemic of primary aldosteronism? (Con). Hypertension 2007;50:454–8.

19. Schwartz GL, Turner ST. Screening for primary aldosteronism in essential hyper-tension: diagnostic accuracy of the ratio of plasma aldosterone concentration to plasma renin activity. Clin Chem 2005;51(2):386–94.

20. Mosso L, Carvajal C, Gonzalez A, et al. Primary aldosteronism and hypertensive disease. Hypertension 2003;42:161–5.

21. Calhoun DA, Nishizaka MK, Zaman MA, et al. High prevalence of primary aldo-steronism among black and white subjects with resistant hypertension. Hyperten-sion 2002;40:892–6.

22. Gallay BJ, Ahmad S, Xu L, et al. Screening for primary aldosteronism without dis-continuing hypertensive medications: plasma aldosterone-renin ratio. Am J Kidney Dis 2001;37:699–705.

23. Eide IK, Torjesen PA, Drolsum A, et al. Low-renin status in therapy-resistant hyper-tension: a clue to efficient treatment. J Hypertens 2004;22:2217–26.

24. Strauch ZT, Hampf M, Bernhardt R, et al. Prevalence of primary hyperaldosteron-ism in moderate to severe hypertension in the central Europe region. J Hum Hypertens 2003;17:349–52.

25. Kaplan NM. Primary aldosteronism. In: Kaplan NM, editor. Clinical hypertension. 8th edition. Baltimore (MD): Lippincott Williams & Wilkins; 2002. p. 459.

26. Sawka AM, Young WF, Thompson GB, et al. Primary aldosteronism: factors asso-ciated with normalization of blood pressure after surgery. Ann Intern Med 2001; 135:258–61.

27. Montori VM, Young WF Jr. Use of plasma aldosterone concentration-to-plasma renin activity ratio as a screening test for primary aldosteronism. A systematic review of the literature. Endocinol Metab Clin North Am 2002;31:619–32.

28. Tanabe A, Natruse M, Takagi G, et al. Variability in the renin/aldosterone profile under random and standardized sampling conditions in primary aldosteronism. J Clin Endocrinol Metab 2003;88:2489–94.

29. Gordon RD. The challenge of more robust and reproducible methodology in screening for primary aldosteronism. J Hypertens 2004;22:251–5.

30. Schwartz GL, Chapman AB, Boerwinkle E, et al. Screening for primary aldosteronism: implications of an increased plasma aldosterone/renin ratio. Clin Chem 2002;48(11):1919–23.

31. Montori VM, Schwartz GL, Chapman AB, et al. Validity of the aldosterone-renin ratio to screen for primary aldosteronism. Mayo Clin Proc 2001;76:877–82.

32. Young WF. Primary aldosteronism: renaissance of a syndrome. Clin Endocrinol 2007;66:607–18.

33. Fogarty J, Engel C, Russo J, et al. Hypertension and pheochromocytoma testing: the association with anxiety orders. Arch Fam Med 1994;3:55.

34. Sawka AM, Gafni A, Thabane L, et al. The economic implications of three biochemical screening algorithms for pheochromocytoma. J Clin Endocrinol Metab 2004;89:2859–66.

35. Pacak K, Linehan WM, Eisenhofer G, et al. NIH Conference. Recent advances in genetics, diagnosis, localization, and treatment of pheochromocytoma. Ann Intern Med 2001;134:315–32.

36. Eisenhofer G, Kopin IJ, Goldstein DS. Catecholamine metabolism: a contemporary view with implications for physiology and medicine. Pharmacol Rev 2004; 56:331–49.

37. Lenders JW, Pacak K, Walther MM, et al. Biochemical diagnosis of pheochromocytoma. Which test is best? JAMA 2002;287:1427–34.

38. Hickman PE, Leong M, Chang J, et al. Plasma free metanephrines are superior to urine and plasma catecholamine metabolites for the investigation of pheochromocytoma. Pathology 2009;41(2):173–7.

39. Pacak K, Eisenhofer G, Ahlman H, et al. Pheochromocytoma: recommendations for clinical practice from the First International Symposium. Nat Clin Pract Endocrinol Metab 2007;3(2):92–102.

40. Peaston RT, Graham KS, Chambers E, et al. Performance of plasma free metanephrines measured by liquid chromatography-tandem mass spectrometry in the diagnosis of pheochromocytoma. Clin Chim Acta 2010;411:546–52.

41. Eisenhofer G, Huysmans F, Pacak K, et al. Plasma metanephrines in renal failure. Kidney Int 2005;67:668–77.

42. Perry CG, Sawka AM, Singh R, et al. The diagnostic accuracy of urinary fractionated metanephrines measured by tandem mass spectrometry in detection of pheochromocytoma. Clin Endocrinol (Oxf) 2007;66:703–8.

43. Grouzmann E, Drouard-Troalen L, Baudin E, et al. Diagnostic accuracy of free and total metanephrines in plasma and fractionated metanephrines in urine of patients with pheochromocytoma. Eur J Endocrinol 2010;162:951–60.

44. Eisenhofer G, Goldstein DS, Walther MM, et al. Biochemical diagnosis of pheochromocytoma: how to distinguish true-from false-positive test results. J Clin Endocrinol Metab 2003;88:2656–66.

45. de Jong WH, Eisenhofer G, Post WJ, et al. Dietary influences on plasma and urinary metanephrines: implications for diagnosis of catecholamine-producing tumors. J Clin Endocrinol Metab 2009;94:2841–9.

46. Algeciras-Schimnich A, Preissner CM, Young WF Jr, et al. Plasma chromogranin A or urine fractionated metanephrines follow-up testing improves the diagnostic accuracy of plasma fractionated metanephrines for pheochromocytoma. J Clin Endocrinol Metab 2008;93:91–5.

Hypertension in Pheochromocytoma: Characteristics and Treatment

Samuel M. Zuber[a,1], Vitaly Kantorovich, MD[b,1], Karel Pacak, MD, PhD, DSc[a,*]

KEYWORDS

- Pheochromocytoma • Paraganglioma • Hypertension
- Sustained • Catecholamine • Cardiovascular diseases

Pheochromocytomas and paragangliomas are tumors derived from chromaffin cells in the adrenal medulla or extra-adrenal paraganglia.[1] Pheochromocytomas and sympathetic paragangliomas usually synthesize and secrete norepinephrine and/or epinephrine, whereas 23% of parasympathetic paraganglia-derived tumors secrete only dopamine.[2,3] Adrenal tumors and tumors located in the sympathetic paraganglia are referred to as pheochromocytomas. Pheochromocytomas are found in 0.2% to 0.6% of subjects with hypertension.[4–6] The cost-effectiveness of diagnostic workup of pheochromocytoma is markedly restricted by low specificity of clinical symptoms together with symptoms overlapping within a wide variety of other conditions, including idiopathic hypertension, hyperthyroidism, heart failure, migraine, and anxiety.[7] In a study performed by the Mayo Clinic, out of 54 pheochromocytomas found on autopsy over a 50-year period, only 24% had been diagnosed before death.[8] McNeil and colleagues[9] reported only 1 undiagnosed pheochromocytoma out of 2031 autopsies, which may very well be related to both advances in biochemical and anatomic diagnosis and some degree of referral bias.

The most common sign of pheochromocytoma is hypertension, found in approximately 95% of patients and related to catecholamine excess.[10,11] Clinical characteristics of hypertension vary and may show either a sustained or a paroxysmal pattern.[12]

The authors have nothing to disclose.

[a] Section on Medical Neuroendocrinology, Program in Reproductive and Adult Endocrinology, *Eunice Kennedy Shriver* National Institute of Child Health and Human Development, National Institutes of Health, Building 10/CRC 1East Room 3140, 10 Center Drive, Bethesda, MD 20892-1109, USA

[b] Division of Endocrinology and Metabolism, University of Arkansas for Medical Sciences, Suite 817, 4301 West Markham Street, Little Rock, AR 72205-7199, USA

[1] Equal contribution.

* Corresponding author.

E-mail address: karel@mail.nih.gov

Endocrinol Metab Clin N Am 40 (2011) 295–311
doi:10.1016/j.ecl.2011.02.002
0889-8529/11/$ – see front matter. Published by Elsevier Inc.

In some patients, hypertensive paroxysms occur in the background of sustained hypertension. On the other hand, a small but significant proportion of patients with pheochromocytoma are normotensive. Pathophysiologic mechanisms of phenotypic characteristics of pheochromocytoma-related hypertension are discussed later. Additional symptoms seen in patients with pheochromocytoma include headache, palpitation, anxiety, and sweating.[13]

In addition to being a great mimicker, pheochromocytoma represents one of the most dazzling clinical paradoxes, in which symptoms and signs vary to hardly understandable degrees in seemingly comparable clinical settings. To understand this paradox, the multiple pathophysiologic variables that lead to clinically significant complications must be taken into account. Some of these variables mentioned and discussed later include (1) catecholamine synthesis in different chromaffin cell organs in health and disease, (2) differences in enzymatic machinery involved in catecholamine synthesis, (3) availability of substrate, (4) size/amount of secreting tissue and its metabolic activity, (5) type of secreted catecholamine, (6) amount of secreted catecholamine, (7) pattern of catecholamine secretion, (8) degree of end-organ damage. But most importantly, a certain depth of basic knowledge of catecholamine synthesis and metabolism is imperative in understanding pheochromocytoma clinically.

PHYSIOLOGY OF CATECHOLAMINE BIOSYNTHESIS

Catecholamines are synthesized in and secreted from chromaffin cells located in the adrenal medulla and sympathetic paraganglia, although catecholamine-positive secretory granules are also found in parasympathetic paraganglia. Enzymatic machinery of catecholamine-producing cells is of great importance for synthesis (**Fig. 1**). The first step is rate limiting as L-tyrosine is brought into the cell where it is hydroxylated to L-3,4-dihydroxyphenylalanine (L-dopa) via tyrosine hydroxylase (TH), an enzyme found only in cells that produce catecholamines.[14,15] Normally, molecular oxygen along with tetrahydropteridine (TH4) act as cofactors in this step, and the oxidation of TH4 by catecholamines represents a negative feedback loop, which inhibits TH from functioning.[16] Subsequently, L-dopa is decarboxylated to L-dihydroxyphenylethylamine (dopamine) by aromatic L-amino acid decarboxylase (AADC) in the cytoplasm of the cell, with pyridoxal phosphate acting as a cofactor in the reaction.[2,13] Dopamine then enters the neurosecretory vesicles, where it is hydroxylated by dopamine β-hydroxylase (DBH) to L-norepinephrine. Norepinephrine is further converted into epinephrine by the enzyme phenylethanolamine-N-methyltransferase (PNMT).

The paraganglial content of PNMT is negligible, which means most of the epinephrine is only produced in the adrenal glands. Under normal conditions, norepinephrine is released into the synaptic space through presynaptic exocytosis and reabsorbed through norepinephrine transporters with minimal, if any, systemic spillover. Norepinephrine and epinephrine are also released from the adrenal medulla through exocytosis in response to cholinergic stimulation by the splanchnic nerves.[13,17]

CATECHOLAMINE ACTION

Catecholamines, namely, norepinephrine, epinephrine, and dopamine, act through ubiquitously expressed G protein–coupled adrenergic receptors and play important roles in practically every aspect of human physiology. Norepinephrine signals through α_1, α_2, and β_1 receptors, whereas epinephrine primarily stimulates only β_1 and β_2 receptors. At normal levels, dopamine does not have much of an effect on any of the adrenergic receptors; however, as plasma concentrations increase (eg, dopamine-secreting tumor), dopamine can stimulate both α and β receptors.[13]

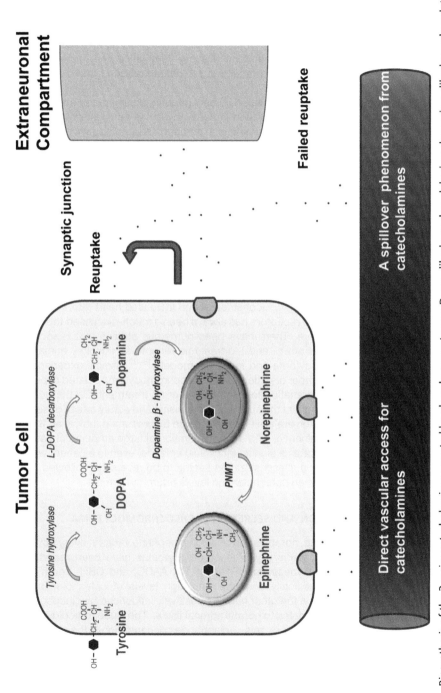

Fig. 1. Biosynthesis of the 3 major catecholamines secreted by pheochromocytomas. Dopa, dihydroxyphenylalanine; dopamine, dihydroxyphenylethylamine; PNMT, phenylethanolamine-*N*-methyltransferase. (*Data from* Eisenhofer G, Lenders JW, Pacak K. Biochemical diagnosis of pheochromocytoma. In: Lehnert H, editor. Pheochromocytoma pathophysiology and clinical management. Front horm res, vol. 31. Basel (Switzerland): Karger; 2004. p. 76–106.)

α_1-Adrenergic receptors are found primarily on smooth muscle tissue, including peripheral (coronary, cerebral, renal,) arteries and veins, causing vasoconstriction on stimulation. This vasoconstriction increases systemic pressure and reduces organ perfusion. It also induces positive inotropic effects in cardiomyocytes. α_2-Adrenergic receptors are located on the presynaptic surface of sympathetic ganglia, acting as a negative feedback loop for norepinephrine release. Stimulation of α_2-adrenergic receptors located on smooth muscles results in arterial vasodilation and coronary vasoconstriction.[13]

β_1-Adrenergic receptors can be stimulated by both norepinephrine and epinephrine. The positive inotropic effect of β_1 activation in cardiomyocytes is significantly more pronounced than that induced by α_1 stimulation. In addition, there is a significant positive chronotropic effect through stimulation of the cardiac pacemaker. Stimulation of β_1 receptors also results in the release of renin, which increases mean arterial blood pressure (BP) by converting angiotensinogen to angiotensin I. β_2-Adrenergic receptors are stimulated mainly by epinephrine and induce vasodilation of muscular arteries, as well as increase norepinephrine release from the sympathetic ganglia.[13]

Dopamine targets D_1 and D_2 dopaminergic receptors. Activation of D_1 receptors results in vasodilation of the renal arteries, whereas D_2 activation inhibits norepinephrine secretion from sympathetic nerve terminals and has a mild negative inotropic effect on the heart. The signaling net result would explain the clinical phenomenon of lack of hypertension and palpitations in patients with dopamine-secreting pheochromocytomas. On the other hand, pharmacologically high levels of dopamine stimulate α and β_1 receptors, causing vasoconstriction and increased heart rate.[13]

Desensitization of adrenergic receptors has always been a much-discussed topic in both research and clinical care. There have been numerous studies that reported significant desensitization of both α- and β-adrenergic receptors in healthy humans or patients with pheochromocytoma and in animal models.[18–22] Clinical experience suggests that a significant number of patients with pheochromocytoma-related hypercatecholaminemia are asymptomatic, despite minimal or no treatment. On the other hand, it should be remembered that the specific mechanisms and actual rate of desensitization in the individual person are still unknown. It can be presumed, however, that paroxysmal hypercatecholaminemia, with a rapid secretion of large amounts of catecholamines, probably precipitates a significant clinical episode, even in a patient with some degree of desensitization. Desensitization seems to be reversible, followed by resensitization of receptors when catecholamine levels return to normal.

CATECHOLAMINE PRODUCTION AND SECRETION IN PHEOCHROMOCYTOMA

The concentration of dopamine, norepinephrine, and epinephrine varies in every tumor depending on its enzymatic machinery. Pheochromocytomas have been reported to express very high levels of messenger RNA for TH, AADC, and DBH. The high levels of TH expression specifically correlate with high levels of catecholamines production.[23] PNMT activity, on the other hand, is positively influenced by glucocorticoids and is predominantly restricted to normal adrenal tissue. The glucocorticoids can increase PNMT activity and, therefore, raise epinephrine concentration in the cell.[24,25] PNMT levels have been recorded to be lower in pheochromocytomas than in normal adrenal tissue, although the prevalence of PNMT in adrenal pheochromocytomas is higher than in extra-adrenal tumors because of the proximity to the adrenal cortex.[16,25]

The secretory profile of pheochromocytomas can be useful as a clinical diagnostic tool. Extra-adrenal tumors tend to predominantly secrete norepinephrine and rarely dopamine.[26,27] Adrenal pheochromocytomas, especially those associated with multiple endocrine neoplasia (MEN) 2, primarily secrete epinephrine or a combination of norepinephrine and epinephrine. Tumors associated with von Hippel-Lindau disease secrete only norepinephrine.[13] Dopamine-secreting tumors are found on rare occasions and only in extra-adrenal pheochromocytomas.[27] These tumors show decreases in DBH expression, which would result in decreases in norepinephrine production and accumulation of dopamine.[28]

Pheochromocytomas can also produce other hormones and peptides, including adrenomedullin, vasoactive intestinal polypeptide, corticotropin, neuropeptide Y, endothelin-1, somatostatin, atrial natriuretic factor, and parathyroid hormone–related peptide. The clinical picture related to the secretion of either one or several additional neuroendocrine products depends on vasoconstrictive versus vasodilatory properties of the substance, superimposed on baseline hypercatecholaminemia.[13,29–34]

The pattern of catecholamine secretion from the tumor can be continuous, episodic, or both, and the hypertensive paroxysm can be precipitated by physical activity (exercise, postural change) or tumor manipulation.[13,35] However, it is still unknown and, therefore, difficult to predict when and how much catecholamines each particular tumor secretes during each secretory episode.

Evidence suggests a correlation between biochemical phenotype and characteristics of hypertension. Patients with tumors that produce high concentrations of norepinephrine are likely to incur sustained hypertension, whereas patients with significantly elevated levels of epinephrine often have paroxysmal and orthostatic hypertension.[36] Patients with dopamine-secreting tumors are most often normotensive.[27]

CLINICAL PATTERN OF PHEOCHROMOCYTOMA-RELATED HYPERTENSION

Hypertension occurs in about 80% to 90% of patients with pheochromocytoma. About half of these patients develop sustained hypertension, and another 45% present with paroxysmal hypertension, whereas 5% to 15% are normotensive.[6,37] The triad of headaches, palpitations, and sweating represent the classic clinical complex seen in patients with pheochromocytoma. Other symptoms may include tachycardia, anxiety, and pallor.[36] Most patients with pheochromocytoma have significantly increased systemic catecholamine levels, with norepinephrine and epinephrine levels reaching 5 to 10 times the upper reference limit; normotension is seen mostly in patients with relatively small amounts of catecholamines in circulation. The clinical phenotype of hypertensive syndrome depends on multiple factors including adrenal content of catecholamines and the pattern and nature of catecholamine secretion. Although the cellular content is enormous, intracellular processing diverts significant amounts into metabolites, an apparent clinical paradox of normal or near-normal plasma catecholamine concentrations and significantly elevated metanephrine levels.[38]

Sustained hypertension strongly correlates with high levels of plasma norepinephrine continuously released from a tumor. Moreover, patients with tumors that predominantly and continuously secreted norepinephrine had higher 24-hour, daytime, and nighttime BP than patients with tumors that secreted only epinephrine.[39] Patients with sustained hypertension were found to have high plasma levels of catecholamines during every measurement, suggesting a continuous rather than paroxysmal secretory pattern.[13] It is not uncommon, however, to observe a patient with baseline sustained hypertension presenting with fluctuating BP levels as a result of short-term changes in catecholamine concentrations in circulation.[13] Children are also significantly more likely to present with sustained hypertension than paroxysmal hypertension. Evidence suggests that excess norepinephrine is stored in the axon terminals of the sympathetic ganglia and is released with activation of sympathetic nervous system, causing continuous vasoconstriction and sustained hypertension.[40] Orthostatic hypotension may also develop in patients with sustained hypertension (especially in those who also have elevated circulating epinephrine levels) and much less commonly in those who have normotension or paroxysmal hypertension.[13] Decreased blood volume caused by consistent vasoconstriction and diminished sympathetic reflex may be important contributing factors for postural hypotension.[41] Postural tachycardia combined with postural hypotension can cause dizziness, palpitations, and syncope when a patient shifts from a supine to an upright position.[42]

Paroxysmal hypertension occurred mostly in patients with high levels of plasma epinephrine and is highly typical for MEN 2–related pheochromocytoma.[13] Episodes of paroxysmal hypertension result from the sudden release of catecholamines by tumors and can be induced by multiple factors including physical activity, smoking, abdominal pressure, postural changes, and anxiety.[13,43] Certain foods or beverages with high concentrations of tyramine (cheese, beer, and wine), drugs (histamine, phenothiazine, or tricyclic antidepressants), and operative procedures performed with or without anesthesia can cause paroxysmal hypertension in patients with pheochromocytoma.[12,34,44] However, most episodes are unpredictable and their frequency can vary from several times in one day to once in several months, with episodes lasting for several minutes to more than an hour. The sporadic release of epinephrine from these tumors may contribute to the fluctuation in BP. Patients with paroxysmal hypertension exhibit dramatic increases in both systolic and diastolic BPs during the paroxysm.[13]

Rarely, patients rapidly cycle between hypertension and hypotension. In one case, the patient's BP fluctuated every 14 minutes, with a BP ranging from 52/34 to 242/129 mm Hg.[45] As with paroxysmal hypertension, these patients had tumors that secreted primarily epinephrine.[46] Although the pathophysiology for this event is unclear, it is suggested that baroreceptors respond to a rapid increase in BP during acute paroxysm with activation of the negative feedback loop via both the sympathetic and parasympathetic systems, causing a rapid decrease in BP.[45,46]

Normotension mostly occurs in patients with familial pheochromocytoma, tumors that may be too small to secrete high levels of catecholamines, or dopamine-secreting tumors. Patients may have no typical symptoms of pheochromocytoma, and some tumors are detected incidentally by a palpable abdominal mass or imaging studies performed to seek the cause of abdominal pain. A study by the Adrenal Incidentaloma Study Group of the Italian Endocrinology Society showed that about half the incidentalomas, later found to be pheochromocytomas, were normotensive. The remaining patients experienced only slight elevations in BP, and none had paroxysmal hypertension.[47] Parasympathetic paragangliomas of the head and neck usually do not secrete catecholamines, and about 25% are associated with some degree of hypertension.[48] About 10% of patients with mutations in the B subunit of succinate dehydrogenase complex (SDHB) may have biochemically silent pheochromocytomas because of the lack of TH.[49] This group is especially concerning because patients with mutation of SDHB are prone to develop metastatic disease. Pheochromocytomas that synthesize and secrete predominantly dopamine also commonly present with normotension or hypotension. These tumors are found to be extra-adrenal and often malignant. The measurement of plasma levels of free methoxytyramine, the metabolite of dopamine, in addition to dopamine and urinary dopamine levels, is necessary for detection and diagnosis of dopamine-secreting pheochromocytomas.[50]

Special cases of pheochromocytoma-related hypertension include pediatric and obstetric cases. Children are more susceptible to sustained hypertension than adults: 60% to 90% of children have sustained hypertension; a small percentage, paroxysmal hypertension; and about 20%, normotension.[51] It is important to note that children usually have secondary rather than primary hypertension caused by renal deformities, renal artery disease, and congenital aortic coarctation.[52] Only after excluding these conditions, should children be screened for pheochromocytoma.[53] About 80% of children with pheochromocytomas are found to have orthostatic hypotension alternating with hypertensive episodes.[54] As in adults, signs and symptoms can vary greatly in children with pheochromocytoma, with headache and sweating being most common.[13,55]

Because of the lack of pheochromocytoma-specific signs and symptoms and the possible adverse effect to both mother and fetus, pregnancy represents an important diagnostic challenge. One of the most common misdiagnoses is preeclampsia.[56] In both pregnancy and preeclampsia, hypertension is usually the telling sign; however, preeclampsia also brings about other symptoms not normally seen in patients with pheochromocytoma, including weight gain, proteinuria, pedal edema, and HELLP syndrome (hemolysis, elevated liver enzymes, and low platelet count).[12] In addition, hypertension associated with preeclampsia usually develops after the 20th week of gestation, but is present throughout the gestation period in patients with pheochromocytoma.[57] Excess catecholamine release in pregnant patients can arise because of a change in intra-abdominal pressure following normal delivery, the compression of the tumor during labor, and postural changes.[13,58] Patients experiencing paroxysmal hypertension, headaches, and resistance to traditional antihypertensive therapy be should strongly suspected of having pheochromocytoma.[56] Undiagnosed pheochromocytoma can lead to fatal consequences for both mother and fetus via hypertensive crises; complications that can arise include hemorrhage, congestive heart failure, ischemia, infarction, and intrauterine growth restriction, which can cause hypoxia and death of the fetus.[57] To avoid complications, tumor resection should take place in the first or second trimester (optimal) or after cesarean delivery when the fetus comes to term.[59] It is important to have close medical management of the patient during the gestation period.

ORGAN-SPECIFIC HYPERTENSIVE COMPLICATIONS OF HYPERCATECHOLAMINEMIA

Pheochromocytoma is known for life-threatening acute hypertensive emergencies and clinical consequences of long-lasting hypertension (**Table 1**).

Cardiovascular

A large number of cardiovascular complications are caused by hypertension. It is suggested that catecholamines, mainly norepinephrine, are capable of structurally changing the vasculature, leading to increased arterial stiffness.[60] Zelinka and colleagues[61] found that the degree of arterial stiffness correlated with high levels of urinary norepinephrine in patients with pheochromocytoma. It was also seen that higher BP variability could increase arterial stiffness. Studies suggest that an increase in α-adrenergic receptor stimulation is capable of increasing extracellular matrix protein production, including collagen and fibronectin, which can result in hypertrophy and can lead to further cardiovascular complications.[62]

Activation of α- and β-adrenergic receptors can also cause vasoconstriction of the coronary arteries and stimulate positive inotropic effects in the heart resulting in tachyarrhythmia. The increase in cardiac contractility along with myocardial hypoxia can result in acute or chronic ischemia and myocardial infarction.[63] Unlike myocardial infarction caused by heart disease, patients with pheochromocytoma with no medical

Table 1
Organ-specific complications of pheochromocytoma-related hypertension

Organ	Syndrome	Mechanism	Receptor	Receptor Action
Heart	Angina Myocardial infarction Cardiomyopathies[a] Myocarditis Acute failure Arrhythmias	Coronary spasm Positive inotropic effect Positive chronotropic effect Unmatched O_2 demand Hypoperfusion	Coronary α_1, β_2 Conducting system β_1, β_2 Conducting system β_1, β_2 Cardiomyocyte β_1, β_2	Constriction Increased conduction Increased automaticity Increased contractility
Brain	Stroke Encephalopathy	Vasoconstriction Unmatched O_2 demand Hypoperfusion	Cerebral arterioles α_1	Mild constriction Most effects related to systemic hypertension
Vascular	Shock Postural hypotension Aortic dissection Organ ischemia Limb ischemia	Vasoconstriction Unmatched O_2 demand Hypoperfusion	Skeletal muscle α_1, α_2, β_2	Arteriolar constriction Arteriolar dilation Venous dilation
Kidneys	ARF Hematuria	Vasoconstriction Unmatched O_2 demand Hypoperfusion	Vascular α_1, α_2, β_1, β_2	Dilation > constriction renin secretion
Lungs	Pulmonary edema ARDS Fibrosis (?) Pulmonary hypertension (?)	Cardiac decompensation Increased permeability	Vascular α_1, β_2 Smooth muscle β_2	Dilation > constriction bronchodilation
GI Tract	Intestinal ischemia (necrosis, peritonitis)	Vasoconstriction Unmatched O_2 demand Hypoperfusion	Visceral arterioles α_1, β_2	Constriction
Ocular	Acute blindness Retinopathy	Vasoconstriction	?	—
AMF	All of the above	—	—	—

Abbreviations: AMF, acute multiorgan failure; ARDS, acute respiratory distress syndrome; ARF, acute renal failure; GI, gastrointestinal; ?, uncertain/unclear.
[a] Including acute (dilated, tako-tsubo) and chronic (hypertrophic, ischemic, obstructive).
Data from Refs.[60–68,87]

history of heart disease seem to have normal coronary arteries on angiography along with normal levels of cardiac enzymes.[64] Long-standing hypertension, chronic myocardial hypoxia, and metabolic myocarditis of hypercatecholaminemia are known to cause cardiomyopathy that, in the case of pheochromocytoma, can be chronic (hypertrophic, dilated, obstructive) or acute (ischemic, tako-tsubo).

Peripheral vascular disease can be acute and caused by intense vasoconstriction resulting in limb ischemia, necrosis, and gangrene or aortic dissection.[63,65,66] On the other hand, chronic disease resembles peripheral arterial insufficiency, presenting with limb pallor, pain, and intermittent claudication.[67]

Cerebrovascular

Pheochromocytoma can also be associated with neurologic complications including hypertensive encephalopathy and stroke.[68] In a healthy person, increased systemic BP causes activation of the α_1-adrenergic receptors located in the cerebral resistance vessels, which constrict.[69] This autoregulation, called Bayliss response, is set to maintain cerebral blood flow. In pheochromocytoma, continuously elevated BP "breaks through" this autoregulation and causes vasodilation, resulting in hypoperfusion and ischemia, which leads to hypertensive encephalopathy.[70] In addition, paroxysmal hypertension can cause hemorrhagic stroke, whereas postural hypotension can result in acute ischemic stroke.[71] Signs and symptoms of hypertensive encephalopathy include headache, papilledema, altered mental status, and even cerebral infarction.[69,72,73]

Renal

Pheochromocytoma is found to be associated with renal complications, including renal failure. A study reports that a patient with a norepinephrine-secreting tumor and hypertension also developed renal failure, which resolved after tumor removal.[74]

Vasoconstriction can cause muscle ischemia in patients with pheochromocytoma. As a result of the lack of oxygen flow to skeletal muscles, the patient can develop rhabdomyolysis and acute tubular necrosis caused by myoglobinuria.[63] High serum levels of creatine kinase together with high levels of urinary myoglobin may be reported in these patients.[75]

Renal artery stenosis can develop in patients with pheochromocytoma and hypertension. Vasoconstriction of the renal artery caused by high levels of catecholamines may lead to impaired kidney function and perhaps renal failure. Most tumors that cause renal artery stenosis have been found to be extra-adrenal and are derived from sympathetic tissue.[76] Such tumors have been found mostly in adults and have been reported as benign pheochromocytomas.[77]

Gastrointestinal

Pheochromocytoma can cause gastrointestinal complications, including intestinal ischemia. Patients with intestinal ischemia usually present with severe, sharp, radiating pain in the abdomen.[78] These tumors are usually large and secrete high amounts of catecholamines, resulting in vasospasm in the visceral arterioles, which causes decreased blood flow and visceral ischemia.[78,79]

Ocular

Patients with pheochromocytoma who have arterial hypertension may also present with hypertensive retinopathy caused by retinal vasoconstriction, increased vascular permeability, and secondary arteriosclerosis.[80,81] A retinal examination may reveal retinal microaneurysms, hemorrhages, cotton-wool spots, and venous bleeding.[82]

Patients with malignant hypertension more commonly show signs of vision problems than other groups.[81]

Multisystem Organ Failure

Patients with pheochromocytoma rarely present with cardiogenic shock, which occurs mainly with epinephrine-secreting tumors.[83–85] β-Receptor downregulation, caused by continuously increased catecholamine levels, can lead to a decrease in contractility, which results in cardiogenic shock.[86]

Patients can also display pheochromocytoma multisystem crisis (PMC). Different from cardiogenic shock, this complication consists of multisystem organ failure, a fever with a temperature of more than 40°C, encephalopathy, and severe hypertension and/or hypotension.[87] PMC can be masked to present as sepsis, which can delay surgery. Surgery and resection of the tumor has been proved to be the ideal choice in regard to treatment.[88] Although the specific cause of PMC is unknown, all the previously discussed complications in this section may present in PMC, and it is therefore important to mention them.

DIAGNOSTIC APPROACH

Pheochromocytoma has been called by many names, from a friendly "great mimicker" to a treacherous "cold-blooded killer" (the associated hypermetabolic state would actually make it rather "warm-blooded") and whatever fits in between, which mostly translates into the fear of missing it, because of the highly feasible fatal complications. Although the most important part of pheochromocytoma diagnosis still remains timely clinical suspicion, the level of its threshold continues to fluctuate. So it is not just "think about it" but rather "think about it, when ...," with the latter being a subject of debate. It is probably reasonable to perform workup on hypertensive patients who do not respond to an appropriate therapeutic trial (the key word being appropriate) or have paroxysmal episodes, rapidly progressive or resistant hypertension, severe hypertension, systemic hypertension (sweating, pallor), or postural reactions (hypotension or tachycardia). Although this selection criteria significantly reduce the number of hypertensive patients who need workup for pheochromocytoma, the addition of a criterion of presenting adrenal incidentalomas with elevation in BP increases the number of workups exponentially. The cost-effectiveness of the current approach is still to be established. Diagnostic workup includes measurement of plasma or urinary metanephrine levels with or without catecholamines and chromogranin A, followed, if positive, by imaging studies. A detailed diagnostic approach is beyond the scope of this article and can be found elsewhere.[12,89–91]

PHARMACOLOGIC TREATMENT OF PHEOCHROMOCYTOMA

Although the ultimate treatment option of pheochromocytoma is surgery, pharmacologic therapy still remains of vital significance in preoperative and operative control of BP, as well as in cases of inoperable metastatic disease (**Table 2**). It is also important to remember that tumor manipulations during surgery may associate with the release of tremendous amounts of catecholamines into circulation, which might be capable of overpowering the pharmacologic blockade. To control hypertension before an operation, even in preoperative normotensive patients, it is recommended that patients undergo preoperative pharmacologic treatment.[92] Phenoxybenzamine (Dibenzyline) is a noncompetitive α_1- and α_2-blocker that reduces BP fluctuation and eases vasoconstriction, preventing an intraoperative hypertensive crisis.[93–95] Patients are usually

Table 2
Approach to treatment of pheochromocytoma-related hypertension

Stage	Goal	Primary Rx	Supplementary/ Alternative Rx
Initial Trx (A)	Normalization of BP Minimal organ complications	In the following order Phenoxybenzamine, po β-Blocker, po Metyrosine, po	Alternative α-blocker (see text) Calcium channel blocker Labetalol, po
Preoperative Trx	Normal BP Normovolemia Optimized cardiac performance	As in (A) Fluids to normovolemia	As in (A)
Intraoperative Trx	Prevention of the following Severe hypercatecholaminemia Severe hypertension Severe hypotension	Nitroprusside, IV β-Blocker, IV Aggressive fluid replacement	Labetalol, IV Nitroprusside, IV
Postoperative Trx	Prevention of hypotension Prevention of hypoglycemia	Aggressive fluid replacement Glucose replacement	—
Trx of Inoperable Disease	Maintenance of normal BP Treatment of metastatic disease	Chemotherapy Radiotherapy Debulking	Experimental therapy

Abbreviations: Alternative Rx, alternative treatment based on center-specific preferences; IV, intravenously; Metyrosine, α-methyl-L-tyrosine (α-MPT, Demser); Supplementary Rx, added to meet the goal for BP control; Trx, treatment.
Data from Refs.[34,92–98]

prescribed 10 to 30 mg twice daily until BP and other symptoms have stabilized, which normally takes 10 to 14 days.[34,95]

An alternative preoperative approach is to avoid the use of phenoxybenzamine, while aggressively using potent, short-acting, intravenous, antihypertensive agents, such as sodium nitroprusside (Nitropress) and nitroglycerin (Nitrostat), to control sudden changes in BP during surgery.[93,96] This approach is based on several reports of the seeming inefficacy of phenoxybenzamine during surgery, as well as the well-known development of postoperative hypotension and tachycardia related to its use.[7,97] On the other hand, it should be remembered that in the event of incomplete alpha-adrenergic receptor blockade and massive release of catecholamines during surgery, phenoxybenzamine would be only partially efficient. It could also be speculated that treatment with phenoxybenzamine was only in part to due to a case of postoperative hypovolemia and rapid cessation of hypercatecholaminemia, with associated hypotension and tachycardia.

Specific α_1-adrenergic receptor blockers, such as prazosin hydrochloride (Minipress), terazosin (Hytrin), and doxazosin (Cardura), can be used instead of phenoxybenzamine to prevent the occurrence of tachycardia by allowing the natural negative feedback mechanism through the unopposed α_2-adrenergic receptors. They also are of a shorter duration of action, which decreases the length of postoperative hypotension.

Calcium channel blockers, such as diltiazem (Cardizem), are effective vasodilators and can be used in patients with pheochromocytoma to control BP.[98] Unlike phenoxybenzamine, calcium channel blockers do not cause dangerous hypotension and are relatively short acting. It is especially useful for normotensive patients or those with very mild hypertension. Combination of calcium channel blockers with prazosin, doxazosin, or another α_1-adrenergic receptor blocker would complement each other well during tumor resection.

Beta-blockade can be used concomitantly with any of the alpha-adrenergic receptor blockades, especially when used with phenoxybenzamine, to prevent reflex tachycardia.[94] It is important, however, that beta-blockade be only used after an alpha-blockade because unopposed beta-blockade can result in a significant increase in arterial pressure.

Metyrosine (Demser) has been proved to be useful in decreasing the synthesis of catecholamines by preoccupying TH with a substrate that is hydroxylated to an inactive metabolite. It is effective in preoperative treatment and in treatment of patients with metastatic and inoperable disease.[97] The latter group is also treated with adrenergic blockers for symptomatic disease, as well as with chemotherapy and radiotherapy.

SUMMARY

Pheochromocytoma is a tumor of the chromaffin cells in the adrenal medulla and sympathetic paraganglia, which synthesizes and secretes catecholamines. Norepinephrine, epinephrine, and dopamine all act on their target receptors, which causes a physiologic change in the body. High circulating levels of catecholamines can lead to severe hypertension and can have devastating effects on multiple body systems (eg, cardiovascular, cerebrovascular), and can lead to death if untreated. Although surgical treatment represents the only modality of ultimate cure, pharmacologic preoperative treatment remains the mainstay of successful outcome.

REFERENCES

1. DeLellis RA, Lloyd RV, Heitz PU, et al. World Health Organization classification of tumours. Pathophysiology and genetics of tumours of endocrine organs. Lyon (France): IARC Press; 2004.
2. Lehnert H. Pheochromocytoma. Pathophysiology and clinical management, vol. 31. Basel (Switzerland): Karger; 2004.
3. van Duinen N, Steenvoorden D, Kema IP, et al. Increased urinary excretion of 3-methoxytyramine in patients with head and neck paragangliomas. J Clin Endocrinol Metab 2010;95(1):209–14.
4. Omura M, Saito J, Yamaguchi K, et al. Prospective study on the prevalence of secondary hypertension among hypertensive patients visiting a general outpatient clinic in Japan. Hypertens Res 2004;27(3):193–202.
5. Ariton M, Juan CS, AvRuskin TW. Pheochromocytoma: clinical observations from a Brooklyn tertiary hospital. Endocr Pract 2000;6(3):249–52.
6. Manger WM. The protean manifestations of pheochromocytoma. Horm Metab Res 2009;41(09):658–63.
7. Lenders JW, Eisenhofer G, Mannelli M, et al. Phaeochromocytoma. Lancet 2005; 366(9486):665–75.
8. Sutton M, Sheps SG, Lie JL. Prevalence of clinically unsuspected pheochromocytoma. Review of a 50-year autopsy series. Mayo Clin Proc 1981;56(6):354–60.

9. McNeil AR, Blok BH, Koelmeyer TD, et al. Phaeochromocytomas discovered during coronial autopsies in Sydney, Melbourne and Auckland. Intern Med J 2000;30(6):648–52.
10. Calhoun DA, Jones D, Textor S, et al. Resistant hypertension: diagnosis, evaluation, and treatment: a scientific statement from the American Heart Association Professional Education Committee of the Council for High Blood Pressure Research. Hypertension 2008;51(6):1403–19.
11. Guérin M, Guillemot J, Thouënnon E, et al. Granins and their derived peptides in normal and tumoral chromaffin tissue: implications for the diagnosis and prognosis of pheochromocytoma. Regul Pept 2010;165(1):21–9.
12. Manger WM. An overview of pheochromocytoma: history, current concepts, vagaries, and diagnostic challenges. Ann N Y Acad Sci 2006;1073:1–20.
13. Manger W, Gifford RW. The clinical and experimental pheochromocytoma. 2nd edition. Malden (MA): Blackwell Science; 1996.
14. Nagatsu T, Levitt M, Udenfriend S. Tyrosine hydroxylase. J Biol Chem 1964; 239(9):2910–7.
15. Kaufman S, Friedman S. Dopamine-β-hydroxylase. Pharmacol Rev 1965;17(2): 71–100.
16. Lehnert H. Regulation of catecholamine synthesizing enzyme gene expression in human pheochromocytoma. Eur J Endocrinol 1998;138(4):363–7.
17. Jameson JL, DeGroot LJ. Endocrinology: adult and pediatric. 6th edition. Philadelphia: Saunders; 2010.
18. Greenacre J, Conolly M. Desensitization of the beta-adrenoceptor of lymphocytes from normal subjects and patients with phaeochromocytoma: studies in vivo. Br J Clin Pharmacol 1978;5(3):191–7.
19. Tsujimoto G, Manger W, Hoffman B. Desensitization of beta-adrenergic receptors by pheochromocytoma. Endocrinology 1984;114(4):1272–8.
20. Tsujimoto G, Honda K, Hoffman B, et al. Desensitization of postjunctional alpha 1- and alpha 2-adrenergic receptor-mediated vasopressor responses in rat harboring pheochromocytoma. Circ Res 1987;61(1):86–98.
21. Krause M, Reinhardt D, Kruse K. Phaeochromocytoma without symptoms: desensitization of the alpha- and beta-adrenoceptors. Eur J Pediatr 1988;147(2): 121–2.
22. Jones C, Hamilton C, Whyte K, et al. Acute and chronic regulation of alpha 2-adrenoceptor number and function in man. Clin Sci 1985;68(Suppl 10):129–32.
23. Isobe K, Nakai T, Yukimasa N, et al. Expression of mRNA coding for four catecholamine-synthesizing enzymes in human adrenal pheochromocytomas. Eur J Endocrinol 1998;138(4):383–7.
24. Wurtman RJ, Axelrod J. Control of enzymatic synthesis of adrenaline in the adrenal medulla by adrenal cortical steroids. J Biol Chem 1966;241(10):2301–5.
25. Betito K, Diorio J, Meaney MJ, et al. Adrenal phenylethanolamine N-methyltransferase induction in relation to glucocorticoid receptor dynamics: evidence that acute exposure to high cortisol levels is sufficient to induce the enzyme. J Neurochem 1992;58(5):1853–62.
26. Brown WJ, Barajas L, Waisman J, et al. Ultrastructural and biochemical correlates of adrenal and extra-adrenal pheochromocytoma. Cancer 1972;29(3):744–59.
27. Proye C, Fossati P, Fontaine P, et al. Dopamine-secreting pheochromocytoma: an unrecognized entity? Classification of pheochromocytomas according to their type of secretion. Surgery 1986;100(6):1154–62.
28. Yasunari K, Kohno M, Minami M, et al. A dopamine-secreting pheochromocytoma. J Cardiovasc Pharmacol 2000;36:S75–7.

29. Letizia C, De Toma G, Caliumi C, et al. Plasma adrenomedullin concentrations in patients with adrenal pheochromocytoma. Horm Metab Res 2001;33(5):290–4.
30. Sano T, Saito H, Inaba H, et al. Immunoreactive somatostatin and vasoactive intestinal polypeptide in adrenal pheochromocytoma an immunochemical and ultrastructural study. Cancer 1983;52(2):282–9.
31. Nijhoff MF, Dekkers OM, Vleming LJ, et al. ACTH-producing pheochromocytoma: clinical considerations and concise review of the literature. Eur J Intern Med 2009; 20(7):682–5.
32. deS Senanayake P, Denker J, Bravo EL, et al. Production, characterization, and expression of neuropeptide Y by human pheochromocytoma. J Clin Invest 1995;96(5):2503–9.
33. Oishi S, Sasaki M, Sato T. Elevated immunoreactive endothelin levels in patients with pheochromocytoma. Am J Hypertens 1994;7(8):717–22.
34. Manger W, Eisenhofer G. Pheochromocytoma: diagnosis and management update. Curr Hypertens Rep 2004;6(6):477–84.
35. Bravo EL. Pheochromocytoma: current perspectives in the pathogenesis, diagnosis, and management. Arq Bras Endocrinol Metabol 2004;48:746–50.
36. Ito Y, Fuimoto Y, Obara T. The role of epinephrine, norepinephrine, and dopamine in blood pressure disturbances in patients with pheochromocytoma. World J Surg 1992;16(4):759–63.
37. Zelinka T, Eisenhofer G, Pacak K. Pheochromocytoma as a catecholamine producing tumor: implications for clinical practice. Stress 2007;10(2):195–203.
38. Pacak K. Preoperative management of the pheochromocytoma patient. J Clin Endocrinol Metab 2007;92(11):4069–79.
39. O'Rourke MF, Staessen JA, Vlachopoulos C, et al. Clinical applications of arterial stiffness; definitions and reference values. Am J Hypertens 2002;15(5):426–44.
40. Bravo E, Tarazi R, Fouad F, et al. Blood pressure regulation in pheochromocytoma. Hypertension 1982;4(3):193–9.
41. Engleman K, Zelis R, Waldmann T, et al. Mechanism of orthostatic hypotension in pheochromocytoma. Circulation 1968;38(Suppl 6):71–2.
42. Streeten DH, Anderson GH. Mechanisms of orthostatic hypotension and tachycardia in patients with pheochromocytoma. Am J Hypertens 1996;9(8):760–9.
43. Widimský J Jr. Recent advances in the diagnosis and treatment of pheochromocytoma. Kidney Blood Press Res 2006;29(5):321–6.
44. Bittar D. Innovar-induced hypertensive crises in patients with pheochromocytoma. Anesthesiology 1979;50(4):366–9.
45. Ionescu CN, Sakharova OV, Harwood MD, et al. Cyclic rapid fluctuation of hypertension and hypotension in pheochromocytoma. J Clin Hypertens 2008;10(12): 936–40.
46. Kobal SL, Paran E, Jamali A, et al. Pheochromocytoma: cyclic attacks of hypertension alternating with hypotension. Nat Clin Pract Cardiovasc Med 2008;5(1): 53–7.
47. Mantero F, Albiger N. A comprehensive approach to adrenal incidentalomas. Arq Bras Endocrinol Metabol 2004;48:583–91.
48. Erickson D, Kudva YC, Ebersold MJ, et al. Benign paragangliomas: clinical presentation and treatment outcomes in 236 patients. J Clin Endocrinol Metab 2001;86(11):5210–6.
49. Timmers HJ, Kozupa A, Eisenhofer G, et al. Clinical presentations, biochemical phenotypes, and genotype-phenotype correlations in patients with succinate dehydrogenase subunit B-associated pheochromocytomas and paragangliomas. J Clin Endocrinol Metab 2007;92(3):779–86.

50. Eisenhofer G, Goldstein DS, Sullivan P, et al. Biochemical and clinical manifestations of dopamine-producing paragangliomas: utility of plasma methoxytyramine. J Clin Endocrinol Metab 2005;90(4):2068–75.
51. Barontini M, Levin G, Sanso G. Characteristics of pheochromocytoma in a 4- to 20-year-old population. Ann N Y Acad Sci 2006;1073:30–7.
52. Londe S. Causes of hypertension in the young. Pediatr Clin North Am 1978;25(1):55–65.
53. Ross JH. Pheochromocytoma: special considerations in children. Urol Clin North Am 2000;27(3):393–402.
54. Beltsevich DG, Kuznetsov NS, Kazaryan AM, et al. Pheochromocytoma surgery: epidemiologic peculiarities in children. World J Surg 2004;28(6):592–6.
55. Ludwig AD, Feig DI, Brandt ML, et al. Recent advances in the diagnosis and treatment of pheochromocytoma in children. Am J Surg 2007;194(6):792–7.
56. Oliva R, Angelos P, Kaplan E, et al. Pheochromocytoma in pregnancy: a case series and review. Hypertension 2010;55(3):600–6.
57. Dugas G, Fuller J, Singh S, et al. Pheochromocytoma and pregnancy: a case report and review of anesthetic management. Can J Anesth 2004;51(2):134–8.
58. Ahlawat SK, Jain S, Kumari S, et al. Pheochromocytoma associated with pregnancy: case report and review of the literature. Obstet Gynecol Surv 1999;54(11):728.
59. George J, Tan JYL. Pheochromocytoma in pregnancy: a case report and review of literature. Obstet Med 2010;3(2):83–5.
60. Petrak O, Strauch B, Zelinka T, et al. Factors influencing arterial stiffness in pheochromocytoma and effect of adrenalectomy. Hypertens Res 2010;33(5):454–9.
61. Zelinka TA, Strauch BA, Petrak OA, et al. Increased blood pressure variability in pheochromocytoma compared to essential hypertension patients. J Hypertens 2005;23(11):2033–9.
62. O'Callaghan CJ, Williams BB. The regulation of human vascular smooth muscle extracellular matrix protein production by [alpha]- and [beta]-adrenoceptor stimulation. J Hypertens 2002;20(2):287–94.
63. Brouwers FM, Lenders JW, Eisenhofer G, et al. Pheochromocytoma as an endocrine emergency. Rev Endocr Metab Disord 2003;4(2):121–8.
64. Brilakis ES, Young WF Jr, Wilson JW, et al. Reversible catecholamine-induced cardiomyopathy in a heart transplant candidate without persistent or paroxysmal hypertension. J Heart Lung Transplant 1999;18(4):376–80.
65. Tack CJ, Lenders JW. Pheochromocytoma as a cause of blue toes. Arch Intern Med 1993;153(17):2061.
66. Januszewicz W, Wocial B. Clinical and biochemical aspects of pheochromocytoma. Cardiology 1985;72(Suppl 1):131–6.
67. Radtke WE, Kazmier FJ, Rutherford BD, et al. Cardiovascular complications of pheochromocytoma crisis. Am J Cardiol 1975;35(5):701–5.
68. Kwong YL, Yu YL, Lam KS, et al. CT appearance in hypertensive encephalopathy. Neuroradiology 1987;29(2):215.
69. Dinsdale H. Hypertensive encephalopathy. Stroke 1982;13(5):717–9.
70. Strandgaard S, Olesen J, Skinhoj E, et al. Autoregulation of brain circulation in severe arterial hypertension. Br Med J 1973;1(5852):507–10.
71. Lin P, Hsu J, Chung C, et al. Pheochromocytoma underlying hypertension, stroke, and dilated cardiomyopathy. Tex Heart Inst J 2007;34(2):244–6.
72. Campellone JV, Kolson DL, Wells GB, et al. Cerebral infarction during hypertensive encephalopathy: case report with pathologic and atypical radiographic findings. J Stroke Cerebrovasc Dis 1995;5(2):66–71.

73. Majic T, Aiyagari V. Cerebrovascular manifestations of pheochromocytoma and the implications of a missed diagnosis. Neurocrit Care 2008;9(3):378–81.
74. Fujiwara M, Imachi H, Murao K, et al. Improvement in renal dysfunction and symptoms after laparoscopic adrenalectomy in a patient with pheochromocytoma complicated by renal dysfunction. Endocrine 2009;35(1):57–62.
75. Shemin D, Cohn PS, Zipin SB. Pheochromocytoma presenting as rhabdomyolysis and acute myoglobinuric renal failure. Arch Intern Med 1990;150(11):2384–5.
76. Hill FS, Jander HP, Murad T, et al. The coexistence of renal artery stenosis and pheochromocytoma. Ann Surg 1983;197(4):484–90.
77. Crowe A, Jones N, Carr P. Five ways to be fooled by phaeochromocytoma-renal and urological complications. Nephrol Dial Transplant 1997;12(2):337–40.
78. Salehi A, Legome EL, Eichhorn K, et al. Pheochromocytoma and bowel ischemia. J Emerg Med 1996;15(1):35–8.
79. Carr ND, Hulme A, Sheron N, et al. Intestinal ischaemia associated with phaeochromocytoma. Postgrad Med J 1989;65(766):594–6.
80. Chatterjee S, Chattopadhyay S, Hope-Ross M, et al. Hypertension and the eye: changing perspectives. J Hum Hypertens 2002;16(10):667–75.
81. Petkou D, Petropoulos IK, Kordelou A, et al. Severe bilateral hypertensive retinopathy and optic neuropathy in a patient with pheochromocytoma. Klin Monbl Augenheilkd 2008;225(5):500–3.
82. Schubert HD. Ocular manifestations of systemic hypertension. Curr Opin Ophthalmol 1998;9(6):69–72.
83. Bergland BE. Pheochromocytoma presenting as shock. Am J Emerg Med 1989;7(1):44–8.
84. Galetta F, Franzoni F, Bernini G, et al. Cardiovascular complications in patients with pheochromocytoma: a mini-review. Biomed Pharmacother 2010;64(7):505–9.
85. Olson SW, Deal LE, Piesman M. Epinephrine-secreting pheochromocytoma presenting with cardiogenic shock and profound hypocalcemia. Ann Intern Med 2004;140(10):849–51.
86. Cryer P. Physiology and pathophysiology of the human sympathoadrenal neuroendocrine system. N Engl J Med 1980;303(8):436–44.
87. Newell KA, Prinz RA, Pickleman J, et al. Pheochromocytoma multisystem crisis: a surgical emergency. Arch Surg 1988;123(8):956–9.
88. Moran ME, Rosenberg DJ, Zornow DH. Pheochromocytoma multisystem crisis. Urology 2006;67(4):846.e819–20.
89. Barron J. Phaeochromocytoma: diagnostic challenges for biochemical screening and diagnosis. J Clin Pathol 2010;63(8):669–74.
90. Eisenhofer G, Siegert G, Kotzerke J, et al. Current progress and future challenges in the biochemical diagnosis and treatment of pheochromocytomas and paragangliomas. Horm Metab Res 2008;40(5):329–37.
91. Adler JT, Meyer-Rochow GY, Chen H, et al. Pheochromocytoma: current approaches and future directions. Oncologist 2008;13(7):779–93.
92. Pacak K, Eisenhofer G, Ahlman H, et al. Pheochromocytoma: recommendations for clinical practice from the first international symposium. Nat Clin Pract Endocrinol Metab 2007;3(2):92–102.
93. Bravo EL, Tagle R. Pheochromocytoma: state-of-the-art and future. Endocr Rev 2003;24(4):539–53.
94. Ross E, Prichard B, Kaufman L, et al. Preoperative and operative management of patients with phaeochromocytoma. Br Med J 1967;1(5534):191–8.
95. Desmonts JM, Marty J. Anaesthetic management of patients with phaeochromocytoma. Br J Anaesth 1984;56(7):781–9.

96. Ulchaker JC, Goldfarb DA, Bravo EL, et al. Successful outcomes in pheochromocytoma surgery in the modern era. J Urol 1999;161(3):764–7.
97. Bravo EL. Evolving Concepts in the pathophysiology, diagnosis, and treatment of pheochromocytoma. Endocr Rev 1994;15(3):356–68.
98. Tokioka H, Takahashi T, Kosogabe Y, et al. Use of diltiazem to control circulatory fluctuations during resection of a phaeochromocytoma. Br J Anaesth 1988;60(5): 582–7.

Diagnosis and Treatment of Primary Aldosteronism

Gian Paolo Rossi, MD*

KEYWORDS

- Arterial hypertension • Aldosterone • Primary aldosteronism
- Diagnosis

The first report of an adrenocortical adenoma causing arterial hypertension and hypo-kalemia that were cured by adrenalectomy appeared in a journal published in Polish in 1953 by Litynski, and therefore remained unnoticed by the medical community.[1] The discovery of aldosterone-producing adenoma (APA) causing primary aldosteronism (PA) is therefore commonly attributed to Jerome Conn[2] in 1955, who must be credited for painstaking studies that lasted decades and led to the full characterization of the syndrome. After his pioneering work,[3] knowledge of the causes of PA has expanded, but from the practical standpoint the most useful classification is that presented in **Box 1**, which has the merit of distinguishing the surgically curable from the surgically incurable causes.[4]

Early identification of surgically curable causes is of paramount importance because adrenalectomy cures PA and can avoid its ominous consequences. Compelling evidence exists that PA is associated with prominent target organ damage, which translates into an excess rate of cardiovascular events.

CONSEQUENCES OF PRIMARY ALDOSTERONISM

When salt intake is not decreased hyperaldosteronism implies oxidant stress,[5,6] oxidative damage to DNA,[7] inflammation,[8] cardiovascular remodeling, hypertrophy, and fibrosis.[9,10] It has been found that PA impairs left ventricular filling and diastolic function,[11] prolongs the electrocardiographic PQ interval,[12] and induces fibrosis of the left ventricular wall,[13] endothelial dysfunction,[14–16] stiffening of the large

---

This work was supported by Grant No. PRIN 2007PRELCC_002 from the Ministry of University and Scientific Research (MIUR) and from FORICA (The FOundation for advanced Research In Hypertension and CArdiovascular diseases) and the Società Italiana dell'Ipertensione Arteriosa. The author has nothing to disclose.
Molecular Hypertension Laboratory, Dipartimento di Medicina Clinica e Sperimentale (DMCS) 'G. Patrassi' - Internal Medicine 4, University of Padua, University Hospital Padua, Via Giustiniani, 2, 35126 Padua, Italy
* DMCS - Clinica Medica 4, Policlinico Universitario, Via Giustiniani, 2, 35126 Padua, Italy.
E-mail address: gianpaolo.rossi@unipd.it

Box 1
Surgically curable and incurable forms of mineralocorticoid excess, including PA

Surgically curable:

    Aldosterone-producing adenoma (aldosteronoma, APA)

        Unilateral

        Bilateral

    Primary unilateral adrenal hyperplasia (PAH)

    Multinodular unilateral adrenocortical hyperplasia (MUAN)

    Ovary aldosterone-secreting tumor

    APA or bilateral hyperplasia (BAH) with concomitant pheochromocytoma

    Aldosterone-producing carcinoma (APC)

    Familial type II hyperaldosteronism (FH-II)

Surgically incurable:

    BAH

    Unilateral APA with BAH:

        Familial type I (FH-I) hyperaldosteronism, also known as GRA

    Apparent mineralocorticoid excess (AME):

        Chronic licorice intake

        Use of carbenoxolone (antacid)

---

arteries,[17,18] remodeling of resistance arteries,[18] and microalbuminuria.[19–22] These changes ultimately translate into an excess rate of cardiovascular events, including atrial fibrillation, ischemic stroke,[23] cerebral hemorrhage,[24] "flash" pulmonary edema, and myocardial infarction.[25]

In patients with lateralized aldosterone secretion, unilateral adrenalectomy corrects the aldosterone excess and thereby permits a tapering of the antihypertensive therapy and/or even provides the long-term normalization of blood pressure despite withdrawal of drugs in up to 82% of the patients. Moreover, it also prevents the development of the adverse cardiovascular changes, or induces the regression of these changes if already present, in most patients.[26,27] Regression of target organ damage can be achieved with antihypertensive treatment, but this requires life-long drug treatment with often multiple antihypertensive agents.[28] This regimen should include mineralocorticoid receptor blockade with spironolactone or eplerenone. These drugs may have side effects and incur cost. Because of these considerations, the author supports exploiting an aggressive strategy aimed at an early diagnosis and a specific treatment of PA. A precise diagnosis will be particularly rewarding for the patients eventually found to have an APA, who in the long term will be cured with adrenalectomy.

PREVALENCE OF PA

In 1965 Conn[29–31] himself pointed out that in many cases of PA hypokalemia was absent, and therefore PA can "masquerade as essential hypertension." Notwithstanding this, most doctors continue to consider hypokalemia the hallmark of the disease, which means that they are prompted to search for PA only in hypokalemic hypertensive patients. It is therefore conceivable that the lack of hypokalemia has led to underdiagnosis of PA and thus to marked underestimation of its prevalence among hypertensive patients.

This proposition partly explains why the debate on the prevalence of PA in hypertensive patients went on for almost two decades. In 1970, Conn[32] conceded that a realistic estimate of the prevalence of PA could be around 7%. However, subsequent studies continued to report rates of prevalence that ranged widely (from 1.4% to 32%, median 8.8%) for the reasons discussed elsewhere.[33,34] The wide range of these figures indicated that the true prevalence rate was uncertain. However, the general consensus among the experts was that PA might be far more prevalent than previously held.[35–52]

In 2006 the first large prospective survey, the PAPY (PA Prevalence in hYpertensives) study, designed to furnish solid data on PA prevalence, was eventually reported.[53] In this study, after a screening test based on the ARR, that is, the aldosterone to renin ratio (measured as plasma aldosterone concentration [PAC]/plasma renin activity [PRA]), the patients underwent a thorough workup aimed to unequivocally establish not only the presence or absence of PA but also to identify the PA subtype. To this end a rigorous set of criteria for diagnosing an APA, based on adrenal vein sampling, pathology, and follow-up data, was introduced (reviewed by Rossi and colleagues[34]). PA patients without lateralization of aldosterone excess were presumed to have idiopathic hyperaldosteronism (IHA), a condition that is generally thought not to be cured by adrenalectomy.

The study conclusively showed that PA involves at least 11.2% of consecutive newly diagnosed hypertensive patients referred to hypertension centers. Most important was the finding that almost half of the PA patients, eg, 4.8% of all the 1125 patients who were screened, had a surgically curable subtype. Therefore, the investigators concluded that PA is by far the most common curable endocrine form of hypertension.

IMPLICATIONS OF THE HIGH PREVALENCE OF PA FOR THE SCREENING STRATEGY

The high prevalence of PA documented in the PAPY study[53] and in other surveys[35,37–48,50–52] has a profound impact on the strategy to be used in the investigation of hypertensive patients. This is because experience has shown that in general the incremental gain of any diagnostic test is maximized when the patient's prior probability of a disease, which can be estimated by the prevalence rate of the disease in the population at risk and by the individual patient assessment, is between 10% and 30%.[54] Hence, given a starting prevalence of PA of 11.2% and by applying the recommendations of the recent Practice Guidelines concerning the categories of patients (**Box 2**) in whom the screening is obligatory,[55] one could enrich the PA prevalence and therefore make cost-effective use of the diagnostic tests.

SCREENING STRATEGY

The strategy of case detection suggested in the Endocrine Society guidelines for the screening of patients[55] was based on the aforementioned considerations on the incremental diagnostic gain (reviewed by Rossi and colleagues[54]). The screening tests should be performed in patients with a higher pretest probability of PA (see **Box 2**). However, some experts favor systematically excluding PA in most newly found hypertensive patients because of the high prevalence rate of PA,[53] and the excess rate of cardiovascular damage and complications that can be prevented with an accurate early diagnosis followed by adrenalectomy. The reason for this is that adrenalectomy provides long-term cure of the biochemical picture of PA in almost all patients, and can correct arterial hypertension in the vast majority of them.[27]

> **Box 2**
> **Conditions that make the search for PA mandatory in a hypertensive patient**
>
> - Unexplained hypokalemia (spontaneous or diuretic-induced)
> - Resistant hypertension and Grade 2 or 3 hypertension
> - Early onset (juvenile) hypertension and/or stroke (<50 years)
> - Incidentally discovered apparently nonfunctioning adrenal mass ("incidentaloma")
> - Evidence of organ damage (left ventricular hypertrophy, diastolic dysfunction, atrioventricular block, carotid atherosclerosis, microalbuminuria, endothelial dysfunction), particularly if disproportionate for the severity of hypertension
> - Overweight/obesity
> - Obstructive sleep apnea syndrome

Implementation of broad screening strategies for PA needs to be reconciled with available health care resources that vary from country to country. Consensus favors screening for screening in certain categories of patients (see **Box 2**) and particularly in those with resistant hypertension, provided that they are reasonable candidates for adrenalectomy. Three categories of patients that were not included in the guidelines have been added to this list because accumulating evidence indicates that these patients might carry a higher risk of PA. These patients include those with evidence of target organ damage that is disproportionate for the degree of blood pressure elevation, those with obstructive sleep apnea syndrome and those with hypertension and overweight/obesity.[56,57]

In the patients enlisted in **Box 2**, the first step for the diagnosis of PA requires the demonstration of an excess aldosterone secretion that is autonomous from the renin-angiotensin system (RAS). To this end the ARR, as proposed by Hiramatsu and colleagues,[58] is used as a simplified approach to the case detection, but its use requires careful consideration to several issues, as described in **Table 1** and discussed further here.

First, the ARR depends on PAC but also on renin; those with suppressed renin will have an increased ARR even with normal PAC. Therefore, the ARR must be interpreted in the light of the PAC itself, which should be higher than 15 ng/dL, and of the lowest detectable level of the renin assay that is being used (see later discussion).[59] Regarding this latter point, it must be mentioned that current assays for PRA and also for direct active renin (DRA) lose their precision in the low range. To avoid over-inflating the ratio ARR, it is common to arbitrarily fix the lowest value at a minimum (which is 0.2 ng/mL/h for PRA and 0.6 mIU/dL [0.36 ng/mL] for DRA).[34,53] These precautions are even more important in the subgroups of patients, such as the elderly and the African American population, who usually exhibit low PRA values. Thus, the combination of PAC of more than 15 ng/dL and an increased ARR, rather than an increased ARR alone, should be used as the screening test for PA.

WHICH RENIN ASSAY SHOULD BE USED?

The DRA assay is recently gaining wide popularity and is actually replacing the PRA assay, for several reasons, including the possibility of handling the samples at room temperature.[54,60] The DRA and PRA assays are differentially affected by pretest handling of the samples. Owing to cryoactivation, freezing or handling of the samples at low temperatures can raise the DRA value artificially.[61,62] On the other hand,

Table 1
Factors affecting the value and suggestions for the correct performance and interpretation of the aldosterone renin ratio (ARR) as a screening test

Factors Affecting ARR	Suggestion
Serum potassium levels	Hypokalemia should be corrected before performing the test to avoid false negative ARR values
PAC	High PAC might originate from low salt intake or diuretics. Prepare patient with adequate salt intake, measure 24-h urinary sodium excretion. Withdraw diuretics at least 4 wk before; MR antagonists at least 6 wk before
Renin assay	Because of low precision of the assay for low PRA values, the lowest level of renin should be fixed arbitrarily at a minimum value to be used in the ARR (see text for explanation)
Patient position and blood sampling	Preparation of the patient and sampling conditions should be standardized at each center
Handling of the samples	Be aware that handling and storage of plasma samples differ for PRA and DRA assays
Drugs	α_1-Receptor blocker doxazosin and long-acting calcium channel blocker are allowed. For other agents, see text
ARR sensitivity and specificity	The cutoff value that provides the best combination of sensitivity and specificity should be identified at each center

Abbreviations: DRA, direct active renin; MR, mineralocorticoid receptor; PAC, plasma aldosterone concentration; PRA, plasma renin activity.

collection of plasma at room temperature can lead to angiotensin-I generation (high blank values) and to angiotensinogen consumption, and therefore to underestimation of renin when the PRA assay is used. However, when the samples are properly collected for each assay, the DRA and PRA values show a good correlation, as recently confirmed in a multicenter study.[63] This correlation is weak in the low-range values, but is stronger when renin is stimulated, for example after captopril challenge.[64] Conversely, the precision of either assay tends to be lower when the values of renin are low or very low, as is usually the case in PA patients. Hence, to increase the accuracy of renin estimation an option could be to use the DRA after stimulation of renin secretion with captopril, as recently suggested.[64]

In addition to these considerations, it has to be acknowledged that the usefulness of DRA in the calculation of the ARR for identifying aldosterone-producing adenoma has been investigated only in one prospective study thus far.[64] Even though this study suggested the feasibility of using the ARR based on the DRA for identifying APA, further experience should be gained before replacement of the PRA could be generally recommended.

PREPARATION OF THE PATIENT

Careful preparation of the patient is of utmost importance, in the author's view, before ordering the screening test. Many antihypertensive drugs affect the PAC and renin values, and thereby the ARR, albeit to markedly different extents (**Table 2**). Drug treatment must therefore be modified before measuring these hormones.

β-Blockers lower renin but affect PAC relatively less, thus raising the ARR.[53] In the author's experience it is better to stop them at least 3 to 4 weeks before the assay, as failure to do so increases markedly the false-positive rate and therefore the number of useless further tests. Conversely, drugs that raise the PRA more than PAC, such as

Table 2
Medications that affect the plasma levels of aldosterone and renin and therefore the aldosterone renin ratio (ARR) as a screening test

Drugs	Effect on PAC	Effect on PRA	Effect on ARR	Notes
ACEIs	↓	↑	↓↓	Increase FN rate. If feasible, withdraw 3–4 wk before
α$_1$-Blockers	→	→	→	Neutral
ARBs	↓	↑	↓↓	Increase FN rate. If feasible, withdraw 3–4 wk before
β-Blockers	↓	↓↓	↑↑	Increase FP rate. If feasible, withdraw 3–4 wk before
CCBs:	↑	↑	↓	Increase FN rate
Short-acting	↘	→	↘	Neutral (minimal effect on FN rate). If
Long-acting				necessary combine with α$_1$-blockers
Centrally acting α$_2$-agonists	↘	↓↓	↑	Increase FP rate
Diuretics	↑	↑↑	↓	Increase FN rate. If feasible, withdraw 3–4 wk before
MR antagonists	↑	↑↑	↓	Increase FN rate. If feasible, withdraw 6 wk before
NSAIDs	↓	↓↓	↑	Increase FP rate. Withdraw for at least 1 wk
Renin inhibitors	↓	↑	↓	Increase FN rate. Experience still limited and effect on the ARR can be dependent on the assay used for estimating renin

Abbreviations: ACEIs, angiotensin-converting enzyme inhibitors; ARBs, angiotensin receptor blockers; CCBs, calcium channel blockers; FN, false negative; FP, false positive; MR, mineralocorticoid receptor; PAC, plasma aldosterone concentration; PRA, plasma renin activity.

diuretics and mineralocorticoid receptor (MR) antagonists, should be withdrawn (at least 3 and 6 weeks before, respectively), to lower the rate of false-negative diagnoses. If diuretics cannot be stopped the finding of a low renin level, and therefore of an elevated ARR, is a strong clue to the presence of PA, while the finding of an unsuppressed renin does not allow PA to be ruled out. Moreover, it should be considered that among the diuretics those causing more likely to cause prominent hypokalemia, such as chlorthalidone, can blunt aldosterone secretion thus inducing a factitious decrease of the ARR, particularly if renin is stimulated.

Angiotensin-converting enzyme (ACE) inhibitors and angiotensin II receptor blockers (ARBs) have an effect that is even worse not only because they raise the PRA but also because they blunt aldosterone secretion. Therefore, these agents reduce the ARR and increase the false-negative results. Theoretically both ACE inhibitors and ARBs could be helpful in unraveling the autonomy of hyperaldosteronism from the RAS, and therefore in reducing false-positive tests in PA. However, the fact that many cases of APA and even more of IHA are angiotensin-responsive markedly limits the usefulness of this strategy. Because of this, whenever feasible these agents should be withdrawn at least 3 to 4 weeks before performing the ARR.

Of importance, other agents have negligible effects on the ARR: the α$_1$-receptor blocker doxazosin does not affect significantly the renin–angiotensin-aldosterone system, whereas the long-acting calcium channel blockers (CCBs) have a small blunting effect on aldosterone secretion.[53,65,66] Hence, these agents can be used to control blood pressure during the screening test whenever it is harmful to interrupt antihypertensive treatment. In those hypertensive individuals in whom blood pressure levels are not satisfactorily reduced by either an α_1-blocker or a CCB alone, a combination of the two agents is a valuable treatment option.[53]

If the patient has severe and/or resistant hypertension and/or evidence of target organ damage and/or previous cardiovascular events, it is unsafe to withdraw medications. Under these conditions, which are not uncommon at referral centers, the ARR must be performed while the patient is on treatment. Even under treatment there are, however, some hints that can assist in making the correct diagnosis. The finding of a high PAC while the patient is on drugs that should lower aldosterone, and/or the discovery of a blunted renin value on agents that are expected to raise renin, are strong clues to the presence of PA that, therefore, should be investigated aggressively by means of adrenal vein sampling (AVS). Hence, knowledge of the effect of the different drugs on the ARR and its components can allow one to support or exclude the diagnosis of PA (see **Table 2**).

CAVEATS ON USE OF THE ARR AS A SCREENING TEST

There are some additional issues concerning the use of the ARR as a screening test that should be acknowledged. First, as for all tests, the choice of more or less stringent cutoff values affects its sensitivity and specificity: as the cutoff value for the ARR becomes more stringent, the number of false positives decreases.

Second, the choice of the optimal cutoff values has a profound impact on the diagnostic performance of the ARR, but has been based on a careful evaluation of the performance of the test by use of the receiver operator characteristics curves only in a few studies.[40,53,67] In the aforementioned PAPY study the use of a cutoff of 40 (where PAC was in ng/dL and PRA in ng/mL/h) was initially chosen based on the findings of a small retrospective study.[68] When used prospectively it resulted in a high specificity (87%) but a low sensitivity (68%).[53] Of note, this is exactly the opposite of what one would like to achieve with a screening test. Using the diagnosis of APA as reference, the investigators were thereafter able to determine experimentally that the optimal cutoff was 26, which corresponded to a higher sensitivity (of 80.5%) without an appreciable loss of specificity (84.5%).[53] Therefore, use of a liberal cutoff such as 26 is advised to maximize sensitivity.

If the patient has been adequately prepared and if the minimum value of renin has been fixed as described, a markedly elevated ARR, in the author's view 100 or more, usually represents a strong indication of the presence of PA. Moreover, in a recent study where the ARR was repeated twice in the same patient the author's group showed that the ARR was reproducible, when performed under carefully standardized conditions.[69] This finding was unexpected, given the known variability of PAC and renin.

Nonetheless, the crucial importance of preparing the patient from the pharmacologic standpoint (see above) and of standardizing the conditions for blood sampling and sample handling (see **Table 1**) cannot be overlooked.

Finally, in essence the ARR is a crude bivariate analysis of variables that furthermore have a skewed distribution. Because of this logistic multivariate discriminant analysis strategies have been proposed to achieve a more accurate identification of PA,[40] based on the awareness that they can adjust for the skewed distribution of PAC and renin. These approaches take into consideration multiple variables and convey quantitative information provided by the absolute values of all these variables altogether, rather than just relying on a ratio of 2 variables. These strategies have the additional advantage of furnishing an estimate of the probability of PA in individual patients, which enables clinicians to make their own decision on whether to proceed with further testing. When tested prospectively, they performed well in the identification of APA.[53] Regardless of the use of the ARR or the logistic discriminant score, the sampling conditions at screening should be standardized to avoid fluctuation of the hormones with ensuing difficulties in interpreting the values. Ideally the ARR or the logistic score should be center-based, with normal ranges established for salt intake in the local population and the type of assay used for aldosterone and renin.

EXCLUSION OF PA

By definition, the screening tests must be highly sensitive to avoid missing any PA case (**Fig. 1**). Hence, they usually carry false-positive cases that need to be identified

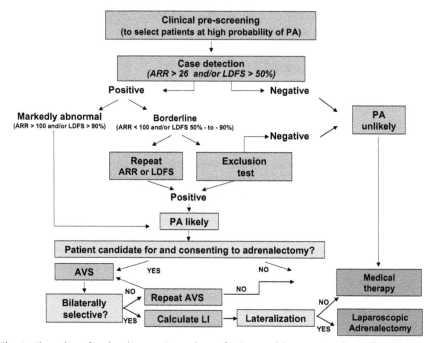

Fig. 1. Flow chart for the diagnostic workup of primary aldosteronism (PA). The diagnostic workup includes a clinical prescreening aimed at identifying patients with a higher pretest probability of PA (see **Box 2**), followed by a strategy that is directed to identifying excess aldosterone secretion and to determining the cause (unilateral or bilateral). By definition the screening tests should be endowed with a high sensitivity, which implies a high false-positive rate. Hence, tests aimed at identification of the false-positive cases are usually suggested. These tests, commonly referred to as "confirmatory tests," have some limitations, as discussed in the text. Moreover, in the patients with high plasma aldosterone concentration/plasma renin activity ratio (ARR) referred to specialized centers they are more useful for exclusion of, rather than confirmation of the diagnosis of PA. Therefore they are indicated here as exclusion tests. A markedly elevated ARR makes PA highly likely and no further testing is required, whereas borderline values of the ARR, for example, between 26 and 100, or of the logistic discriminant function score (LDFS, between 50% and 90%) need to be further evaluated by repeating the ARR or performing an exclusion test. If the ARR and/or the LDFS are repeatedly abnormal, the patient should be further evaluated to establish the need for adrenalectomy, provided that he or she is a candidate for general anesthesia and is willing to undergo surgery. Medical treatment is advised if these conditions are not present. AVS, adrenal vein sampling; LI, lateralization index.

and excluded before selecting the patient for AVS. The tests available to this goal are oral sodium loading test, the saline infusion test, the fludrocortisone with salt loading test, and the captopril challenge.[35,40,70,71] The following considerations need to be made with respect to these tests. First of all, if the screening test results are markedly abnormal, for example, the ARR is greater than 100, there is no need, in the author's view, to perform any exclusion test.

Second, all these tests rely on the assumption that PA is autonomous from the RAS, which is not often the case.[72,73] Moreover, based on this assumption they are aimed at demonstrating a nonsuppressible aldosterone excess after blunting the RAS. Third, as they are intended to show a decrease of PAC, given that and because hypokalemia blunts aldosterone secretion (and therefore might prevent detection of the blunting effect of each test), they must be performed only after correction of the hypokalemia (with oral or intravenous potassium supplementation).

Fourth, it has to be appreciated that relying on these tests can lead to missing several curable APAs. Therefore at the author's institution, once a markedly elevated ARR has been found and/or a second ARR has confirmed it with a value of the ARR greater than 26, one proceeds directly with AVS.[69]

If one would like to rely on the exclusion tests, the following issues need to be considered. The oral sodium loading is widely used in the United States, but less commonly so in Europe because it gives inconsistent results due to the poor standardization and the variable adherence of the patients to the protocol.[70] The most popular tests in Europe are the saline infusion test[70,74] and the captopril test,[40,52,71] which have a moderate sensitivity and a high specificity in patients on an adequate sodium intake, for example, greater than 133 mEq/d (6.3 g NaCl/d).[75] In the author's experience, at a lower sodium intake the saline infusion is more accurate than the captopril test which, therefore, should be used only after sodium repletion.[75]

At the optimal cutoff values both the saline infusion and the captopril test are more specific than sensitive. Because of this, at the prevalence rates that are commonly encountered at referral centers after a positive screening test, the negative predictive value markedly exceeds the positive predictive value for both the saline and the captopril test.[75]

This finding means that these tests are more useful in excluding rather than confirming the presence of PA, and therefore should be regarded as "exclusion" rather than "confirmatory" tests.[75] Physicians will thus avoid mistakenly attributing to these tests a confirmatory role that they do not have. Finally, according to some experts the fludrocortisone and salt loading test would be the most specific,[35] but these tests require costly hospitalization for careful surveillance of the patients owing to the risk of worsening hypertension and possible severe hypokalemia, so that their use is limited to few centers.

IMAGING OF PA

High-resolution computed tomography (CT) with fine (2–3 mm) cuts of the upper abdomen currently represent, in the author's experience, the best available technique for the identification of adrenal nodules.[66,76,77] The nodules may be APAs. However, large nodules of adrenal hyperplasia may also be seen, as in PAH[78] and BAH (see **Box 1** for definitions of these conditions). Magnetic resonance imaging can be slightly more sensitive, but is less specific and more susceptible to motion artifacts.[79]

Fatal aldosterone-producing carcinomas are usually large.[80,81] At variance, nearly 50% of the APAs currently identified are smaller than 20 mm in diameter or less. In some series up to 42% of the APAs are less than 6 mm.[46,82] The nodules of PAH and MUAN are most often smaller than 10 mm, which makes them undetectable by imaging with available technologies.

It has been appreciated that a nonfunctioning adrenal mass can coexist by chance in a hypertensive patient with a biochemical picture of PA with a small CT-undetectable APA. Furthermore, an adrenal nodule in a patient with PA can be an APA but also a macronodule of hyperplasia in a patient with IHA,[83,84] a micronodule in a patient with PAH,[78,82] or an apparently nonfunctioning incidentally discovered adenoma ("incidentaloma"), found in 2% to 10% of adults at autopsy regardless of the presence of hypertension.[85]

Adrenal imaging is inadequate to achieve discrimination between APA and IHA, as shown by a study of 194 patients with PA who underwent both CT and AVS, in whom AVS was used as gold standard for the diagnosis. CT mistakenly suggested an APA in 24.2% of the patients; identified correctly a unilateral or bilateral aldosterone excess only in 53%; falsely suggested a BAH in 21.2% of the patients with a unilateral source of aldosterone excess; and showed the presence of an APA in the wrong adrenal in 12 patients.[86] Similar data on the fallibility of CT for diagnosing the surgically curable subtypes of PA have been reported by others,[84] and by the results of a recent meta-analysis.[87] Overall, CT results alone are misleading in about half of the patients, and can lead to useless and/or inappropriate adrenalectomy in nearly 25% of cases or to exclusion from adrenalectomy of about 25% who are potentially curable with this procedure.

ADRENAL VEIN SAMPLING

Because of the fallacies of imaging tests, the guidelines from the Endocrine Society[55] advocate the use of adrenal vein catheterization in the establishment of the diagnosis of unilateral production of aldosterone for patients who have a high likelihood of cure after adrenalectomy. Not all agree that AVS should be the gold standard for diagnosis of APA in identifying surgical candidates.[88] Many experts, however, form a current consensus that AVS is the gold standard, and necessary, test for demonstrating the lateralization of aldosterone secretion through the measurement of PAC and plasma cortisol concentration (PCC) in adrenal venous blood[89] prior to surgery. Measurements of PCC is used to confirm placement of the catheter and correct for dilutions that might occur during sampling via calculation of the selectivity index,[89] on both sides. Assessment of this index is crucial, as most centers make use only of AVS data that are bilaterally selective. However, the cutoff for defining selectivity has been a matter of debate, largely because most centers perform bilateral simultaneous AVS without any stimulation. Some centers still use the sequential technique during stimulation with adrenocorticotropic hormone (ACTH; cosyntropin) that markedly increases the PCC step-up (see later discussion). The most common cutoff used to define selectivity is 3, but this mostly pertains to values obtained after ACTH,[86,90] which increases the PCC step-up markedly between blood in each adrenal vein and in the inferior vena cava.[91,92] However, some have used a ratio as low as 1.1 with no apparent loss of diagnostic accuracy, and with a marked increase of the proportion of AVS studies that could be used for diagnostic purposes.[89,93]

In patients with bilaterally selective AVS results, the data should be systematically assessed not by relying on absolute hormone values but by calculating the lateralization index, as defined by the author's group.[89] This index provides an accurate diagnosis,[89,93] but again there is still no consensus on the cutoff values to be used.[94,95] Common cutoffs to differentiate unilateral production from bilateral aldosterone excess range between 3 and 5,[86,96,97] but variable cutoffs have also been proposed based on the concurrence of contralateral suppression (see later discussion).[98] Use of a higher or tight cutoff while selecting a subgroup of patients that are most likely to benefit from adrenalectomy can preclude curative surgery for many patients. In fact the author's group has used a ratio as low as 2.0 with strong documentation of success in the only studies that have formally assessed the performance of different cutoffs by using low cutoff values.[89,93] The fact that in a more recent study 20.5% of the patients were cured despite having a lateralization index below 2.0[89] provides evidence that the use of a restriction can result in denying curative adrenalectomy to a substantial proportion of the patients. Hence these observations, along with the recent report that even patients with bilateral aldosterone excess can benefit from adrenalectomy,[99] would support the use of a low cutoff value for the lateralization index.

Variation in the criteria and ratios among different centers has limited consensus[100,101] and has led to the suggestion that the use of a higher cutoff would provide more consistent results.[95] However, these studies were affected by a selection bias, because only the more difficult cases that required repeated AVS were analyzed, and by the circular reasoning that AVS findings were used as a reference for assessing the AVS diagnostic performance itself. The most likely cause of the variation in the cutoff values of the lateralization index used is the difficulty in catheterization of the right adrenal vein, resulting in the mixing of blood from renal capsular veins or hepatic veins, diluting the aldosterone from the adrenal. For catheterization of the hepatic vein or sampling whereby the hepatic vein opens into the adrenal vein causes a dilution of aldosterone, in fact the values of steroids might be lower than peripheral values, as they represent liver metabolism of steroids.[102] The problem has been addressed by using super-selective catheterization after identifying the hepatic vein and advancing the catheter until it is secure in the adrenal vein,[102] or by rapid measurement of cortisol in the adrenal vein to confirm the localization of the catheter and making the adjustments as needed.[103,104]

Expressing the results as lateralization index, for example, as ratio, though very useful in predicting response to surgical removal of the affected side, ignores a widely recognized finding that is seldom reported and discussed. Whatever criteria for lateralization are used, the contralateral adrenal gland is seldom suppressed to levels similar to peripheral values, and these are most often higher than the peripheral values, especially when stimulated with ACTH.[105] To the author's knowledge there are no reports of adrenal vein PAC and PCC levels in normal individuals. Plasma and urinary aldosterone is suppressed to very low levels by the administration of deoxycorticosterone to normal humans,[106] but there is no information about the adrenal production or the responsiveness to stimulation in this setting. Such data in subjects whose adrenal production of aldosterone is suppressed by an exogenous mineralocorticoid would be valuable for determining the "normal" level of aldosterone production to be used for establishing normal range, and thereby for choosing the cutoff to ascertain lateralization.

Some investigators have proposed an index of contralateral suppression, calculated as a PAC/PCC in the contralateral vein lower than the PAC/PCC in the peripheral vein.[98] However, no study has convincingly shown the accuracy of this index for the identification of unilateral causes of PA thus far. Moreover, experimental studies have shown that even during prominent sodium loading aldosterone secretion persists, and clinical studies using in situ hybridization and immunohistochemistry have evidenced persistent aldosterone synthesis even in the adrenal cortex surrounding an APA.[107,108]

AVS is expensive and technically demanding, and carries a tiny risk of adrenal vein rupture.[109] Because of this and because AVS is aimed at posing the indication for adrenalectomy, it should be reserved only for patients in whom there is a strong biochemical evidence of PA and, moreover, are low-risk candidates for general anesthesia and surgery who are willing to undergo adrenalectomy. These issues should be discussed with the patient before offering AVS and, conversely, AVS should be proposed to all patients before surgery. At the author's institution adrenalectomy is no longer undertaken without evidence of lateralized aldosterone secretion.

Some centers reserve AVS only for those who are older than 40 years, based on the premise that the prevalence of nonfunctioning adenoma (so-called incidentaloma) increases with age, and therefore an adrenal mass in a patient younger than 40 with PA "must be an APA."[86,110] This strategy runs the risk that unnecessary or even wrong-sided adrenalectomies will be performed, as PA can be attributable to BAH or to a small contralateral APA invisible on CT.

AVS should be performed only in patients with normokalemia, for example, after correction of the hypokalemia and after confounding drugs have been discontinued. Because both the performance and the interpretation of AVS require considerable experience, this test should be performed only at referral centers thoroughly familiar with the necessary procedures. Use of bilaterally simultaneous catheterization during AVS[91] avoids generating artificial differences between sides owing to the different timing of the blood sampling under the stressful condition represented by AVS.

The previous assessment of right adrenal vein drainage anatomy by CT with 3-dimensional reconstruction can allow planning of super-selective catheterization, which is necessary to obviate the dilution of adrenal blood with blood derived from the liver.[102]

ACTH stimulation, which is being systematically used at some centers to abolish stress-related differences between sides,[86] increases the selectivity index,[89,91,92,111,112] but is unnecessary when bilateral simultaneous AVS[91] is used. Moreover, it exerts a confounding effect on the lateralization index, therefore the author and others do not support its use.[89,91,92,111,112]

To address the several issues that remain controversial and/or unresolved,[101] an international multicenter study, the Adrenal Vein sampling International Study (AVIS), has been recently launched and is ongoing. The first results of this study on more than 2500 patients have shown that the rate of major complications of AVS is 0.57%, thus proving that the procedure is safe in experienced hands.

An alternative approach to the demonstration of lateralized aldosterone excess entails the administration of ^{131}I-labeled cholesterol analogues such as [6β-^{131}I]-methyl-19-norcholesterol (NP59) after blunting during the preceding week the ACTH drive to the adrenocortical zona fasciculata with dexamethasone (1 mg every day). This technique is intrinsically insensitive and therefore is able to demonstrate only large (>1.5 cm) and markedly hypersecreting APA which, as mentioned earlier, do not make up the majority of the tumors currently identified.[82,113–115] Current shortage in the supply of the radiotracer has also led to the abandonment of the use of NP59.

A further approach that is being tested entails ^{11}C-methomidate positron emission tomography, which requires a facility for the preparation of the tracer and therefore could be developed only at large tertiary referral centers. Whether it could identify the majority of APAs that are small remains to be demonstrated.

DIFFERENTIAL DIAGNOSIS

Some rare forms of mineralocorticoid excess or low renin hypertension, which need to be considered in the differential diagnosis of PA before selecting the patients for AVS, are listed in **Box 3**. Patients with these conditions will gain no benefit from adrenalectomy and therefore should not be submitted to AVS. For a detailed discussion of other forms the reader is referred elsewhere.[4,34]

TREATMENT

In patients who are candidates for general anesthesia and are willing to undergo surgery, demonstration of lateralized aldosterone secretion is crucial for the choice of the most appropriate treatment strategy (see **Fig. 1**). Laparoscopic adrenalectomy,

---

Box 3
Forms of low renin hypertension that need to be considered in the differential diagnosis of PA

- Low renin primary (essential) hypertension
- Familial hyperaldosteronism:

  Type I (FH-I), also known as glucocorticoid-remediable aldosteronism (GRA)

  Type II (FH-II)
- Apparent mineralocorticoid excess (AME)
- Chronic consumption of licorice
- Liddle syndrome

---

which can be performed with a 2-day hospital stay at a very low operative risk,[116–118] is currently the best treatment that can be offered. In general, with adrenalectomy hypertension is cured in approximately 33% to 72% of cases and is markedly ameliorated in 40% to 50% of cases.[26,119] However, in the author's experience, when the diagnosis stands on demonstration of lateralized aldosterone excess, as determined above, the cure rate of PA, defined as the normalization of PAC and renin and the correction of hypokalemia if present, is close to 100% and that of hypertension is about 30%. An additional 52% of the patients showed a marked improvement, in that the number and/or doses of antihypertensive drugs can be markedly decreased, and/or their hypertension is no longer resistant to treatment.[27] Attempts to identify the predictors of blood pressure outcome have given consistent results only for duration of hypertension,[120] and more recently for the presence of vascular remodeling.[27] Hence, overall these data support the concept that the sooner the diagnosis is made and adrenalectomy is performed, the better in terms of outcome.

Failure to cure hypertension can be attributed to an inaccurate diagnosis, lack of performing or correctly interpreting AVS results, the development of bilateral APA over time, or more commonly to the concurrence of primary hypertension. Given the high prevalence of primary (essential) hypertension, it can be anticipated that from 20% to 30% of the patients with PA can have concurrent primary hypertension.[121] This estimate implies that cure of the biochemical picture of PA, but not of hypertension, occurs.

Patients who are not candidates for surgery or who do not show lateralized aldosterone excess may be effectively treated with MR receptor antagonists such as spironolactone, canrenone, potassium canrenoate, or eplerenone. The latter drug may be a more specific but less potent MR antagonist. Hypokalemia can be corrected, but additional medications, such as CCBs for control of hypertension, are often needed. Amiloride can also be a valuable option to correct hypokalemia for patients who develop side effects with the MR receptor antagonists. Often a RAS blocker is also useful in controlling the counter-regulatory stimulation of the RAS that is associated with use of MR receptor antagonists.

Additional potent and specific MR antagonists are also being developed.[7] Pilot studies suggest that they can effectively control blood pressure in PA patients and decrease left ventricular mass, but whether they are as effective as adrenalectomy in providing regression of target organ damage remains to be conclusively proved. The occurrence of gynecomastia and impotence, which can occur with the oldest MR receptor antagonists (especially spironolactone), is dose dependent, which suggests the use of lower doses in combination, if necessary, with other agents such as long-acting CCBs, some of which also have MR antagonistic properties,[122] ACE inhibitors, or ARBs. Both the latter drugs can be particularly useful as they effectively control the stimulation of the RAS provoked by the diuretic action of the MR antagonists. Because the MR antagonists, while being effective in controlling the hyperaldosteronism, do not correct it, aldosterone synthase inhibitors are also being developed and tested in phase 3 trials.

SUMMARY

A few simple rules can allow physicians to successfully identify many patients with arterial hypertension caused by PA among the so-called essential hypertensive patients. The hyperaldosteronism and the hypokalemia can be cured with adrenalectomy in practically all of these patients. Moreover, in a substantial proportion of them the blood pressure can be normalized or markedly lowered if a unilateral cause of PA is discovered. Hence, the screening for PA can be rewarding both for the patient and for the clinician, particularly in those cases where hypertension is severe and/or resistant to treatment, in which the removal of an APA can allow blood pressure to be brought under control despite withdrawal of or a prominent reduction in the number and doses of antihypertensive medications.

REFERENCES

1. Kucharz EJ. Forgotten description of primary hyperaldosteronism. Lancet 1991; 337:1490.
2. Conn JW. Presidential address. I. Painting background. II. Primary aldosteronism, a new clinical syndrome. J Lab Clin Med 1955;45:3–17.
3. Conn JW, Knopf RF, Nesbit RM. Clinical characteristics of primary aldosteronism from an analysis of 145 cases. Am J Surg 1964;107:159–72.
4. Rossi GP. Surgically correctable hypertension caused by primary aldosteronism. Best Pract Res Clin Endocrinol Metab 2006;20:385–400.
5. Fritsch NM, Schiffrin EL. Aldosterone: a risk factor for vascular disease. Curr Hypertens Rep 2003;5:59–65.
6. Pu Q, Neves MF, Virdis A, et al. Endothelin antagonism on aldosterone-induced oxidative stress and vascular remodeling. Hypertension 2003;42:49–55.
7. Schupp N, Queisser N, Wolf M, et al. Aldosterone causes DNA strand breaks and chromosomal damage in renal cells, which are prevented by mineralocorticoid receptor antagonists. Horm Metab Res 2010;42(6):458–65.
8. Rocha R, Rudolph AE, Frierdich GE, et al. Aldosterone induces a vascular inflammatory phenotype in the rat heart. Am J Physiol Heart Circ Physiol 2002;283:H1802–10.
9. Brilla CG, Maisch B, Weber KT. Myocardial collagen matrix remodelling in arterial hypertension. Eur Heart J 1992;13(Suppl D):24–32.
10. Brilla CG, Pick R, Tan LB, et al. Remodeling of the rat right and left ventricles in experimental hypertension. Circ Res 1990;67:1355–64.
11. Rossi GP, Sacchetto A, Pavan E, et al. Left ventricular systolic function in primary aldosteronism and hypertension. J Hypertens 1997;19(Suppl 8):S147–51.
12. Rossi GP, Sacchetto A, Pavan E, et al. Remodeling of the left ventricle in primary aldosteronism due to Conn's adenoma. Circulation 1997;95:1471–8.
13. Rossi GP, Di Bello V, Ganzaroli C, et al. Excess aldosterone is associated with alterations of myocardial texture in primary aldosteronism. Hypertension 2002; 40:23–7.

14. Farquharson CA, Struthers AD. Aldosterone induces acute endothelial dysfunction in vivo in humans: evidence for an aldosterone-induced vasculopathy. Clin Sci (Lond) 2002;103:425–31.
15. Nishizaka MK, Zaman MA, Green SA, et al. Impaired endothelium-dependent flow-mediated vasodilation in hypertensive subjects with hyperaldosteronism. Circulation 2004;109:2857–61.
16. Taddei S, Virdis A, Mattei P, et al. Vasodilation to acetylcholine in primary and secondary forms of human hypertension. Hypertension 1993;21:929–33.
17. Muiesan ML, Rizzoni D, Salvetti M, et al. Structural changes in small resistance arteries and left ventricular geometry in patients with primary and secondary hypertension. J Hypertens 2002;20:1439–44.
18. Rizzoni D, Muiesan ML, Porteri E, et al. Relations between cardiac and vascular structure in patients with primary and secondary hypertension. J Am Coll Cardiol 1998;32:985–92.
19. Halimi JM, Mimran A. Albuminuria in untreated patients with primary aldosteronism or essential hypertension. J Hypertens 1995;13:1801–2.
20. Rossi GP, Bernini G, Desideri G, et al. Renal damage in primary aldosteronism: results of the PAPY Study. Hypertension 2006;48:232–8.
21. Rossi GP, Sechi LA, Giacchetti G, et al. Primary aldosteronism: cardiovascular, renal and metabolic implications. Trends Endocrinol Metab 2008;19:88–90.
22. Sechi LA, Novello M, Lapenna R, et al. Long-term renal outcomes in patients with primary aldosteronism. JAMA 2006;295:2638–45.
23. Nishimura M, Uzu T, Fujii T, et al. Cardiovascular complications in patients with primary aldosteronism. Am J Kidney Dis 1999;33:261–6.
24. Takeda R, Matsubara T, Miyamori I, et al. Vascular complications in patients with aldosterone producing adenoma in Japan: comparative study with essential hypertension. The Research Committee of Disorders of Adrenal Hormones in Japan. J Endocrinol Invest 1995;18:370–3.
25. Milliez P, Girerd X, Plouin PF, et al. Evidence for an increased rate of cardiovascular events in patients with primary aldosteronism. J Am Coll Cardiol 2005;45:1243–8.
26. Sawka AM, Young WF, Thompson GB, et al. Primary aldosteronism: factors associated with normalization of blood pressure after surgery. Ann Intern Med 2001;135:258–61.
27. Rossi GP, Bolognesi M, Rizzoni D, et al. Vascular remodeling and duration of hypertension predict outcome of adrenalectomy in primary aldosteronism patients. Hypertension 2008;51:1366–71.
28. Catena C, Colussi G, Lapenna R, et al. Long-term cardiac effects of adrenalectomy or mineralocorticoid antagonists in patients with primary aldosteronism. Hypertension 2007;50:911–8.
29. Conn JW. Primary aldosteronism. In: Hypertension: pathophysiology and treatment. New York: McGraw-Hill; 1977.
30. Conn JW. Part I. Painting background. Part II. Primary aldosteronism, a new clinical syndrome. J Lab Clin Med 1990;116:253–67.
31. Conn JW. Plasma renin activity in primary aldosteronism. JAMA 1964;190:222–5.
32. Conn JW. A concluding response. Arch Intern Med 1969;123:154–5.
33. Rossi GP. Primary aldosteronism: a needle in a haystack or a yellow cab on fifth avenue? Curr Hypertens Rep 2004;6:1–4.
34. Rossi GP, Pessina AC, Heagerty AM. Primary aldosteronism: an update on screening, diagnosis and treatment. J Hypertens 2008;26:613–21.

35. Gordon RD, Ziesak MD, Tunny TJ, et al. Evidence that primary aldosteronism may not be uncommon: 12% incidence among antihypertensive drug trial volunteers. Clin Exp Pharmacol Physiol 1993;20:296–8.

36. Anderson GH Jr, Blakeman N, Streeten DH. The effect of age on prevalence of secondary forms of hypertension in 4429 consecutively referred patients. J Hypertens 1994;12:609–15.

37. Gordon RD, Stowasser M, Tunny TJ, et al. High incidence of primary aldosteronism in 199 patients referred with hypertension. Clin Exp Pharmacol Physiol 1994;21:315–8.

38. Abdelhamid S, Muller-Lobeck H, Pahl S, et al. Prevalence of adrenal and extra-adrenal Conn syndrome in hypertensive patients. Arch Intern Med 1996;156: 1190–5.

39. Brown MA, Cramp HA, Zammit VC, et al. Primary hyperaldosteronism: a missed diagnosis in 'essential hypertensives'? Aust N Z J Med 1996;26:533–8.

40. Rossi GP, Rossi E, Pavan E, et al. Screening for primary aldosteronism with a logistic multivariate discriminant analysis. Clin Endocrinol (Oxf) 1998;49: 713–23.

41. Mosso L, Fardella C, Montero J, et al. High prevalence of undiagnosed primary hyperaldosteronism among patients with essential hypertension. Rev Med Chil 1999;127:800–6 [in Spanish].

42. Rayner BL, Opie LH, Davidson JS. The aldosterone/renin ratio as a screening test for primary aldosteronism. S Afr Med J 2000;90:394–400.

43. Loh KC, Koay ES, Khaw MC, et al. Prevalence of primary aldosteronism among Asian hypertensive patients in Singapore. J Clin Endocrinol Metab 2000;85: 2854–9.

44. Denolle T, Hanon O, Mounier-Vehier C, et al. [What tests should be conducted for secondary arterial hypertension in hypertensive patients resistant to treatment?]. Arch Mal Coeur Vaiss 2000;93:1037–9 [in French].

45. Cortes P, Fardella C, Oestreicher E, et al. [Excess of mineralocorticoids in essential hypertension: clinical-diagnostic approach]. Rev Med Chil 2000;128: 955–61 [in Spanish].

46. Nishikawa T, Omura M. Clinical characteristics of primary aldosteronism: its prevalence and comparative studies on various causes of primary aldosteronism in Yokohama Rosai hospital. Biomed Pharmacother 2000;54(Suppl 1):83s–5s.

47. Fardella CE, Mosso L, Gomez-Sanchez C, et al. Primary hyperaldosteronism in essential hypertensives: prevalence, biochemical profile, and molecular biology. J Clin Endocrinol Metab 2000;85:1863–7.

48. Lim PO, Dow E, Brennan G, et al. High prevalence of primary aldosteronism in the Tayside hypertension clinic population. J Hum Hypertens 2000;14: 311–5.

49. Rayner BL, Myers JE, Opie LH, et al. Screening for primary aldosteronism— normal ranges for aldosterone and renin in three South African population groups. S Afr Med J 2001;91:594–9.

50. Calhoun DA, Nishizaka MK, Zaman MA, et al. Hyperaldosteronism among black and white subjects with resistant hypertension. Hypertension 2002;40:892–6.

51. Schwartz GL, Chapman AB, Boerwinkle E, et al. Screening for primary aldosteronism: implications of an increased plasma aldosterone/renin ratio. Clin Chem 2002;48:1919–23.

52. Rossi E, Regolisti G, Negro A, et al. High prevalence of primary aldosteronism using postcaptopril plasma aldosterone to renin ratio as a screening test among Italian hypertensives. Am J Hypertens 2002;15:896–902.

53. Rossi GP, Bernini G, Caliumi C, et al. A prospective study of the prevalence of primary aldosteronism in 1,125 hypertensive patients. J Am Coll Cardiol 2006; 48:2293–300.
54. Rossi GP, Seccia TM, Pessina AC. Clinical use of laboratory tests for the identification of secondary forms of arterial hypertension. Crit Rev Clin Lab Sci 2007;44:1–85.
55. Funder JW, Carey RM, Fardella C, et al. Case detection, diagnosis, and treatment of patients with primary aldosteronism: an endocrine society clinical practice guideline. J Clin Endocrinol Metab 2008;93:3266–81.
56. Goodfriend TL, Calhoun DA. Resistant hypertension, obesity, sleep apnea, and aldosterone: theory and therapy. Hypertension 2004;43:518–24.
57. Rossi GP, Belfiore A, Bernini G, et al. Body mass index predicts plasma aldosterone concentrations in overweight-obese primary hypertensive patients. J Clin Endocrinol Metab 2008;93(7):2566–71.
58. Hiramatsu K, Yamada T, Yukimura Y, et al. A screening test to identify aldosterone-producing adenoma by measuring plasma renin activity. Results in hypertensive patients. Arch Intern Med 1981;141:1589–93.
59. Mulatero P, Dluhy RG, Giacchetti G, et al. Diagnosis of primary aldosteronism: from screening to subtype differentiation. Trends Endocrinol Metab 2005;16: 114–9.
60. Sealey JE. Plasma renin activity and plasma prorenin assays. Clin Chem 1991; 37:1811–9.
61. Roding JH, Weterings T, van der Heiden C. Plasma renin activity: temperature optimum at approximately 45 degrees C. Clin Chem 1997;43:1243–4.
62. Sealey JE, Gordon RD, Mantero F. Plasma renin and aldosterone measurements in low renin hypertensive states. Trends Endocrinol Metab 2005;16:86–91.
63. Campbell DJ, Nussberger J, Stowasser M, et al. Activity assays and immunoassays for plasma renin and prorenin: information provided and precautions necessary for accurate measurement. Clin Chem 2009;55:867–77.
64. Rossi GP, Barisa M, Belfiore A, et al. The aldosterone renin ratio based on the plasma renin activity and the direct renin assay for diagnosing aldosterone-producing adenoma. J Hypertens 2010;28(9):1892–9.
65. Mulatero P, Rabbia F, Milan A, et al. Drug effects on aldosterone/plasma renin activity ratio in primary aldosteronism. Hypertension 2002;40:897–902.
66. Stowasser M, Gordon RD, Rutherford JC, et al. Diagnosis and management of primary aldosteronism. J Renin Angiotensin Aldosterone Syst 2001;2:156–69.
67. Stowasser M, Gordon RD, Gunasekera TG, et al. High rate of detection of primary aldosteronism, including surgically treatable forms, after 'non-selective' screening of hypertensive patients. J Hypertens 2003;21:2149–57.
68. Giacchetti G, Ronconi V, Lucarelli G, et al. Analysis of screening and confirmatory tests in the diagnosis of primary aldosteronism: need for a standardized protocol. J Hypertens 2006;24:737–45.
69. Rossi GP, Seccia TM, Palumbo G, et al. Within-patient reproducibility of the aldosterone: renin ratio in primary aldosteronism. Hypertension 2010;55:83–9.
70. Agharazii M, Douville P, Grose JH, et al. Captopril suppression versus salt loading in confirming primary aldosteronism. Hypertension 2001;37:1440–3.
71. Castro OL, Yu X, Kem DC. Diagnostic value of the post-captopril test in primary aldosteronism. Hypertension 2002;39:935–8.
72. Irony I, Kater CE, Biglieri EG, et al. Correctable subsets of primary aldosteronism. Primary adrenal hyperplasia and renin responsive adenoma. Am J Hypertens 1990;3:576–82.

73. Gordon RD, Gomez-Sanchez CE, Hamlet SM, et al. Angiotensin-responsive aldosterone-producing adenoma masquerades as idiopathic hyperaldosteronism (IHA:adrenal hyperplasia) or low-renin hypertension. J Hypertens Suppl 1987;5(Suppl 5):S103–6.
74. Holland OB, Brown H, Kuhnert L, et al. Further evaluation of saline infusion for the diagnosis of primary aldosteronism. Hypertension 1984;6:717–23.
75. Rossi GP, Belfiore A, Bernini G, et al. Comparison of the captopril and the saline infusion test for excluding aldosterone-producing adenoma. Hypertension 2007;50:424–31.
76. Gordon RD. Primary aldosteronism. J Endocrinol Invest 1995;18:495–511.
77. Mulatero P, Stowasser M, Loh KC, et al. Increased diagnosis of primary aldosteronism, including surgically correctable forms, in centers from five continents. J Clin Endocrinol Metab 2004;89:1045–50.
78. Goh BK, Tan YH, Chang KT, et al. Primary hyperaldosteronism secondary to unilateral adrenal hyperplasia: an unusual cause of surgically correctable hypertension. A review of 30 cases. World J Surg 2007;31:72–9.
79. Rossi GP, Chiesura-Corona M, Tregnaghi A, et al. Imaging of aldosterone-secreting adenomas: a prospective comparison of computed tomography and magnetic resonance imaging in 27 patients with suspected primary aldosteronism. J Hum Hypertens 1993;7:357–63.
80. Rossi GP, Vendraminelli R, Cesari M, et al. A thoracic mass with hypertension and hypokalaemia. Lancet 2000;356:1570.
81. Seccia TM, Fassina A, Nussdorfer GG, et al. Aldosterone-producing adrenocortical carcinoma: an unusual cause of Conn's syndrome with an ominous clinical course. Endocr Relat Cancer 2005;12:149–59.
82. Omura M, Sasano H, Fujiwara T, et al. Unique cases of unilateral hyperaldosteronemia due to multiple adrenocortical micronodules, which can only be detected by selective adrenal venous sampling. Metabolism 2002;51:350–5.
83. Fallo F, Barzon L, Boscaro M, et al. Coexistence of aldosteronoma and contralateral nonfunctioning adrenal adenoma in primary aldosteronism. Am J Hypertens 1997;10:476–8.
84. Magill SB, Raff H, Shaker JL, et al. Comparison of adrenal vein sampling and computed tomography in the differentiation of primary aldosteronism. J Clin Endocrinol Metab 2001;86:1066–71.
85. Mantero F, Terzolo M, Arnaldi G, et al. A survey on adrenal incidentaloma in Italy. Study Group on Adrenal Tumors of the Italian Society of Endocrinology. J Clin Endocrinol Metab 2000;85:637–44.
86. Young WF, Stanson AW, Thompson GB, et al. Role for adrenal venous sampling in primary aldosteronism. Surgery 2004;136:1227–35.
87. Kempers MJ, Lenders JW, van Outheusden L, et al. Systematic review: diagnostic procedures to differentiate unilateral from bilateral adrenal abnormality in primary aldosteronism. Ann Intern Med 2009;151:329–37.
88. Stewart PM, Allolio B. Adrenal vein sampling for primary aldosteronism: time for a reality check. Clin Endocrinol (Oxf) 2010;72:146–8.
89. Rossi GP, Pitter G, Bernante P, et al. Adrenal vein sampling for primary aldosteronism: the assessment of selectivity and lateralization of aldosterone excess baseline and after adrenocorticotropic hormone (ACTH) stimulation. J Hypertens 2008;26:989–97.
90. Stowasser M, Gordon RD. Primary aldosteronism—careful investigation is essential and rewarding. Mol Cell Endocrinol 2004;217:33–9.

91. Rossi GP, Ganzaroli C, Miotto D, et al. Dynamic testing with high-dose adreno-corticotrophic hormone does not improve lateralization of aldosterone oversecretion in primary aldosteronism patients. J Hypertens 2006;24:371–9.

92. Seccia TM, Miotto D, De Toni R, et al. Adrenocorticotropic hormone stimulation during adrenal vein sampling for identifying surgically curable subtypes of primary aldosteronism: comparison of 3 different protocols. Hypertension 2009;53:761–6.

93. Rossi GP, Sacchetto A, Chiesura-Corona M, et al. Identification of the etiology of primary aldosteronism with adrenal vein sampling in patients with equivocal computed tomography and magnetic resonance findings: results in 104 consecutive cases. J Clin Endocrinol Metab 2001;86:1083–90.

94. Rossi GP. New concepts in adrenal vein sampling for aldosterone in the diagnosis of primary aldosteronism. Curr Hypertens Rep 2007;9:90–7.

95. Mulatero P, Bertello C, Sukor N, et al. Impact of different diagnostic criteria during adrenal vein sampling on reproducibility of subtype diagnosis in patients with primary aldosteronism. Hypertension 2010;55:667–73.

96. Young WF, Stanson AW. What are the keys to successful adrenal venous sampling (AVS) in patients with primary aldosteronism? Clin Endocrinol (Oxf) 2009;70:14–7.

97. Letavernier E, Peyrard S, Amar L, et al. Blood pressure outcome of adrenalectomy in patients with primary hyperaldosteronism with or without unilateral adenoma. J Hypertens 2008;26:1816–23.

98. Mulatero P, Bertello C, Rossato D, et al. Roles of clinical criteria, computed tomography scan, and adrenal vein sampling in differential diagnosis of primary aldosteronism subtypes. J Clin Endocrinol Metab 2008;93:1366–71.

99. Sukor N, Gordon RD, Ku YK, et al. Role of unilateral adrenalectomy in bilateral primary aldosteronism: a 22-year single center experience. J Clin Endocrinol Metab 2009;94:2437–45.

100. Harvey A, Kline G, Pasieka JL. Adrenal venous sampling in primary hyperaldosteronism: comparison of radiographic with biochemical success and the clinical decision-making with "less than ideal" testing. Surgery 2006;140:847–53.

101. Auchus RJ, Wians FH Jr, Anderson ME, et al. What we still do not know about adrenal vein sampling for primary aldosteronism. Horm Metab Res 2010;42:411–5.

102. Miotto D, De Toni R, Pitter G, et al. Impact of accessory hepatic veins on adrenal vein sampling for identification of surgically curable primary aldosteronism. Hypertension 2009;54:885–9.

103. Mengozzi G, Rossato D, Bertello C, et al. Rapid cortisol assay during adrenal vein sampling in patients with primary aldosteronism. Clin Chem 2007;53:1968–71.

104. Auchus RJ, Michaelis C, Wians FH Jr, et al. Rapid cortisol assays improve the success rate of adrenal vein sampling for primary aldosteronism. Ann Surg 2009;249:318–21.

105. Carr CE, Cope C, Cohen DL, et al. Comparison of sequential versus simultaneous methods of adrenal venous sampling. J Vasc Interv Radiol 2004;15:1245–50.

106. Shade RE, Grim CE. Suppression of renin and aldosterone by small amounts of DOCA in normal man. J Clin Endocrinol Metab 1975;40:652–8.

107. Enberg U, Volpe C, Hoog A, et al. Postoperative differentiation between unilateral adrenal adenoma and bilateral adrenal hyperplasia in primary aldosteronism by mRNA expression of the gene CYP11B2. Eur J Endocrinol 2004;151:73–85.

108. Nishimoto K, Nakagawa K, Li D, et al. Adrenocortical zonation in humans under normal and pathological conditions. J Clin Endocrinol Metab 2010;95:2296–305.
109. Daunt N. Adrenal vein sampling: how to make it quick, easy, and successful. Radiographics 2005;25(Suppl 1):S143–58.
110. Mulatero P, Milan A, Fallo F, et al. Comparison of confirmatory tests for the diagnosis of primary aldosteronism. J Clin Endocrinol Metab 2006;91(7):2618–23.
111. Rossi GP, Pitter G, Miotto D. To stimulate or not to stimulate: is adrenocorticotrophic hormone testing necessary, or not? J Hypertens 2007;25:481–4.
112. Rossi GP, Pitter G, Miotto D. To stimulate or not to stimulate: is adrenocorticotrophic hormone testing necessary, or not? Round 2. J Hypertens 2007;25:1518–20.
113. Hogan MJ, McRae J, Schambelan M, et al. Location of aldosterone-producing adenomas with [131]I-19-iodocholesterol. N Engl J Med 1976;294:410–4.
114. Nomura K, Kusakabe K, Maki M, et al. Iodomethylnorcholesterol uptake in an aldosteronoma shown by dexamethasone-suppression scintigraphy: relationship to adenoma size and functional activity. J Clin Endocrinol Metab 1990;71:825–30.
115. Mansoor GA, Malchoff CD, Arici MH, et al. Unilateral adrenal hyperplasia causing primary aldosteronism: limitations of I-131 norcholesterol scanning. Am J Hypertens 2002;15:459–64.
116. Toniato A, Bernante P, Rossi GP, et al. Laparoscopic versus open adrenalectomy: outcome in 35 consecutive patients. Int J Surg Investig 2000;1:503–7.
117. Jeschke K, Janetschek G, Peschel R, et al. Laparoscopic partial adrenalectomy in patients with aldosterone-producing adenomas: indications, technique, and results. Urology 2003;61:69–72.
118. Meria P, Kempf BF, Hermieu JF, et al. Laparoscopic management of primary hyperaldosteronism: clinical experience with 212 cases. J Urol 2003;169:32–5.
119. Lumachi F, Ermani M, Basso SM, et al. Long-term results of adrenalectomy in patients with aldosterone-producing adenomas: multivariate analysis of factors affecting unresolved hypertension and review of the literature. Am Surg 2005;71:864–9.
120. Obara T, Ito Y, Okamoto T, et al. Risk factors associated with postoperative persistent hypertension in patients with primary aldosteronism. Surgery 1992;112:987–93.
121. Proye CA, Mulliez EA, Carnaille BM, et al. Essential hypertension: first reason for persistent hypertension after unilateral adrenalectomy for primary aldosteronism? Surgery 1998;124:1128–33.
122. Dietz JD, Du S, Bolten CW, et al. A number of marketed dihydropyridine calcium channel blockers have mineralocorticoid receptor antagonist activity. Hypertension 2008;51:742–8.

Glucocorticoid-remediable Aldosteronism

Florencia Halperin, MD, Robert G. Dluhy, MD*

KEYWORDS

- Glucocorticoid-remediable aldosteronism • Aldosterone
- Hypertension

In 1966, Sutherland described a father and son with hypokalemia and hypertension.[1] Since then, multiple kindreds with clinical and biochemical features of primary aldosteronism (PA) and an autosomal dominant pattern of inheritance have been reported.[2–4] The early literature described affected individuals as having all the classical characteristics of mineralocorticoid excess, including hypertension, hypokalemia, and suppressed plasma renin activity. But Sutherland and colleagues[1] observed that these findings could all be reversed by the administration of exogenous glucocorticoids, such as dexamethasone. Thus, the disorder came to be known as dexamethasone-suppressible aldosteronism, and later glucocorticoid-remediable aldosteronism (GRA) (it is also referred to as familial hyperaldosteronism type I). Almost 30 years later, advances in molecular biology led to the characterization of the genetic basis of GRA.[3,5] We now know that a chimeric gene duplication results from an unequal crossing over between the highly homologous 11β-hydroxylase and aldosterone synthase genes. As a consequence, aldosterone synthase is expressed ectopically in the cortisol-producing *zona fasciculata* of the adrenal gland under the regulation of adrenocorticotropin (ACTH).[3] Genetic screening techniques have facilitated the identification of at-risk individuals and families. Understanding the molecular pathophysiology of GRA has permitted the use of directed therapy for effective antihypertensive treatment.

PREVALENCE AND EPIDEMIOLOGY

GRA appears to be the most common monogenic form of hypertension in humans. It accounts for approximately 1% of cases of PA.[6] Although other etiologies of PA are more frequent in women, GRA occurs equally among women and men.[7]

The authors have nothing to disclose.
Division of Endocrinology, Diabetes and Hypertension, Harvard Medical School, Brigham and Women's Hospital, 221 Longwood Avenue, Boston, MA 02115, USA
* Corresponding author.
E-mail address: rdluhy@partners.org

Endocrinol Metab Clin N Am 40 (2011) 333–341
doi:10.1016/j.ecl.2011.01.012
0889-8529/11/$ – see front matter © 2011 Elsevier Inc. All rights reserved.

Cases of GRA have been reported worldwide (**Fig. 1**), including in Canada,[1] the United States,[3] Germany,[8] the United Kingdom,[9,10] Ireland,[10] Italy,[11] China,[12] Taiwan,[13] Japan,[14] Australia,[3] and Chile.[15] Some of the affected individuals described also had Dutch and Ukrainian ancestry.[3] To date, no cases have been reported among blacks.

CLINICAL PRESENTATION

The clinical features of GRA are variable. Typically, the disorder is characterized by early onset hypertension. In one retrospective series, 80% of children who carried the chimeric gene duplication had hypertension by 13 years of age; 50% of the children had moderate-severe hypertension at diagnosis, defined as blood pressure greater than the 99th percentile for age and sex.[16]

Most individuals affected with GRA are severely hypertensive.[10,17,18] However, some have only mild hypertension or may even be normotensive[11]; in one Italian kindred less than one-third of affected subjects had systolic blood pressures in the hypertensive range.[2] Thus, a lack of family history of severe hypertension in first-degree relatives does not exclude the diagnosis of GRA in any individual.

The blood pressure variability in GRA may relate to the multiplicity of hereditary factors that regulate blood pressure within families. Environmental factors, such as variation in dietary sodium intake, may also contribute to phenotypic variance.[19] But even normotensive individuals with GRA have left ventricular structural changes compared with matched controls, and therefore may be at an increased risk for cardiovascular disease despite normal blood pressure.[20] This finding may reflect direct adverse effects of aldosterone excess on the cardiovascular system.[21]

GRA is also characterized by a markedly increased prevalence of early cerebrovascular complications, primarily cerebral hemorrhages, which are often fatal.[22] A retrospective series that reviewed 376 subjects with GRA (in 27 kindreds) revealed that 18% of the subjects (in 48% of the kindreds) suffered a cerebrovascular event. Of these, 70% were hemorrhagic strokes that resulted from ruptured intracranial aneurysms, and the mortality rate was 61%.[22] The mean age at the time of the initial event was 31.7 years. Therefore screening of asymptomatic patients with GRA is recommended with cerebral magnetic resonance angiography beginning at puberty and then every 5 years.[19,22] However, reduction in event rates as a result of screening has not been demonstrated.

Despite the fact that GRA is a mineralocorticoid-excess state, and contrary to what was described in early case reports, spontaneous hypokalemia is uncommon. Most affected individuals are normokalemic,[18] and serum potassium level is therefore not a sensitive screening test for this disorder. However, individuals with GRA are likely to develop hypokalemia if treated with a potassium-wasting diuretic, such as hydrochlorothiazide.[8,18] Why lower rates of spontaneous hypokalemia are seen in GRA compared with other subtypes of PA is not well understood, but renal potassium handling does not seem to be impaired.[23]

PATHOPHYSIOLOGY

Aldosterone is normally synthesized in the *zona glomerulosa* (ZG) of the adrenal gland; its production is restricted to this layer of the adrenal cortex because of zonal-specific expression of aldosterone synthase (CYP11B2), which hydroxylates corticosterone to produce aldosterone. The renin-angiotensin system (RAS) and potassium balance are the principal regulators of aldosterone secretion in the ZG. On the other hand, cortisol is produced only in the *zona fasciculata* of the adrenal cortex. The last step in cortisol

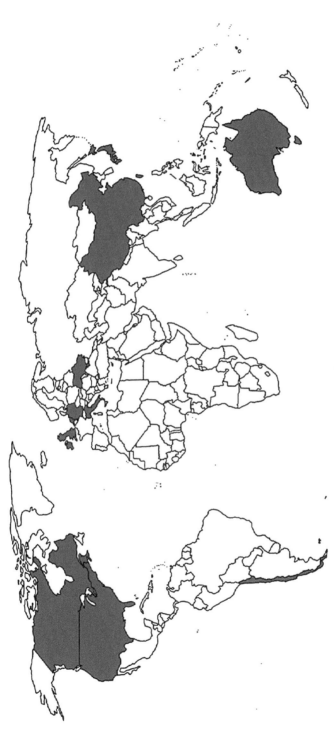

Fig. 1. Geographic distribution of reported cases of GRA. Countries where affected individuals and pedigrees have been reported are shaded in gray.

synthesis depends on 11β-hydroxylase, which hydroxylates 11-deoxycortisol. 11β-hydroxylase and cortisol production are positively regulated by ACTH.[24]

In GRA, chimeric gene duplication results from unequal crossing over between the highly homologous 11β-hydroxylase (CYP11B1) and aldosterone synthase (CYP11B2) genes. The chimera is a gene duplication resulting from the fusion of the 5' ACTH-responsive promoter region of the 11β-hydroxylase gene to the 3' coding sequences of the aldosterone synthase gene (**Fig. 2**). As a consequence, aldosterone is produced ectopically in the *zona fasciculata* and its synthesis is solely under the regulation of ACTH.[25,26]

Biochemically, GRA is a mineralocorticoid excess state; regulation of aldosterone secretion by ACTH, which is not sensitive to sodium homeostasis, leads to hyperaldosteronism and volume expansion. As a result, the RAS is suppressed and the normal regulation of aldosterone by angiotensin II (AII) is not seen. For example, aldosterone secretion does not increase following upright posture[27] or AII infusion.[17] Additionally, the normal potassium-induced rise in aldosterone is absent in GRA.[23] On the other hand, aldosterone regulation by ACTH results in a circadian pattern of aldosterone production that parallels that of cortisol.[14]

GRA is also characterized biochemically by the production of large quantities of the products of the cortisol C-18 oxidation pathway, 18-oxocortisol (18-oxo-F), and 18-hydroxycortisol (18-OH-F).[28–30] Elevated 24-hour urinary and plasma levels of these compounds have high sensitivity and specificity for the diagnosis of GRA.[18,29] Patients with aldosterone-producing adenomas also demonstrate modest overproduction of 18-oxo-F and 18-OH-F, but in GRA the levels are markedly increased.[28,31]

Suppressing ACTH with exogenous glucocorticoids leads to profound suppression of aldosterone levels in GRA and to the reversal of the clinical and biochemical features of hyperaldosteronism.[1,18] Chronic exogenous glucocorticoid therapy also restores aldosterone responsiveness to AII and leads to reactivation of the previously suppressed RAS and ZG.[25]

GENETICS

GRA is inherited as an autosomal dominant trait. In 1992, Lifton and his colleagues[26] first described a large GRA pedigree in which the disease cosegregated with a chimeric gene duplication resulting from an unequal crossing over between the highly homologous 11β-hydroxylase (CYP11B1) and aldosterone synthase (CYP11B2) genes, both located on chromosome 8 in close proximity to one another. In multiple GRA pedigrees, all subjects have proved to have chimeric gene duplications.[3,4,8,14,32] As a consequence of the duplication, aldosterone production occurs ectopically in the *zona fasciculata* and is solely and abnormally regulated by ACTH rather than AII (which is suppressed).[3,26] Subjects with GRA have 2 normal copies of CYP11B1 and CYP11B2 in addition to the chimeric duplication (see **Fig. 2**).

Sequence analysis of DNA from unrelated pedigrees suggests that the crossing over and fusion sites are variable.[3] The variability of the crossover site implies that these mutations did not originate from a single ancestor but rather arose independently in each pedigree.[33] However, in all cases fusion occurs upstream of exon 5 of the aldosterone synthase gene,[3,4] which suggests that exon 5 encodes a region that is essential for aldosterone synthase function. This finding is supported by in vitro experiments demonstrating in chimeric gene constructs that if the fusion occurs downstream of exon 5, aldosterone synthase activity is undetectable.[4]

When inheritance of the chimeric gene is through maternal transmission (vs paternal transmission), affected individuals have significantly higher mean arterial pressure and

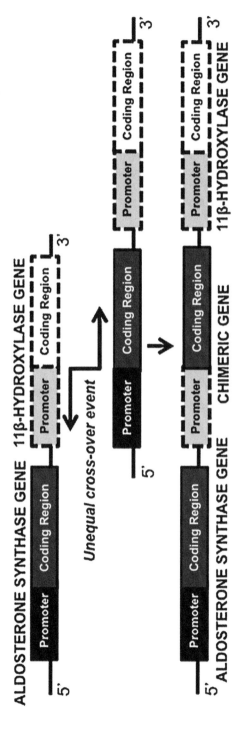

Fig. 2. Chimeric gene formation in GRA results from an unequal crossover event. The 5′ ACTH-responsive promoter region of the 11β-Hydroxylase gene is fused to the 3′ coding sequence of the aldosterone synthase gene. As a result, aldosterone synthesis is abnormally regulated by ACTH rather than by the renin-angiotensin system.

plasma aldosterone concentrations (PAC).[34] Although conclusive evidence is lacking, it has been speculated that in utero exposure to excess mineralocorticoids could alter the programming of blood pressure regulatory mechanisms, such as the expression of genes that regulate aldosterone synthesis.[34]

DIAGNOSIS

Studies of children and adolescents with GRA suggest that severe hypertension with a positive family history of early onset hypertension or hemorrhagic stroke warrant a high index of suspicion for this disorder.[16] The Endocrine Society clinical practice guidelines for the detection, diagnosis, and treatment of patients with PA therefore recommend screening for GRA in patients with confirmed PA who had onset of hypertension at earlier than 20 years of age, or who have a family history of PA or of strokes at less than 40 years of age.[7] All first-degree relatives of patients who have been diagnosed with GRA should be screened.

Establishment of the diagnosis is best accomplished by genetic testing for the presence of the chimeric gene in peripheral blood DNA. A Southern blot technique was initially described by Lifton and colleagues,[3] but a faster polymerase chain reaction-based method has been subsequently developed.[32] Genetic testing is highly sensitive and specific for GRA.

If access to genetic testing is not available, biochemical alternatives include demonstration of profound suppression of PAC (<4 ng/dL) after treatment with 4 days of dexamethasone (at a dosage of 0.5 mg every 6 hours).[23,35,36] Biochemical testing can also be performed by measurement of urinary 18-oxo-F and 18-OH-F as previously described. These biochemical screening methods were used for disease detection before the development of genetic testing and have high sensitivity and specificity.[30,31,36] However, glucocorticoid suppression of aldosterone has more recently been reported to be a misleading diagnostic strategy, as some patients with PA but without the chimeric gene also demonstrated suppression of PAC with dexamethasone treatment.[37]

TREATMENT

In patients with GRA, hypertension is often severe and difficult to control with standard antihypertensive therapies. Particular caution must be taken with the use of potassium-wasting diuretics, as these can induce hypokalemia in affected individuals.[18] Exogenous glucocorticoid administration, which suppresses pituitary ACTH secretion, can improve or normalize blood pressure, and is considered the first-line treatment for GRA.[7]

An exogenous glucocorticoid with a long biologic half-life, such as dexamethasone or prednisone, is most effective at maintaining prolonged ACTH suppression. Dosing should be at nighttime to suppress the physiologic early morning ACTH peak.[7] In adults, the recommended starting doses of dexamethasone and prednisone are 0.125 to 0.25 mg and 2.5 to 5.0 mg daily, respectively.[7] Dosing should take into consideration the body surface area and body mass index of treated patients.

The goal of treatment in GRA is to normalize blood pressure as well as serum potassium if hypokalemia is present. The lowest possible dose of glucocorticoid that achieves these therapeutic goals should be used, and overtreatment should be carefully avoided given the adverse consequences of iatrogenic Cushing's syndrome. Measurement of plasma renin activity and PAC may help the clinician determine the effectiveness of treatment and avoid overtreatment. Of note, biochemical markers of hyperaldosteronism, such as urinary 18-oxosteroid and even PAC, may remain elevated despite achieving normotension.[38]

Partial suppression of ACTH with synthetic glucocorticoid does not always normalize blood pressure, which may be a result of end-organ damage from long-standing, poorly controlled hypertension or of the presence of concomitant essential hypertension. In such cases, the addition of a mineralocorticoid receptor (MR) antagonist should be considered. The 2 currently available MR antagonists are spironolactone and eplerenone. Although spironolactone is the least expensive, it has antiandrogenic effects that usually lead to gynecomastia and erectile dysfunction in men; antiprogesterone actions may result in menstrual irregularities in women. Eplerenone is a second-generation option with greater MR specificity and therefore fewer side effects. Treatment alternatives also include amiloride or triamterene, which inhibit sodium reabsorption by the aldosterone-regulated epithelial sodium channel in the distal nephron; both have been used successfully for management of GRA, but usually in conjunction with other antihypertensive agents.

In children with GRA, impaired linear growth as a result of mild steroid overtreatment has been reported.[16] There are also concerns about the antiandrogenic effects of spironolactone during pubertal development, especially in boys. Therefore, eplerenone may be the preferred first line of treatment in GRA-affected children,[7] but cost of this agent is a limiting factor. Treatment targets for blood pressure in children should be determined from age and gender-specific normative data.[16]

To minimize potassium wasting and help lower blood pressure, all patients with GRA should also follow a sodium-restricted diet of less than 2 g/day.[19]

SUMMARY

GRA is a hereditary form of primary hyperaldosteronism in which the presence of a chimeric gene duplication results in the sole and abnormal regulation of aldosterone by ACTH. Severe hypertension with a family history of early onset hypertension or hemorrhagic stroke should raise suspicion for the presence of the disorder. Elucidation of the genetic basis for GRA has led to the development of genetic testing, which has facilitated early detection as well as the use of directed antihypertensive therapies with glucocorticoids or mineralocorticoid receptor antagonists.

REFERENCES

1. Sutherland DJ, Ruse JL, Laidlaw JC. Hypertension, increased aldosterone secretion and low plasma renin activity relieved by dexamethasone. Can Med Assoc J 1966;95(22):1109–19.
2. Mulatero P, di Cella SM, Williams TA, et al. Glucocorticoid-remediable aldosteronism: low morbidity and mortality in a four-generation Italian pedigree. J Clin Endocrinol Metab 2002;87(7):3187–91.
3. Lifton RP, Dluhy RG, Powers M, et al. Hereditary hypertension caused by chimaeric gene duplications and ectopic expression of aldosterone synthase. Nat Genet 1992;2(1):66–74.
4. Pascoe L, Curnow KM, Slutsker L, et al. Glucocorticoid-suppressible hyperaldosteronism results from hybrid genes created by unequal crossovers between CYP11B1 and CYP11B2. Proc Natl Acad Sci U S A 1992;89(17):8327–31.
5. Lifton RP, Dluhy RG, Powers M, et al. The molecular basis of glucocorticoid-remediable aldosteronism, a mendelian cause of human hypertension. Trans Assoc Am Physicians 1992;105:64–71.

6. Jackson RV, Lafferty A, Torpy DJ, et al. New genetic insights in familial hyperaldosteronism. Ann N Y Acad Sci 2002;970:77–88.

7. Funder JW, Carey RM, Fardella C, et al. Case detection, diagnosis, and treatment of patients with primary aldosteronism: an endocrine society clinical practice guideline. J Clin Endocrinol Metab 2008;93(9):3266–81.

8. Vonend O, Altenhenne C, Buchner NJ, et al. A German family with glucocorticoid-remediable aldosteronism. Nephrol Dial Transplant 2007;22(4):1123–30.

9. Jamieson A, Slutsker L, Inglis G, et al. Clinical, biochemical and genetic features of five extended kindred's with glucocorticoid-suppressible hyperaldosteronism. Endocr Res 1995;21(1–2):463–9.

10. O'Mahony S, Burns A, Murnaghan DJ. Dexamethasone-suppressible hyperaldosteronism: a large new kindred. J Hum Hypertens 1989;3(4):255–8.

11. Fallo F, Pilon C, Williams TA, et al. Coexistence of different phenotypes in a family with glucocorticoid-remediable aldosteronism. J Hum Hypertens 2004;18(1):47–51.

12. Ding W, Liu L, Hu R, et al. Clinical and gene mutation studies on a Chinese pedigree with glucocorticoid-remediable aldosteronism. Chin Med J (Engl) 2002;115(7):979–82.

13. Hsieh CJ, Wang PW, Liu JC, et al. Glucocorticoid-remediable aldosteronism: a case report. Changgeng Yi Xue Za Zhi 1997;20(1):52–7.

14. Yokota K, Ogura T, Kishida M, et al. Japanese family with glucocorticoid-remediable aldosteronism diagnosed by long-polymerase chain reaction. Hypertens Res 2001;24(5):589–94.

15. Carvajal CA, Stehr CB, Gonzalez PA, et al. A de novo unequal cross-over mutation between CYP11B1 and CYP11B2 genes causes Familial Hyperaldosteronism type I. J Endocrinol Invest 2010. [Epub ahead of print].

16. Dluhy RG, Anderson B, Harlin B, et al. Glucocorticoid-remediable aldosteronism is associated with severe hypertension in early childhood. J Pediatr 2001;138(5):715–20.

17. Stowasser M, Bachmann AW, Huggard PR, et al. Severity of hypertension in familial hyperaldosteronism type I: relationship to gender and degree of biochemical disturbance. J Clin Endocrinol Metab 2000;85(6):2160–6.

18. Rich GM, Ulick S, Cook S, et al. Glucocorticoid-remediable aldosteronism in a large kindred: clinical spectrum and diagnosis using a characteristic biochemical phenotype. Ann Intern Med 1992;116(10):813–20.

19. Dluhy RG. Glucocorticoid-remediable aldosteronism. J Clin Endocrinol Metab 1999;84(12):4341–4.

20. Stowasser M, Sharman J, Leano R, et al. Evidence for abnormal left ventricular structure and function in normotensive individuals with familial hyperaldosteronism type I. J Clin Endocrinol Metab 2005;90(9):5070–6.

21. Joffe HV, Adler GK. Effect of aldosterone and mineralocorticoid receptor blockade on vascular inflammation. Heart Fail Rev 2005;10(1):31–7.

22. Litchfield WR, Anderson BF, Weiss RJ, et al. Intracranial aneurysm and hemorrhagic stroke in glucocorticoid-remediable aldosteronism. Hypertension 1998;31(1 Pt 2):445–50.

23. Litchfield WR, Coolidge C, Silva P, et al. Impaired potassium-stimulated aldosterone production: a possible explanation for normokalemic glucocorticoid-remediable aldosteronism. J Clin Endocrinol Metab 1997;82(5):1507–10.

24. Simpson ER, Waterman MR. Regulation of the synthesis of steroidogenic enzymes in adrenal cortical cells by ACTH. Annu Rev Physiol 1988;50:427–40.

25. Dluhy RG, Lifton RP. Glucocorticoid-remediable aldosteronism (GRA): diagnosis, variability of phenotype and regulation of potassium homeostasis. Steroids 1995; 60(1):48–51.
26. Lifton RP, Dluhy RG, Powers M, et al. A chimaeric 11 beta-hydroxylase/ aldosterone synthase gene causes glucocorticoid-remediable aldosteronism and human hypertension. Nature 1992;355(6357):262–5.
27. Ganguly A, Grim CE, Weinberger MH. Anomalous postural aldosterone response in glucocorticoid-suppressible hyperaldosteronism. N Engl J Med 1981;305(17): 991–3.
28. Ulick S, Chan CK, Gill JR. Defective fasciculata zone function as the mechanism of glucocorticoid-remediable aldosteronism. J Clin Endocrinol Metab 1990;71(5): 1151–7.
29. Mosso L, Gomez-Sanchez CE, Foecking MF, et al. Serum 18-hydroxycortisol in primary aldosteronism, hypertension, and normotensives. Hypertension 2001; 38(3 Pt 2):688–91.
30. Gomez-Sanchez CE, Montgomery M, Ganguly A, et al. Elevated urinary excretion of 18-oxocortisol in glucocorticoid-suppressible aldosteronism. J Clin Endocrinol Metab 1984;59(5):1022–4.
31. Ulick S, Blumenfeld JD, Atlas SA, et al. The unique steroidogenesis of the aldos-teronoma in the differential diagnosis of primary aldosteronism. J Clin Endocrinol Metab 1993;76(4):873–8.
32. Jonsson JR, Klemm SA, Tunny TJ, et al. A new genetic test for familial hyperal-dosteronism type I aids in the detection of curable hypertension. Biochem Bio-phys Res Commun 1995;207(2):565–71.
33. Dluhy RG, Williams GH. Glucocorticoid-remediable aldosteronism. Cardiovasc Res 1996;31(6):870–2.
34. Jamieson A, Slutsker L, Inglis GC, et al. Glucocorticoid-suppressible hyperaldos-teronism: effects of crossover site and parental origin of chimaeric gene on phenotypic expression. Clin Sci (Lond) 1995;88(5):563–70.
35. Mulatero P, Veglio F, Pilon C, et al. Diagnosis of glucocorticoid-remediable aldo-steronism in primary aldosteronism: aldosterone response to dexamethasone and long polymerase chain reaction for chimeric gene. J Clin Endocrinol Metab 1998;83(7):2573–5.
36. Stowasser M, Bachmann AW, Jonsson JR, et al. Clinical, biochemical and genetic approaches to the detection of familial hyperaldosteronism type I. J Hypertens 1995;13(12 Pt 2):1610–3.
37. Fardella CE. Genetic study of patients with dexamethasone-suppressible aldo-steronism without the chimeric CYP11B1/CYP11B2 gene. J Clin Endocrinol Metab 2001;86(10):4805–7.
38. Stowasser M, Bachmann AW, Huggard PR, et al. Treatment of familial hyperal-dosteronism type I: only partial suppression of adrenocorticotropin required to correct hypertension. J Clin Endocrinol Metab 2000;85(9):3313–8.

Familial or Genetic Primary Aldosteronism and Gordon Syndrome

Michael Stowasser, MBBS, FRACP, PhD[a,b,]*,
Eduardo Pimenta, MD, FAHA[a,b],
Richard D. Gordon, MD, PhD, FRACP, FRCP[a,b]

KEYWORDS

- Familial • Primary aldosteronism
- Familial hyperaldosteronism type II
- Familial hypertension and hyperkalemia • Genetics
- Gordon syndrome • Pseudohypoaldosteronism type II

Salt-sensitive forms of hypertension have received considerable renewed attention in recent years. Reasons for this include (1) the new awareness that certain varieties (and in particular, the various forms of primary aldosteronism [PA]) are more common than previously realized, (2) the fact that most hypertensive conditions for which underlying genetic mutations have been discovered have been salt-sensitive varieties, (3) the development of animal models of salt-sensitive hypertension and PA, and (4) new insights into regulation of salt status (including the discovery of new molecular pathways) and pathogenesis of salt-sensitive hypertension that have evolved from the discovery of these clinical mutations and development of these animal models.

This article focuses on 2 main forms of salt-sensitive hypertension (familial or genetic PA and Gordon syndrome) and the current state of knowledge regarding their genetic bases. The glucocorticoid-remediable form of familial PA (familial hyperaldosteronism type I [FH-I]) is dealt with only briefly here because it is covered in depth by Robert Dluhy elsewhere in this issue.

This work was supported by the National Health & Medical Research Council of Australia, the National Heart Foundation of Australia and the Irene Hunt Hypertension Research Trust, University of Queensland.
The authors have nothing to disclose.
[a] Endocrine Hypertension Research Center, University of Queensland School of Medicine, Princess Alexandra Hospital, Ipswich Road, Woolloongabba, Brisbane 4102, Australia
[b] Endocrine Hypertension Research Center, University of Queensland School of Medicine, Greenslopes Private Hospital, Newdegate Street, Greenslopes, Brisbane 4102, Australia
* Corresponding author. Hypertension Unit, University of Queensland School of Medicine, Princess Alexandra Hospital, Ipswich Road, Woolloongabba, Brisbane 4102, Australia.
E-mail address: m.stowasser@uq.edu.au

Endocrinol Metab Clin N Am 40 (2011) 343–368
doi:10.1016/j.ecl.2011.01.007
0889-8529/11/$ – see front matter © 2011 Elsevier Inc. All rights reserved.

endo.theclinics.com

PA

In PA, autonomous overproduction of the salt-retaining mineralocorticoid hormone aldosterone by the adrenal cortex leads to suppressed levels of its normal chronic regulator, plasma renin activity (PRA), and angiotensin II (AII).[1] Aldosterone production in excess of normal requirements and not able to be completely suppressed by salt loading results in salt and water retention, which causes hypertension to slowly develop, and urinary potassium wasting, which eventually leads to hypokalemia.[1] Although it was previously believed to be rare, recent evidence has indicated that 5% to 15% of hypertension may be caused by PA, and that most patients are normo-kalemic at presentation.[2–8] This finding has led to the realization that screening approaches relying on the presence of hypokalemia miss most patients with PA. Based on this new understanding, an Endocrine Society clinical guideline on case detection, diagnosis, and management of PA recommended screening for PA amongst all but the mildest hypertensive individuals by measurement of the plasma aldosterone/renin ratio (ARR).[9]

Diagnosis of PA has a major clinical effect on patients found to have this condition.[10] For the 30% to 35% of patients with PA who are found to have unilateral forms, unilateral laparoscopic adrenalectomy leads to cure of hypertension in 50% to 80% (with the remainder improved)[11–14] and a significantly improved quality of life.[14] In the 65% to 70% who have bilateral forms, hypertension usually responds well to medical treatment with aldosterone antagonists (spironolactone, eplerenone, or amiloride)[15] and, in occasional highly selected patients offered surgery because of failure to respond to or tolerate medications, may improve after unilateral adrenalec-tomy (although less predictably than with unilateral PA).[16] There is now abundant evidence to suggest that aldosterone excess in PA leads to adverse cardiovascular and renal outcomes that are independent of its effects on blood pressure (BP).[17–21] Importantly from a management perspective, treatment specifically directed against aldosterone excess protects against the development of these complications more effectively than nonspecific antihypertensive medications,[22] further emphasizing the importance of detection of patients with PA who may then benefit from such directed management.

EVIDENCE FOR A GENETIC BASIS FOR PA

With the exception of FH-I and possibly FH-III (see later discussion and elsewhere in this issue), the cause of PA is unknown. However, several lines of evidence suggest that genetic factors are likely to be involved at least in some, and possibly most, indi-viduals with this condition. First and perhaps the most important of these is the description of (so far) 3 familial varieties (**Table 1**), each of which has shown an autosomal-dominant pattern of inheritance.

Second, in most cases of aldosterone-producing adenoma (APA), histopathologic examination of the remaining gland has revealed diffuse and/or nodular cortical hyperplasia,[23] consistent with an inherent (probably genetic) tendency to hyper-plasia/neoplasia of the entire adrenal cortex. The fact that most cases of PA are bilateral[6] is in keeping with this concept. Such a tendency to diffuse or nodular over-growth is seen in the parathyroid and pancreas in multiple endocrine neoplasia type I (MEN I), which is caused by well-defined genetic mutations of the MEN1 gene encod-ing the tumor suppressing protein menin.[24] PA has been reported to occur in associ-ation with MEN I.[25]

Fourth, recent evidence from the Framingham Offspring Study[26] has provided further support for the importance of aldosterone in the development of hypertension

Table 1
Clinical, biochemical, morphologic, and genetic features of FH types I, II, and III

	FH-I	FH-II	FH-III
Prevalence	Rare (<1% PA)	Unknown (at least 5 times more common than FH-I)	Very rare (only 1 family described)
Mode of inheritance	Autosomal dominant	Autosomal dominant; other modes also possible in some families	Autosomal dominant
Male/female ratio	Approximately 1:1	Approximately 1:1	1:2
Age of onset of HT	Childhood to early adulthood	Usually adulthood	Childhood
Severity of HT	Normotensive to severely hypertensive (causing early death from stroke)	Normotensive to severely hypertensive	Severely hypertensive
% hypokalemic	Approximately 25%	Approximately 25%	100%
Aldosterone response to dexamethasone	Marked, sustained suppression	Minimal	Increase
Hybrid steroid levels (18-hydroxycortisol and 18-oxocortisol)	Increased	Increased (in patients with AII-unresponsive APA) or normal	Markedly increased
Adrenal morphology	Diffuse hyperplasia; occasional nodules	Diffuse or nodular hyperplasia; adenoma	Massive bilateral diffuse and/or nodular hyperplasia
Laterality of adrenal aldosterone production	Bilateral	Unilateral (approximately 30%) or bilateral (70%)	Presumably bilateral
Treatment	Glucocorticoids or medications antagonizing aldosterone action	Unilateral adrenalectomy or medications antagonizing aldosterone action	Bilateral adrenalectomy

Abbreviation: HT, hypertension.

and for the hypothesis that genetic factors are involved. After initially describing significant relationships of aldosterone levels with BP progression and hypertension development among Framingham study participants, these investigators found similar correlations using the ARR,[27] thus adding considerable extra weight to the argument that disturbed aldosterone production, relatively autonomous of its normal chronic regulator (renin-AII), plays a greater role in the development of human hypertension than has been traditionally recognized. The investigators were also able to show significant heritability of the ARR ($h = 0.34$). In a linkage analysis that included 1225 genotyped individuals from 328 families, the most striking locus of linkage for logARR in a model that adjusted for multiple variables (but not for medications) was at chromosome 7p21-22, where the multipoint logarithm of odds (LOD) score was

2.78. As described later, this is the same locus that had previously been reported to show linkage with the second-described familial variety of PA (familial hyperaldosteronism type II [FH-II]). The LOD score fell substantially (to 1.14) after adjusting for angiotensin-converting enzyme (ACE) inhibitor and β-adrenoceptor blocker and was markedly attenuated (to 0.43) when patients taking ACE inhibitors were excluded from the analysis.[27] Nevertheless, the coincidence of these findings with those in FH-II is surprising, and the possibility that the 7p21-22 locus harbors genetic variants predisposing to autonomous aldosterone production and development of hypertension (including, but not limited to FH-II) warrants further exploration.

Fifth, several transgenic and knockout animal models of PA have recently been developed (see later discussion), providing proof of concept that genetic bases (other than that already described for FH-I) could underlie human forms.

FH-I

First described in 1966,[28] FH-I can result in hypertension so severe as to cause early death (usually from hemorrhagic hypertensive stroke), yet is reversible by the administration of glucocorticoids in small doses that partially suppress adrenocorticotrophic hormone (ACTH) without producing steroid side effects.[29,30] Lifton and colleagues[31] showed that patients with FH-I inherit, in addition to the 2 wild-type aldosterone synthase (AS) genes, a hybrid gene in which the regulatory sequences are derived from the 11β-hydroxylase gene (CYP11B1, which is normally regulated by ACTH), whereas most of the coding sequences are from AS (CYP11B2, normally regulated primarily by AII). As a result, expression of the hybrid gene is regulated by ACTH and leads to the synthesis of aldosterone, and therefore aldosterone production in FH-I is also regulated by ACTH rather than by AII (thereby explaining the therapeutic suppressive effect of glucocorticoids).

Unlike wild-type CYP11B2, which is expressed only in zona glomerulosa, the hybrid gene is expressed throughout all layers of the adrenal cortex (by virtue of its CYP11B1 regulatory sequences), including zona fasciculata, where cortisol is available as a substrate for the 18-hydroxylase and 18-oxidase activities of its gene product.[32,33] This characteristic results in excessive formation of so-called hybrid steroids, 18-hydroxycortisol and 18-oxocortisol, urinary levels of which are consistently high in patients with FH-I.[34] For unexplained reasons, high levels are also usually found in patients with the classic, AII-unresponsive variety of APA but not usually in those with AII-responsive APA or bilateral adrenal hyperplasia (BAH).[35]

As in other varieties of PA, most patients with FH-I are normokalemic[36,37] and hence masquerade as having essential hypertension. Patients may even be normotensive[36-39] and hence escape detection (although passing on the gene) if only hypertensive relatives of affected patients are screened. Even screening by ARR testing can occasionally yield normal results. On the other hand, genetic testing for the presence of the hybrid gene, either by Southern blotting[31] or by a faster, polymerase chain reaction (PCR)-based method,[40] reliably permits early detection of FH-I, even at birth. Thus the identification of the hybrid gene has not only advanced our understanding of molecular control of aldosterone secretion and BP but has also led to the development of greatly improved methods of detection of this familial variety of PA, supplanting the more cumbersome and less reliable dexamethasone suppression test (in which marked, persistent suppression of aldosterone during several days of dexamethasone administration confirmed FH-I), and permitting identification at earlier, even normotensive stages of the disease process.[41] Low-dose glucocorticoids, amiloride, or aldosterone receptor antagonists are effective as long-term treatment.

In studies of normotensive individuals with FH-I and age-matched and sex-matched controls, individuals with FH-I showed echocardiographic evidence of abnormal left ventricular structure and function[42] and increased levels of the inflammatory marker interleukin 6[43] even in the absence of hypertension, consistent with aldosterone excess causing cardiovascular inflammation and remodeling independently of its effects on BP. This finding raises the question as to whether patients with FH-I, and perhaps other forms of PA, should be considered for specific treatment even before hypertension develops, and whether treatment in hypertensive individuals should go beyond just normalizing BP and aim instead to more completely reverse aldosterone excess or block its action.

FH-II

A second familial variety of PA, in which aldosterone is not glucocorticoid suppressible, was first described by the Greenslopes Hospital Hypertension Unit (GHHU) in Brisbane, Australia in 1991,[44] and additional families were subsequently also reported from other countries.[45,46] This condition was labeled FH-II[47] to distinguish it from the glucocorticoid-suppressible FH-I. The GHHU and its sister unit, the Princess Alexandra Hospital Hypertension Unit (PAHHU) (also in Brisbane), are now following 42 Australian families (104 patients) with FH-II and have found this condition to be at least 5 times more common than FH-I.[48–50] Mode of transmission of phenotype has followed a dominant pattern in 16 families but remains less certain in the other 26. In each family, PA was confirmed by fludrocortisone suppression testing (FST), and the absence of the hybrid gene (confirmed by genetic testing) and failure of dexamethasone to suppress aldosterone (where performed) excluded FH-I.

These patients have shown substantial diversity in phenotypic expression.[48,49] Among the 104 patients identified so far by our Brisbane group, ages at presentation ranged from 14 to 78 years, 54 (52%) were female, and 26 (25%) were hypokalemic. Twenty-nine (28%) have undergone unilateral adrenalectomy. Of these, 25 had unilateral PA confirmed by preoperative adrenal venous sampling (AVS) and/or postoperative cure of hypertension and biochemical PA, 1 almost lateralized on AVS but with incomplete contralateral suppression, and 3 had bilateral PA but were unable to tolerate aldosterone antagonist treatment in the doses required to control hypertension. Two (2%) other patients have undergone bilateral adrenalectomy, 1 for bilateral giant macronodular hyperplasia causing autonomous adrenal aldosterone and cortisol production, and the other for PA caused by non-giant bilateral nodular hyperplasia. The remaining 73 (70%) patients, in whom hypertension has been treated medically with agents that block aldosterone action, comprise 56 with bilateral PA confirmed by AVS, 1 with unilateral PA who opted for medical treatment, and 18 in whom AVS either has not yet been performed (n = 12) or who gave inconclusive results (n = 6).

Clinical, biochemical, and morphologic characteristics of patients with FH-II do not differ significantly from those with apparently nonfamilial PA.[2,48,49] It is therefore possible that mutations underlying FH-II may be common among the broader PA population.

Unlike in FH-I, the genetic defect(s) underlying FH-II have not yet been elucidated. Identification of such defects would further understanding of the pathogenesis of FH-II, as has occurred in the case of FH-I since elucidation of the hybrid gene defect,[31] and has important implications for patient management. As in apparently nonfamilial PA, detection of FH-II currently involves biochemical screening by ARR testing and confirmation of PA by FST. As has already been observed in FH-I, elucidation of mutations causing FH-II may lead to the development of new genetic screening tests that could greatly simplify diagnosis, prove to be more sensitive and specific than biochemical testing, and thereby facilitate earlier and more frequent detection.

CANDIDATE GENE STUDIES IN FH-II

The search for genetic abnormalities causing FH-II has involved both candidate gene and genome-wide search approaches. We have excluded the hybrid gene mutation responsible for FH-I in all of our patients with FH-II.[48,49] Sequencing studies performed within Yutaka Shizuta's laboratory in Kochi, Japan on peripheral blood leukocyte (PBL) DNA from 1 of our Australian patients with FH-II did not reveal mutations in the coding region of CYP11B2 (Shizuta Y, personal communication, 1992).

It is possible in vitro to introduce point mutations into CYP11B1 that confer AS activity to its gene product.[51] Theoretically, such mutations might be expected to result in ACTH-regulated aldosterone overproduction (as in FH-I), but escape detection by methods currently used to detect the hybrid CYP11B1/CYP11B2 gene. However, Fallo and colleagues[46] found no evidence of such mutations in PBL DNA from patients with FH-II or in DNA extracted from 10 APAs from patients with apparently sporadic PA whose aldosterone levels decreased by at least 50% in response to dexamethasone[52] and more recently in PBL DNA from 10 Australian patients (4 families) with FH-II from the GHHU/PAHHU series (Fallo F, unpublished observations, 2006). This group also sought, but did not find, either the −344T or the intron conversion alleles of CYP11B2 (which have been implicated in PA) to be present in any of their 4 patients with FH-II.[46]

PCR single-strand conformation polymorphism analysis of the p53 tumor suppressor gene revealed no evidence of mutations in either PBL or tumor DNA from 24 patients with aldosterone-producing tumors (7 of whom had FH-II) or in PBL from an additional 7 with FH-II.[53]

LINKAGE ANALYSIS STUDIES IN FH-II

Linkage studies performed in collaboration with Stratakis and colleagues (National Institutes of Health, Bethesda, MD, USA), involving 1 large, informative family from the GHHU series revealed no evidence of cosegregation of phenotype with polymorphisms within either the CYP11B2, the AT1, or MEN1 loci.[54,55] However, a genome-wide search in this family showed linkage between FH-II and a locus at chromosome 7p22 with a maximum paired LOD score of 3.26.[56] Subsequent work involving a second Australian family and a South American family identified by Dr Maria New (New York Presbyterian Hospital) increased the multipoint LOD score for the locus to 4.61.[57] Recombination events in our largest Australian family of 8 affected individuals narrowed the locus by 1.8 Mbp, allowing the exclusion of almost half the candidate genes in the original locus.[57] Linkage to 7p22 has also been recently verified in 2 Italian families with FH-II identified by Dr Paolo Mulatero (University of Torino). The combined multipoint LOD score for the 5 families that are informative for the 7p22 locus (2 Australian, 1 South American, and 2 Italian) seems to have put the LOD score beyond reasonable doubt at 5.22.[58]

Although Fallo and colleagues[59] were unable to show loss of heterozygosity (LOH) at the 7p22 locus in APAs removed from patients with FH-II, this would not exclude causative mutations unable to be detected by the LOH approach.

SEQUENCING AT CHROMOSOME 7p22 IN FH-II

There are approximately 50 genes residing within the linked 7p22 locus. Initial sequencing efforts were directed toward the more likely candidates among these genes including *PRKAR1B*,[60] *RBaK*,[61,62] *PMS2*,[61] and *GNA12*,[61] and more recently *ZNF12*, *RPA3*, and *GLCCI* (Sukor N, unpublished data, 2009). All 7 genes were relevant because they are involved either in cell cycle control or steroid action, and adrenal cortical hyperplasia and neoplasia and abnormal steroid regulation are characteristic features of FH-II. In each case, gDNA from 2 affected and 2 unaffected individuals from our largest 7p22-linked family with FH-II was used to sequence the gene followed by further genotyping of interesting single-nucleotide polymorphisms in additional affected and unaffected individuals from families with FH-II, as well as unrelated normotensive controls. However, no mutations likely to be causative for FH-II were identified by this approach.[60–62] Intensive examination of this region using more streamlined methodology is under way.

GENETIC HETEROGENEITY IN FH-II

For 2 additional Australian families with FH-II, linkage at the 7p22 region could not be shown.[57] Hence FH-II, and PA in general, is likely to be genetically heterogeneous. This finding is not surprising given the high degree of clinical and biochemical phenotypic diversity observed in FH-II and other forms of PA. Genetic heterogeneity has been reported in other inherited forms of hypertension such as Liddle syndrome[63] and Gordon syndrome.[64]

FAMILIAL HYPERALDOSTERONISM TYPE III

In 2008, Geller and colleagues[65] described a father and 2 daughters with severe, childhood-onset hypertension, hyperaldosteronism (with increased urinary or serum aldosterone levels), markedly suppressed PRA, and severe hypokalemia. Measurement of serum and urinary hybrid steroids (18-hydroxycortisol and 18-oxocortisol) in the daughters yielded markedly increased levels that were considerably higher than those usually encountered in FH-I or AII-unresponsive APA. Unlike in FH-I, genetic testing for the hybrid gene was negative, and BP and serum aldosterone levels progressively increased (rather than decreased) in response to dexamethasone administration. The persistence of cortisol secretion during dexamethasone treatment, and the suppression of basal levels of ACTH, suggested that dysregulation of adrenal steroid biosynthesis was not confined to aldosterone in these patients.

In all 3 individuals, hypertension and hypokalemia responded poorly to aldosterone antagonist agents, but were corrected by bilateral adrenalectomy. Histopathologic examination revealed markedly enlarged adrenals, accounted for by diffuse and/or nodular hyperplasia of zona fasciculata.[65]

The investigators seem to have excluded mutations in *CYP11B1* or *CYP11B2* as being causative, and did not find mutations in coding regions of several other candidates, including the AII and ACTH receptors.

Very recently, Choi and co-workers reported the affected (but not the unaffected) members of this pedigree to harbor a mutation in the potassium channel *KCNJ5*.[66] When this mutation was expressed in a cell line, it resulted in increased sodium conductance and cell depolarization, which in adrenal glomerulosa cells results in calcium entry, the principal signal for aldosterone production. The authors also proposed that chronic increased calcium entry might also be the stimulus for the marked adrenocortical hyperplasia seen in these individuals, but evidence supporting this hypothesis is less convincing.

The investigators seem to have described a new familial form of hyperaldosteronism, which has prompted introduction of the term familial hyperaldosteronism type III.[67,68] Absence of the hybrid gene mutation and of suppressibility of aldosterone by dexamethasone distinguishes it from FH-I. The very early age of onset, markedly increased hybrid steroid levels, and lack of efficacy of aldosterone antagonist agents are not typical for FH-II. Failure of cortisol to suppress with dexamethasone and the presence of marked bilateral cortical hyperplasia are not characteristic of either FH-I or FH-II, although we have previously described a 46-year-old man with FH-II, giant macronodular hyperplasia affecting both adrenals, and autonomous adrenal overproduction of both aldosterone and cortisol.[69] Although a few other cases sharing some (but not all) features with members of this family have been reported,[70,71] this condition seems to be rare.

GENETIC STUDIES IN APPARENTLY NONFAMILIAL PA

Studies aimed at shedding light on the molecular basis of PA in patients without known affected family members have used a variety of approaches. The roles of various candidate genes have been examined by way of direct sequencing, association studies, and examination of tissue expression in removed adrenal tissues.

Davies and colleagues[72] reported associations of hypertension with 2 polymorphisms at the CYP11B2 locus, a C-344T transition within the promoter region and an intron 2 CYP11B2/CYP11B1 gene conversion. The −344T allele was also associated with higher urinary aldosterone excretion rates.[72] These investigators subsequently reported an excess of the −344T allele among hypertensive patients with raised versus those with normal ARRs,[73] and in patients with APA versus normotensive controls.[74] Although several other groups have similarly found evidence of association of these alleles with aldosterone excess,[75,76] others have reported conflicting results.[77,78] Differences in ethnicity may help to explain these discrepant findings, but it has also been postulated that these alleles may be markers of other, more functionally relevant genetic variants with which they are in linkage disequilibrium. As an extension of this hypothesis, Connell and colleagues[79] have proposed that excessive aldosterone production, autonomous of renin-AII, may result from loss-of-function mutations in CYP11B1. According to their hypothesis, these mutations would lead to reduced 11β-hydroxylase activity and therefore reduced cortisol production, resulting in a chronic state of subtle ACTH activation, and in turn to ACTH-induced simulation of aldosterone. Although these investigators were able to report that the −344T allele was associated with impaired adrenal 11β-hydroxylase efficiency,[80] a study of 8 novel CYP11B1 missense mutations found that none accounted for hypertension and/or an increased ARR among a population of 160 subjects.[81]

Carroll and colleagues[82] found no evidence of the hybrid gene mutation within APAs. Takeda and colleagues[83] found no CYP11B2 coding region mutations in PBL DNA from patients with apparently nonfamilial APA or BAH, and Hampf and colleagues[84] found no mutations in the promoter region in patients with apparently nonfamilial BAH. Mutations of AT1 (AII type 1 receptor gene) were sought but not found in patients with apparently nonfamilial APA.[85,86]

LOH at the MEN 1 locus was shown by restriction fragment length polymorphism analysis in 5 of 11 informative aldosterone-producing tumors removed from patients with PA from our series (2 with FH-II),[87] and by microsatellite marker analysis in 7 of

33 tumors[88] (which we later extended to 10 of 62 tumors). Beckers and colleagues[25] reported LOH at the MEN 1 locus in an APA from a patient with MEN 1. However, the true pathogenetic significance of these findings remain unclear.

KCNH2 (or HERG [human-ether-a-go-go-related gene]) encodes HERG protein, the α-subunit (pore-forming region) of a homotetrameric potassium channel.[89] Because potassium is a principal regulator of aldosterone synthesis and KCNH2 is expressed in normal adrenal tissue,[90] Sarzani and colleagues[91] proposed KCNH2 as a candidate for PA. These investigators observed expression of KCNH2 in all of 17 APAs studied, and found the 897T variant of this gene to be significantly more common among patients with APA than in patients with moderate to severe essential hypertension or in normotensive. However, KCNH2 somatic mutations were not detected within APA tissues.[91]

Williams and colleagues[92] recently reported on the use of transcriptional screening, comparing gene expression in APA versus normal adrenal tissue, to identify genes showing differential expression as potential candidates in the pathogenesis of APA. This novel approach led to the identification of several differentially expressed genes, the most conspicuous of which (teratocarcinoma-derived growth factor 1 [TDGF-1]) was upregulated in APA 14-fold by microarray and 21-fold by real-time PCR. Subsequent in vitro transfection studies using an adrenocortical carcinoma cell line (H295R) showed that TDGF-1 mediated an increase in aldosterone secretion by these cells and protected them from apoptosis.[92] A similar approach was used by Giuliani and colleagues[93] to compare expression of urotensin II (a widely expressed vasoactive peptide) and its receptor in APA, pheochromocytoma, and normal adrenal tissues. Although urotensin II was expressed in lower levels in APA than the other tissues, the receptor was markedly overexpressed. The investigators subsequently showed urotensin II infusion to increase zona glomerulosa CYP11B2 expression and plasma aldosterone levels in normotensive rats.[93] Although the clinical relevance of these findings has yet to be ascertained, this new approach is showing promising potential toward the elucidation of the molecular bases and pathways involved in the development of APA and possibly other forms of PA.

Even more recently, Choi and colleagues, using high-throughput whole exomic sequencing techniques on paired tumor and peripheral blood DNA samples, were able to demonstrate somatic mutations in the potassium channel gene, KCNJ5, in 8 of 22 APAs.[66] As described above, they subsequently showed a germline mutation in the same gene to be present in affected members of a family with FH-III. Confirmation of these results in other APA series is awaited with interest.

GENETIC ANIMAL MODELS OF PA

Recently reported genetically modified animal models of PA have provided molecular hints about potential mechanisms of autonomous aldosterone secretion in humans (**Table 2**). Billet and colleagues[94] created a knockin mouse model with a gain-of-function mutation of the AII type 1A receptor gene that impaired the internalization and desensitization of the receptor. This genetic modification resulted in constitutive activation of the AT1A receptor, leading to renin suppression, modest hypertension, and cardiac, vascular, and renal fibrosis. These sequelae resembled the phenotype of nongenetic murine models of PA induced by administering high doses of mineralocorticoid to salt-fed uninephrectomized animals. Aldosterone levels remain unchanged in these animals (and were therefore inappropriately normal in the face of low renin levels), which is also the case for many patients with PA.

Deletion of Kcnma1, which encodes the α-subunit of the large-conductance, voltage-activated and Ca^{2+}-activated potassium (BK) channel, in mice induced

Table 2
Genetic animal models of PA

Name of Model	Species	Description	Proposed Mechanism of Hyperaldosteronism	References
AT_{1A}MUT	Mouse	Knockin, gain-of-function mutation of the AII type 1A (AT_{1A}) receptor gene	Constitutive activation of the AT_{1A} receptor leading to direct stimulation of aldosterone production by zona glomerulosa (ZG) cells	[94]
$Kcnma1^{-/-}$	Mouse	Knockout of the large-conductance, voltage-activated and Ca^{2+}-activated K^+ (BK) channel α-subunit gene	Loss of BK-mediated control of calcium influx in ZG cells	[95]
$Kcnmb1^{-/-}$	Mouse	Knockout of the BK channel β1-subunit gene	Reduced renal BK activity leading to renal K^+ retention and hyperkalemia but also possibly reduced ZG BK activity causing serum K^+-independent (primary) adrenal aldosterone hypersecretion	[96]
Adβarr1-treated	Rat	Overexpression of βarrestin-1 (βarr1) induced by adrenal-targeted adenoviral-mediated gene delivery	Direct activation of a G protein-independent aldosterone synthetic pathway in ZG cells by βarr1	[97]
Cry-null	Mouse	Knockout of the cryptochrome (Cry)-1 and 2 genes	Overexpression of type VI 3β-hydroxysteroid dehydrogenase in ZG cells caused by loss of regulation by Cry	[98]
$TASK^{-/-}$	Mouse	Knockout of the TWIK-related acid sensitive potassium (TASK) channel type 1 and 3 subunit genes	Loss of TASK-mediated control of depolarization and calcium influx in ZG cells	[99]
$apc^{Min/+}$	Mouse	Loss-of-function mutation in the adenomatous polyposis coli (APC) gene	Loss of APC-mediated regulation of aldosterone release by an as yet undefined pathway	[100]
$AS^{hi/hi}$	Mouse	Gain-of-function mutation of the AS gene	Increased expression of AS	[101]

hypertension, hyperaldosteronism, and decreased potassium levels.[95] However, increased BP might have been secondary not only to aldosterone excess but also to increased myogenic vessel tone induced by BK channel dependent vascular abnormalities.[95] Renin levels were only slightly and not significantly lower than in wild-type animals, unlike in clinical PA, but were nevertheless not increased and hence the hyperaldosteronism was believed more likely to be of a primary than a secondary nature. The fact that the BK α-subunit was expressed in high levels within wild-type zona glomerulosa cells was consistent with that concept. A potential mechanism for PA in these animals proposed by the investigators involved loss of BK-mediated control of calcium influx through calcium channels in glomerulosa cells. In a different study, Grimm and colleagues[96] reported that the previously described hypertension in *Kcnmb1* (β1-subunit of BK) knockout mice is associated with volume expansion and is aldosterone dependent. Treatment with eplerenone induced correction of the fluid imbalance and reduced BP. However, unlike Kcnma1 knockout mice (which have reduced serum potassium levels), these animals showed increased serum potassium, leading the investigators to propose that the aldosterone hypersecretion might have been mainly secondary to renal potassium retention and hyperkalemia (unlike in PA). Nevertheless, the fact that these investigators were able to show expression of the BK β1-subunit in the adrenal glands of wild-type mice raised the possibility that at least some of the hyperaldosteronism may have been primary in nature.[96]

The discovery of a new, G protein-independent, β-arrestin-1 (βarr1)-mediated signaling pathway of AT1 receptor-induced aldosterone secretion has also resulted in the creation of a genetic animal model of PA.[97] Human zona glomerulosa cells, when treated with AII, secreted aldosterone and expressed high levels of βarr1, a universal receptor adapter/scaffolding protein.[97] These cells also secreted aldosterone when treated with SII, an AII analogue that induces βarr (but not G protein) coupling to the AT1 receptor. In rats, adrenal gland-specific overexpression of βarr1 also led to an increase in aldosterone production.[97]

Aldosterone production has also been linked to malfunction of the circadian clock. Salt-sensitive hypertension caused by abnormally high synthesis of aldosterone has been reported in *Cry*-null mice, a genetically modified animal model that shows a functionally impaired circadian clock and shows arrhythmic behavior, physiology, and metabolism.[98] A molecular search to explain the abnormal steroidogenesis in these animals led to the identification of type VI 3β-hydroxyl-steroid dehydrogenase (*Hsd3b6*) as a new hypertension candidate gene in mice.[98] *Hsd3b6*, which is expressed exclusively in aldosterone-producing cells and is under transcriptional control of the circadian clock, is functionally similar to the *HSD3B1* gene that is expressed in aldosterone-producing cells in the human adrenal gland.

Potassium current and membrane potential in adrenal zona glomerulosa cells are dependent on the expression of TWIK-related acid-sensitive potassium (TASK) channels. Genetic deletion of subunits TASK-1 and TASK-3 channels from mice caused zona glomerulosa membrane depolarization and elicited autonomous overproduction of aldosterone, suggesting another possible genetic mechanism for PA.[99]

Mice carrying a defective adenomatous polyposis coli gene were found to exhibit reduced urinary sodium excretion and increased plasma aldosterone, plasma volume, and BP levels.[100] However, because renin was not measured, the possibility that this finding represented a model of secondary (rather than primary) hyperaldosteronism cannot be excluded.

The effects of genetic mutations leading to overexpression of AS have also been studied. Mice (*AS^hi/hi*) with modestly increased expression of AS, induced by replacing the 3' untranslated region of AS mRNA with that from a stable mRNA, showed similar BP and aldosterone levels to wild-type mice while fed a normal-salt diet.[101] However, when fed a high-salt diet, *AS^hi/hi* mice had higher BP and plasma aldosterone levels, lower plasma potassium, and greater expression of the α-subunit of the epithelial sodium channel (an aldosterone-induced gene) compared with wild-type mice.

Furthermore, on a low-salt diet, $AS^{hi/hi}$ maintained normal BP (unlike wild-type mice) and showed less activation of the renin-angiotensin-aldosterone system. These results provide a potential mechanism by which the reported interaction between aldosterone and salt in experimental models and the increased salt sensitivity observed in some patients can at least be partially explained.

THE FUTURE FOR PA

Elucidating the genetic basis of some familial forms of PA has already provided a new and exciting perspective, encompassing the possibility of unequivocal early diagnosis of the inherited tendency to develop PA, with the enhanced management possibilities that follow. These include close follow-up of children identified as carrying the mutation, with institution of dietary salt restriction early, before BP-independent effects of hyperaldosteronism can develop. Taking a careful family history and encouraging appropriate investigation of other hypertensive family members assumes greater importance. The development of a variety of animal models for PA and their molecular genetic documentation will continue to open up new areas of investigation and understanding of salt and BP homeostasis in mammals, including humans. The definition of PA is already broadening, and will continue to do so as our understanding increases.

GORDON SYNDROME

The consistent, unique clinical characteristic of Gordon syndrome is chronic hyperkalemia despite normal renal glomerular function. This characteristic is accompanied by varying degrees of hyperchloremia and acidemia, and in the most severely affected, by muscle weakness, short stature, and even intellectual disability. The biochemical abnormalities have been completely reversed by dietary sodium restriction in some, and by thiazide diuretics in all. Hypertension is an important feature, more frequent and more severe in males, often absent in young patients but almost invariably present in adults. With both apparently sporadic but more usually dominant familial distribution, variability in phenotype can sometimes be explained by variability in genotype, which is currently the focus of intense investigations that reveal complex interactions between WNK kinases and their targets, which include the well-established channels for ion transport in the kidney and elsewhere. The WNK kinases, discovered as a result of seeking the genetic basis of Gordon syndrome, are proving to be widely distributed with actions in a diverse range of tissues in addition to renal tubules, where mutations studied in animal models frequently lead to hypertension and hence generate hope for new therapeutic strategies.

EARLY CLINICAL PRESENTATIONS AND PATHOPHYSIOLOGIC INTERPRETATIONS

The initial reports of hypertension with hyperkalemia despite normal glomerular filtration rate were in severely affected patients from Australia and appeared to be sporadic cases, because other affected family members were sought but not found. A 15-year-old male presented in Sydney in 1964 with severe hypertension and hyperkalemia (7.0–8.2 mmol/L).[102] In the absence of renin or aldosterone measurements, hypertension was attributed to a renal tubular abnormality causing hyperkalemia, which then stimulated aldosterone to cause hypertension.[102,103] A 10-year-old female presented in Adelaide in 1967 with short stature and high BP (160/100 mm Hg), potassium 8.5 mmol/L, and undetectable renin.[104] Because of extremely suppressed renin and pressor hyperreactivity, Gordon and colleagues[104] proposed a primary renal tubular lesion proximal to where aldosterone achieves kaliuresis, but causing sodium retention and volume expansion as the hypertensive mechanism, with extremely suppressed renin preventing normal responsiveness of aldosterone to potassium, and contributing to reduced potassium excretion. A rapid improvement on a low-salt diet and eventual correction of all abnormal features by prolonged dietary sodium restriction provided support for this hypothesis. Biochemical features the mirror image of Barrter syndrome[105] suggested to Gordon the possibility of a deficiency of the yet to be identified natriuretic hormone, the action of which had been discovered by de Wardener and colleagues[106] during cross-circulation experiments in dogs, volume expansion in 1 dog causing natriuresis in the other. This possibility also appealed to Hugh de Wardener,[107] who named the condition Gordon syndrome in the fourth edition of *Diseases of the Kidney*. After the discovery[108] of an atrial natriuretic hormone (ANH) and the development of assays to measure it, levels were found to be paradoxically lower than expected in Gordon syndrome, and not as responsive to saline infusion as expected, and higher than expected in Barrter syndrome.[109,110] Further evidence suggesting atypical regulation of ANH in Gordon syndrome and Barrter syndrome followed.[111–114] Tubular resistance to ANH was reported in a patient with Gordon syndrome,[115] but was not confirmed in others.[114] The question of altered regulation of ANH in Gordon syndrome remains open, and it is possible that the recently recognized wide distribution of the WNK system, including the cardiovascular system, may explain this. Other proposed pathophysiologic bases for Gordon syndrome have included a problem with prostaglandin synthesis and a generalized cell membrane defect.[116–118]

IS PHENOTYPIC HETEROGENEITY EXPLAINED BY GENETIC HETEROGENEITY?

Although there may be subgroups in Gordon syndrome in respect of regulation of ANH secretion, this seems more certain in respect of renal calcium handling, which may be based on genetic heterogeneity,[114] caused by mutations occurring in either WNK1 or WNK4.[119] On the other hand, apparently differing renal tubular responsiveness to aldosterone and aldosterone antagonists may depend on whether aldosterone is suppressed or not at the time of administration of spironolactone, as it does in Liddle syndrome, with the tubule unresponsive to spironolactone before any treatment, but normally responsive when aldosterone is unsuppressed by a low-salt diet and triamterene or amiloride.[120] Similarly, the tubular kaluretic responsiveness (or lack of it) to sodium chloride and sodium sulfate infusion in Gordon syndrome seems to depend on the presence of low, normal, or increased levels of aldosterone at the time of study (eg, increased by dietary salt restriction or diuretics). This characteristic has varied widely in different reports of Gordon syndrome, leading to differing assertions, documented and discussed in reviews of up to 69 reported cases.[120–123] Another example of apparent phenotypic variability likely fully explained by prevailing conditions or previous treatment without the need to invoke genetic variation is degree of suppression of renin and of aldosterone, and BP level, which depend critically on previous exposure to treatment with diuretics, the effects of which can take many months to completely disappear. There has been heterogeneity in the magnitude of the therapeutic response to dietary sodium restriction,[120–123] which in some cases rapidly reversed some or all of the presenting abnormalities.[104,124,125]

DIAGNOSIS

Because hyperkalemia despite normal renal glomerular function (serum creatinine or creatinine clearance) is the most consistent clinical feature of hyperkalemic hypertension, reliable assessment of potassium level in the blood is essential, but not so easily achieved. Plasma potassium is more reliable than serum potassium, because the clotted red cells release potassium and higher levels result. Delay in separation of plasma from cells also falsely increases plasma levels because failing cell membrane pumps allow potassium to escape into the plasma. Hemolysis is the most serious contributor to falsely high potassium levels, and occurs if vacuum tubes are used to collect the sample, or if the veins are difficult to access. Closing the fist to activate forearm muscles results in potassium leaving the cells and reaching the veins to falsely increase levels. Hence the common sampling problems all lead to false-positive results. However, as has been discussed, a low-salt diet lowers potassium levels in Gordon syndrome, and any exposure to potassium-wasting diuretics such as thiazides or loop diuretics can lead to false-negative results at least partly explained by aldosterone stimulation leading to kaliuresis. With the advent of precise genetic identification of affected members of families with this condition, it becomes possible by repeated measurement on liberal salt diets without medications to establish whether there is any overlap in plasma potassium levels between affected and unaffected family members.

Hypertension is most often the abnormality leading to presentation. Chronic hyperkalemia without renal failure in Gordon syndrome seems surprisingly well tolerated, perhaps because it has been relatively stable and present in utero and from birth. Although the potential for cardiac arrhythmias exists, in their absence it may be safest to not attempt to correct the hyperkalemia as rapidly as would be indicated if this was a new development. Immediate institution of a low-salt diet begins to ameliorate the abnormalities.[104,124,125]

Because patients with Gordon syndrome are unusually responsive to thiazide diuretics, it is desirable to commence them on a dose 50% of standard for a patient of that age and weight. Many patients with Gordon syndrome have been treated for decades with thiazide diuretics with excellent results, including resumption of normal growth rate when short stature was a presenting feature,[118,120–123] and correction of hypercalciuria when that is a feature. Gordon's original patient has been followed for 43 years and remains well, with normal BP and plasma potassium and creatinine levels and taking chlorthalidone 25 mg and atenolol 25 mg daily.

APPROPRIATE ALTERNATIVE TITLES

The name Gordon syndrome persists, possibly because it is shorter that the term pseudohypoaldosteronism type II used by Schambelan and colleagues[126] after studying an apparently sporadic case, and proposing a renal distal tubule chloride shunt. Probably the most appropriate name for the syndrome, familial hyperkalemia and hypertension (FHH or FHHt), followed the description of familial cases, firstly by Farfel and associates[118] from Tel Aviv University Medical School in Israel. These investigators initially proposed, after apparent failure of glucose and insulin infusion to adequately lower potassium, a generalized cell membrane defect affecting potassium transfer. This remarkable family has been carefully followed, with a series of reports detailing new observations as the family has grown in size, including hypercalciuria and reduced bone mineral density (see later discussion). Pregnancy was associated with disappearance of hypertension, but persistence of hyperkalemia and associated biochemical abnormalities.[127] We have encountered no reports elucidating whether potassium levels at birth differ depending on whether the condition has been inherited from the mother or the father. It is possible that a normokalemic mother might have an ameliorating effect on potassium levels before and immediately after birth, in which case a potassium level increasing for the first time might be more likely to have untoward effects.

ELUCIDATION OF A GENETIC BASIS PERMITS UNEQUIVOCAL SEPARATION OF
AFFECTED FROM UNAFFECTED FAMILY MEMBERS, AND LEADS TO DISCOVERY OF
A NEW GROUP OF KINASES INVOLVED IN ION TRANSPORT IN THE KIDNEY AND MANY
OTHER TISSUES

After showing linkage of the syndrome to chromosomes 17 and 1,[128,129] and then to chromosome 12 as well,[130] the large Israeli family, a large French family, and many others were used in a collaboration that uncovered the genetic basis of the syndrome.[131,132] Apart from a variety of effects shown in the renal tubule and elsewhere, mutations in WNK (with no lysine) kinases are involved in a complicated control system for the Na and Cl cotransporter (NCCT) where thiazides act, and this may explain the marked sensitivity to thiazide diuretics that most patients with Gordon syndrome show.[120–123] It may also explain why these patients display clinical and biochemical features that are the opposite of those seen in the Gitelman variant of Barrter syndrome[133] in which there are mutations leading to loss of function in the NCCT. A variety of mutations in WNK1 on chromosome 12 and in WNK4 on chromosome 17 have been described, but the location of the WNK gene on chromosome 1 suggested by the linkage studies[128] remains elusive.[132]

Characterization of the particular mutation involved in the Israeli family permitted affected members to be decisively separated from unaffected members and the 2 groups compared. This strategy made it possible to unequivocally show the presence of hypercalciuria, hypocalcemia, and decreased bone mineral density in those affected.[134] At least 46 members of this family are now being carefully followed (**Fig. 1**), equally divided between affected and unaffected individuals.[135] This situation represents an invaluable resource for further insights into the clinical expression of this particular mutation in WNK4. The disturbances of both sodium and calcium homeostasis from which these patients suffer seem to be opposite to those of Gitelman syndrome, which is caused by inactivating mutations in the thiazide-sensitive NCCT.[133] Only 1 of the hypercalciuric patients reported by the Israeli group[118,134] had an episode of renal colic (before commencing treatment with thiazide diuretic), and 1 who was diagnosed late in life had a stag-horn renal calculus. There have been few reports of patients with FHH and renal calculi.[136,137] The failure to document hypocalcemia in most reported cases[120–123] may sometimes have been because of failure to look, but is consistent with clinical, secondary to genetic, heterogeneity.

LITHIUM CLEARANCE AS AN INDEX OF RENAL TUBULAR SODIUM REABSORPTION

A recent report from the Israeli group[135] includes studies based on endogenous lithium clearance as a supposed negative index of proximal renal tubular sodium reabsorption. Expecting to find it increased, because all the molecular genetic evidence on the WNK kinases in FHH suggested enhanced distal tubular sodium reabsorption, which should lead to reduced proximal tubular sodium reabsorption and increased lithium clearance, as Klemm and colleagues[138] had found earlier in a smaller study using exogenous lithium clearance, lithium clearance was reduced, as is expected in increased proximal sodium reabsorption. One of the reported patients with FHH (a 7-year-old boy) presenting with nephrolithiasis had indices consistent with an increase in both proximal and distal sodium reabsorption. As well, an increased serum phosphate was reported in several patients with FHH consistent with increased proximal sodium reabsorption.[120–123] However, the most likely explanation for apparently increased proximal tubule sodium reabsorption is that under the conditions of study, particularly in those patients who had experienced previous exposure to thiazide diuretics, lithium clearance was reflecting either distal alone, or distal plus proximal

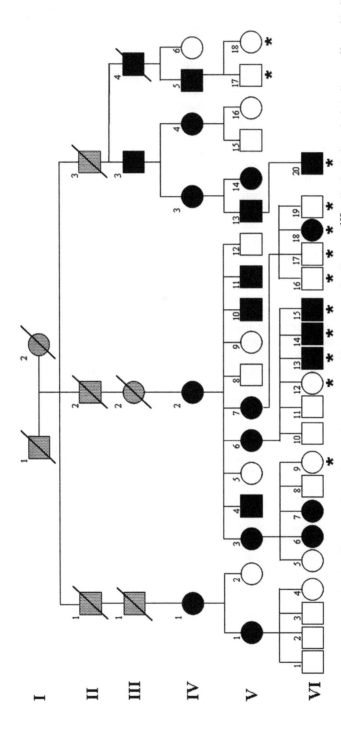

Fig. 1. Pedigree of an Israeli family affected with Gordon syndrome reported by Mayan and colleagues.[135] Fully shaded symbols indicate affected individuals, open symbols unaffected individuals, and half-shaded symbols family members not examined by the reporting investigators. Square symbols indicate males, circles females, and diagonal lines deceased individuals. (*From* Mayan H, Melnikov S, Novikov I, et al. Familial hyperkalemia and hypertension: pathogenetic insights based on lithium clearance. J Clin Endocrinol Metab 2009;94:3011; with permission.)

sodium reabsorption.[139] In support of excessive activity of the NCCT in Gordon syndrome, the Israeli group have recently reported increased urinary NCCT protein in patients with FHH.[140]

STUDIES ESTABLISHING A WIDER ROLE FOR WNK KINASES THAN SIMPLY THE RENAL TUBULE

Findings consistent with the WNK kinases having a significant role in tissues other than the renal tubules include altered sodium and/or chloride transport in many epithelia both from laboratory studies[141,142] and from studies in patients with FHH.[143,144]

Using a reporter gene to monitor expression of L-WNK1 in mice during development and adulthood revealed unexpected early expression in the vessels and primitive heart and generalized cardiovascular expression in adulthood, raising the possibility of the WNK system influencing BP by mechanisms independent of the kidney.[145] A second unexpected finding was expression in the granular layer and Purkinje cells of the cerebellum.[145] Such unexpected developments and new directions are the subject of intense discussion.[132]

Families with FHH in whom examination of DNA seeking the currently recognized mutations is negative have been encountered by groups in France, England, Australia, and the United States, consistent with at least 1 more currently unrecognized mutation, and probably many more.

A ROLE FOR WNK KINASES IN SO-CALLED ESSENTIAL HYPERTENSION?

The locus for WNK4 lies in a large area on chromosome 17 where there is linkage to BP variation in the Framingham Heart Study population.[146] There have been no other convincing findings linking WNK4 to hypertension in the general population, and only contradictory findings in population studies seeking relationships between WNK1 variants and BP.[147] It may be important that in none of these studies was urinary sodium measured as a surrogate for dietary salt intake.

THE FUTURE FOR GORDON SYNDROME

Gordon syndrome is both clinically and genetically diverse. Inherited in an autosomal-dominant fashion, its frequency seems to be rare, but it masquerades as essential hypertension if it is not considered before thiazide diuretics are commenced. If hyperkalemia is detected in a hypertensive patient, potassium levels should be checked in all family members, and not only in those with increased BP. Some affected families have the currently recognized most common causative mutations in WNK genes, making detection of affected members certain, but others do not.

In part because of Gordon syndrome, detailed examination of the many processes involved in renal tubular ion transfer is an area of more intense research activity, stimulated by the discovery of a previously unsuspected system of WNK kinases that influences and interacts with previously known ion-transporting mechanisms.[148] Many of the animal models used are based on molecular genetic understanding of Gordon and Gitelman syndromes, which have many opposing features. Significant alterations in BP are often seen in these models, and it is possible that a more complete understanding could lead to the development of new agents capable of lowering BP, with possible eventual clinical application. In this way, perhaps, we will observe the full circle leading from clinical observation to molecular understanding that finally delivers useful clinical applications.

REFERENCES

1. Conn JW. The evolution of primary aldosteronism: 1954–1967. Harvey Lect 1966;62:257–91.
2. Gordon RD, Klemm SA, Tunny TJ, et al. Primary aldosteronism: hypertension with a genetic basis. Lancet 1992;340:159–61.
3. Gordon RD, Stowasser M, Tunny TJ, et al. High incidence of primary aldosteronism in 199 patients referred with hypertension. Clin Exp Pharmacol Physiol 1994;21:315–8.
4. Lim PO, Dow E, Brennan G, et al. High prevalence of primary aldosteronism in the Tayside hypertension clinic population. J Hum Hypertens 2000;14:311–5.
5. Loh KC, Koay ES, Khaw MC, et al. Prevalence of primary aldosteronism among Asian hypertensive patients in Singapore. J Clin Endocrinol Metab 2000;85: 2854–9.
6. Mulatero P, Stowasser M, Loh KC, et al. Increased diagnosis of primary aldosteronism, including surgically correctable forms, in centers from five continents. J Clin Endocrinol Metab 2004;89:1045–50.
7. Rossi GP, Bernini G, Caliumi C, et al. A prospective study of the prevalence of primary aldosteronism in 1,125 hypertensive patients. J Am Coll Cardiol 2006; 48:2293–300.
8. Young WF. Primary aldosteronism: update on diagnosis and treatment. Endocrinologist 1997;7:213–21.
9. Funder JW, Carey RM, Fardella C, et al. Case detection, diagnosis, and treatment of patients with primary aldosteronism: an endocrine society clinical practice guideline. J Clin Endocrinol Metab 2008;93:3266–81.
10. Stowasser M, Gordon RD. Primary aldosteronism–careful investigation is essential and rewarding. Mol Cell Endocrinol 2004;217:33–9.
11. Celen O, O'Brien MJ, Melby JC, et al. Factors influencing outcome of surgery for primary aldosteronism. Arch Surg 1996;131:646–50.
12. Rutherford JC, Taylor WL, Stowasser M, et al. Success of surgery for primary aldosteronism judged by residual autonomous aldosterone production. World J Surg 1998;22:1243–5.
13. Stowasser M, Gordon RD, Gunasekera TG, et al. High rate of detection of primary aldosteronism, including surgically treatable forms, after 'non-selective' screening of hypertensive patients. J Hypertens 2003;21:2149–57.
14. Sukor N, Kogovsek C, Gordon RD, et al. Improved quality of life, blood pressure, and biochemical status following unilateral laparoscopic adrenalectomy for unilateral primary aldosteronism. J Clin Endocrinol Metab 2010;95:1360–4.
15. Lim PO, Young WF, MacDonald TM. A review of the medical treatment of primary aldosteronism. J Hypertens 2001;19:353–61.
16. Sukor N, Gordon RD, Ku YK, et al. Role of unilateral adrenalectomy in bilateral primary aldosteronism: a 22-year single center experience. J Clin Endocrinol Metab 2009;94:2437–45.
17. Milliez P, Girerd X, Plouin PF, et al. Evidence for an increased rate of cardiovascular events in patients with primary aldosteronism. J Am Coll Cardiol 2005;45:1243–8.
18. Rossi GP, Bernini G, Desideri G, et al. Renal damage in primary aldosteronism: results of the PAPY Study. Hypertension 2006;48:232–8.
19. Rossi GP, Cesari M, Pessina AC. Left ventricular changes in primary aldosteronism. Am J Hypertens 2003;16:96–8.
20. Weber KT, Brilla CG. Pathological hypertrophy and cardiac interstitium. Fibrosis and renin-angiotensin-aldosterone system. Circulation 1991;83:1849–65.

21. Young MJ, Funder JW. Mineralocorticoid receptors and pathophysiological roles for aldosterone in the cardiovascular system. J Hypertens 2002;20:1465–8.
22. Catena C, Colussi G, Nadalini E, et al. Cardiovascular outcomes in patients with primary aldosteronism after treatment. Arch Intern Med 2008;168:80–5.
23. Neville AM, O'Hare MJ. Histopathology of the human adrenal cortex. Clin Endocrinol Metab 1985;14:791–820.
24. Skogseid B, Eriksson B, Lundqvist G, et al. Multiple endocrine neoplasia type 1: a 10-year prospective screening study in four kindreds. J Clin Endocrinol Metab 1991;73:281–7.
25. Beckers A, Abs R, Willems PJ, et al. Aldosterone-secreting adrenal adenoma as part of multiple endocrine neoplasia type 1 (MEN1): loss of heterozygosity for polymorphic chromosome 11 deoxyribonucleic acid markers, including the MEN1 locus. J Clin Endocrinol Metab 1992;75:564–70.
26. Vasan RS, Evans JC, Larson MG, et al. Serum aldosterone and the incidence of hypertension in nonhypertensive persons. N Engl J Med 2004;351:33–41.
27. Newton-Cheh C, Guo CY, Gona P, et al. Clinical and genetic correlates of aldosterone-to-renin ratio and relations to blood pressure in a community sample. Hypertension 2007;49:846–56.
28. Sutherland DJ, Ruse JL, Laidlaw JC. Hypertension, increased aldosterone secretion and low plasma renin activity relieved by dexamethasone. Can Med Assoc J 1966;95:1109–19.
29. Fallo F, Sonino N, Armanini D, et al. A new family with dexamethasone-suppressible hyperaldosteronism: aldosterone unresponsiveness to angiotensin II. Clin Endocrinol (Oxf) 1985;22:777–85.
30. Stowasser M, Bachmann AW, Huggard PR, et al. Treatment of familial hyperaldosteronism type I: only partial suppression of adrenocorticotropin required to correct hypertension. J Clin Endocrinol Metab 2000;85:3313–8.
31. Lifton RP, Dluhy RG, Powers M, et al. A chimaeric 11 beta-hydroxylase/aldosterone synthase gene causes glucocorticoid-remediable aldosteronism and human hypertension. Nature 1992;355:262–5.
32. Lifton RP, Dluhy RG, Powers M, et al. Hereditary hypertension caused by chimaeric gene duplications and ectopic expression of aldosterone synthase. Nat Genet 1992;2:66–74.
33. Pascoe L, Jeunemaitre X, Lebrethon MC, et al. Glucocorticoid-suppressible hyperaldosteronism and adrenal tumors occurring in a single French pedigree. J Clin Invest 1995;96:2236–46.
34. Gomez-Sanchez CE, Montgomery M, Ganguly A, et al. Elevated urinary excretion of 18-oxocortisol in glucocorticoid-suppressible aldosteronism. J Clin Endocrinol Metab 1984;59:1022–4.
35. Stowasser M, Bachmann AW, Tunny TJ, et al. Production of 18-oxo-cortisol in subtypes of primary aldosteronism. Clin Exp Pharmacol Physiol 1996;23:591–3.
36. Rich GM, Ulick S, Cook S, et al. Glucocorticoid-remediable aldosteronism in a large kindred: clinical spectrum and diagnosis using a characteristic biochemical phenotype. Ann Intern Med 1992;116:813–20.
37. Stowasser M, Bachmann AW, Huggard PR, et al. Severity of hypertension in familial hyperaldosteronism type I: relationship to gender and degree of biochemical disturbance. J Clin Endocrinol Metab 2000;85:2160–6.
38. Fallo F, Pilon C, Williams TA, et al. Coexistence of different phenotypes in a family with glucocorticoid-remediable aldosteronism. J Hum Hypertens 2004;18:47–51.

39. Stowasser M, Huggard PR, Rossetti TR, et al. Biochemical evidence of aldosterone overproduction and abnormal regulation in normotensive individuals with familial hyperaldosteronism type I. J Clin Endocrinol Metab 1999;84:4031–6.

40. Jonsson JR, Klemm SA, Tunny TJ, et al. A new genetic test for familial hyperaldosteronism type I aids in the detection of curable hypertension. Biochem Biophys Res Commun 1995;207:565–71.

41. Mulatero P, Veglio F, Pilon C, et al. Diagnosis of glucocorticoid-remediable aldosteronism in primary aldosteronism: aldosterone response to dexamethasone and long polymerase chain reaction for chimeric gene. J Clin Endocrinol Metab 1998;83:2573–5.

42. Stowasser M, Sharman J, Leano R, et al. Evidence for abnormal left ventricular structure and function in normotensive individuals with familial hyperaldosteronism type I. J Clin Endocrinol Metab 2005;90:5070–6.

43. Staermose S, Marwick TH, Gordon RD, et al. Elevated serum interleukin 6 levels in normotensive individuals with familial hyperaldosteronism type 1. Hypertension 2009;53:e31–2.

44. Gordon RD, Stowasser M, Tunny TJ, et al. Clinical and pathological diversity of primary aldosteronism, including a new familial variety. Clin Exp Pharmacol Physiol 1991;18:283–6.

45. London N, Swales J, Hollinrake K, et al. Familial Conn's syndrome. Postgrad Med J 1992;68:976–7.

46. Fallo F, Veglio F, Mulatero P, et al. Genetic studies in familial aldosteronism not suppressible by dexamethasone. J Endocr Genet 2000;1:159–64.

47. Stowasser M, Gordon RD, Tunny TJ, et al. Familial hyperaldosteronism type II: five families with a new variety of primary aldosteronism. Clin Exp Pharmacol Physiol 1992;19:319–22.

48. Stowasser M, Gordon RD. Familial hyperaldosteronism. J Steroid Biochem Mol Biol 2001;78:215–29.

49. Stowasser M, Gordon RD. Primary aldosteronism: from genesis to genetics. Trends Endocrinol Metab 2003;14:310–7.

50. Gordon RD, Stowasser M. Familial forms broaden horizons in primary aldosteronism. Trends Endocrinol Metab 1998;9:220–7.

51. Curnow KM, Mulatero P, Emeric-Blanchouin N, et al. The amino acid substitutions Ser288Gly and Val320Ala convert the cortisol producing enzyme, CYP11B1, into an aldosterone producing enzyme. Nat Struct Biol 1997;4: 32–5.

52. Pilon C, Mulatero P, Barzon L, et al. Mutations in CYP11B1 gene converting 11beta-hydroxylase into an aldosterone-producing enzyme are not present in aldosterone-producing adenomas. J Clin Endocrinol Metab 1999;84: 4228–31.

53. Ballantine DM, Klemm SA, Tunny TJ, et al. PCR-SSCP analysis of the p53 gene in tumours of the adrenal gland. Clin Exp Pharmacol Physiol 1996;23:582–3.

54. Torpy DJ, Gordon RD, Lin JP, et al. Familial hyperaldosteronism type II: description of a large kindred and exclusion of the aldosterone synthase (CYP11B2) gene. J Clin Endocrinol Metab 1998;83:3214–8.

55. Torpy DJ, Stratakis CA, Gordon RD. Linkage analysis of familial hyperaldosteronism type II–absence of linkage to the gene encoding the angiotensin II receptor type 1. J Clin Endocrinol Metab 1998;83:1046.

56. Lafferty AR, Torpy DJ, Stowasser M, et al. A novel genetic locus for low renin hypertension: familial hyperaldosteronism type II maps to chromosome 7 (7p22). J Med Genet 2000;37:831–5.

57. So A, Duffy DL, Gordon RD, et al. Familial hyperaldosteronism type II is linked to the chromosome 7p22 region but also shows predicted heterogeneity. J Hypertens 2005;23:1477–84.
58. Sukor N, Mulatero P, Gordon RD, et al. Further evidence for linkage of familial hyperaldosteronism type II at chromosome 7p22 in Italian as well as Australian and South American families. J Hypertens 2008;26:1577–82.
59. Fallo F, Pilon C, Barzon L, et al. Retention of heterozygosity at chromosome 7p22 and 11q13 in aldosterone-producing tumours of patients with familial hyperaldosteronism not remediable by glucocorticoids. J Hum Hypertens 2004; 18:829–30.
60. Elphinstone MS, Gordon RD, So A, et al. Genomic structure of the human gene for protein kinase A regulatory subunit R1-beta (PRKAR1B) on 7p22: no evidence for mutations in familial hyperaldosteronism type II in a large affected kindred. Clin Endocrinol (Oxf) 2004;61:716–23.
61. Jeske YW, So A, Kelemen L, et al. Examination of chromosome 7p22 candidate genes RBaK, PMS2 and GNA12 in familial hyperaldosteronism type II. Clin Exp Pharmacol Physiol 2008;35:380–5.
62. So A, Jeske YW, Gordon RD, et al. No evidence for coding region mutations in the retinoblastoma-associated Kruppel-associated box protein gene (RBaK) causing familial hyperaldosteronism type II. Clin Endocrinol (Oxf) 2006;65: 829–31.
63. Warnock DG. Liddle syndrome: genetics and mechanisms of Na+ channel defects. Am J Med Sci 2001;322:302–7.
64. Cope G, Golbang A, O'Shaughnessy KM. WNK kinases and the control of blood pressure. Pharmacol Ther 2005;106:221–31.
65. Geller DS, Zhang J, Wisgerhof MV, et al. A novel form of human mendelian hypertension featuring nonglucocorticoid-remediable aldosteronism. J Clin Endocrinol Metab 2008;93:3117–23.
66. Choi M, Scholl UI, Björklund P, et al. K+ channel mutations in adrenal aldosterone-producing adenomas and hereditary hypertension. Science 2011;331:768–72.
67. Mulatero P. A new form of hereditary primary aldosteronism: familial hyperaldosteronism type III. J Clin Endocrinol Metab 2008;93:2972–4.
68. Quack I, Vonend O, Rump LC. Familial hyperaldosteronism I-III. Horm Metab Res 2010;42:424–8.
69. Stowasser M, Gordon RD. Primary aldosteronism: learning from the study of familial varieties. J Hypertens 2000;18:1165–76.
70. Greco RG, Carroll JE, Morris DJ, et al. Familial hyperaldosteronism, not suppressed by dexamethasone. J Clin Endocrinol Metab 1982;55:1013–6.
71. Malagon-Rogers M. Non-glucocorticoid-remediable aldosteronism in an infant with low-renin hypertension. Pediatr Nephrol 2004;19:235–6.
72. Davies E, Holloway CD, Ingram MC, et al. Aldosterone excretion rate and blood pressure in essential hypertension are related to polymorphic differences in the aldosterone synthase gene CYP11B2. Hypertension 1999;33: 703–7.
73. Lim PO, Macdonald TM, Holloway C, et al. Variation at the aldosterone synthase (CYP11B2) locus contributes to hypertension in subjects with a raised aldosterone-to-renin ratio. J Clin Endocrinol Metab 2002;87:4398–402.
74. Inglis GC, Plouin PF, Friel EC, et al. Polymorphic differences from normal in the aldosterone synthase gene (CYP11B2) in patients with primary hyperaldosteronism and adrenal tumour (Conn's syndrome). Clin Endocrinol (Oxf) 2001;54: 725–30.

75. Nicod J, Bruhin D, Auer L, et al. A biallelic gene polymorphism of CYP11B2 predicts increased aldosterone to renin ratio in selected hypertensive patients. J Clin Endocrinol Metab 2003;88:2495–500.
76. Komiya I, Yamada T, Takara M, et al. Lys(173)Arg and -344T/C variants of CYP11B2 in Japanese patients with low-renin hypertension. Hypertension 2000;35:699–703.
77. Mulatero P, Schiavone D, Fallo F, et al. CYP11B2 gene polymorphisms in idiopathic hyperaldosteronism. Hypertension 2000;35:694–8.
78. Pojoga L, Gautier S, Blanc H, et al. Genetic determination of plasma aldosterone levels in essential hypertension. Am J Hypertens 1998;11:856–60.
79. Connell JM, MacKenzie SM, Freel EM, et al. A lifetime of aldosterone excess: long-term consequences of altered regulation of aldosterone production for cardiovascular function. Endocr Rev 2008;29:133–54.
80. Davies E, Holloway CD, Ingram MC, et al. An influence of variation in the aldosterone synthase gene (CYP11B2) on corticosteroid responses to ACTH in normal human subjects. Clin Endocrinol (Oxf) 2001;54:813–7.
81. Barr M, MacKenzie SM, Wilkinson DM, et al. Functional effects of genetic variants in the 11beta-hydroxylase (CYP11B1) gene. Clin Endocrinol (Oxf) 2006;65:816–25.
82. Carroll J, Dluhy R, Fallo F, et al. Aldosterone-producing adenomas do not contain glucocorticoid-remediable aldosteronism chimeric gene duplications. J Clin Endocrinol Metab 1996;81:4310–2.
83. Takeda Y, Furukawa K, Inaba S, et al. Genetic analysis of aldosterone synthase in patients with idiopathic hyperaldosteronism. J Clin Endocrinol Metab 1999;84: 1633–7.
84. Hampf M, Widimsky J, Bernhardt R. Aldosterone synthase gene in patients suffering from hyperaldosteronism. Endocr Res 1998;24:877–80.
85. Klemm SA, Ballantine DM, Tunny TJ, et al. PCR-SSCP analysis of the angiotensin II type 1 receptor gene in patients with aldosterone-producing adenomas. Clin Exp Pharmacol Physiol 1995;22:457–9.
86. Davies E, Bonnardeaux A, Plouin PF, et al. Somatic mutations of the angiotensin II (AT1) receptor gene are not present in aldosterone-producing adenoma. J Clin Endocrinol Metab 1997;82:611–5.
87. Iida A, Blake K, Tunny T, et al. Allelic losses on chromosome band 11q13 in aldosterone-producing adrenal tumors. Genes Chromosomes Cancer 1995; 12:73–5.
88. Gordon R, Gartside M, Tunny T, et al. Different allelic patterns at chromosome 11q13 in paired aldosterone-producing tumours and blood DNA. Clin Exp Pharmacol Physiol 1996;23:594–6.
89. Charpentier F, Merot J, Loussouarn G, et al. Delayed rectifier K(+) currents and cardiac repolarization. J Mol Cell Cardiol 2010;48:37–44.
90. Wymore RS, Gintant GA, Wymore RT, et al. Tissue and species distribution of mRNA for the IKr-like K+ channel, erg. Circ Res 1997;80:261–8.
91. Sarzani R, Pietrucci F, Corinaldesi C, et al. The functional HERG variant 897T is associated with Conn's adenoma. J Hypertens 2006;24:479–87.
92. Williams TA, Monticone S, Morello F, et al. Teratocarcinoma-derived growth factor-1 is upregulated in aldosterone-producing adenomas and increases aldosterone secretion and inhibits apoptosis in vitro. Hypertension 2010;55:1468–75.
93. Giuliani L, Lenzini L, Antonello M, et al. Expression and functional role of urotensin-II and its receptor in the adrenal cortex and medulla: novel insights for the pathophysiology of primary aldosteronism. J Clin Endocrinol Metab 2009;94:684–90.

94. Billet S, Bardin S, Verp S, et al. Gain-of-function mutant of angiotensin II receptor, type 1A, causes hypertension and cardiovascular fibrosis in mice. J Clin Invest 2007;117:1914–25.

95. Sausbier M, Arntz C, Bucurenciu I, et al. Elevated blood pressure linked to primary hyperaldosteronism and impaired vasodilation in BK channel-deficient mice. Circulation 2005;112:60–8.

96. Grimm PR, Irsik DL, Settles DC, et al. Hypertension of Kcnmb1-/- is linked to deficient K secretion and aldosteronism. Proc Natl Acad Sci U S A 2009;106: 11800–5.

97. Lymperopoulos A, Rengo G, Zincarelli C, et al. An adrenal beta-arrestin 1-mediated signaling pathway underlies angiotensin II-induced aldosterone production in vitro and in vivo. Proc Natl Acad Sci U S A 2009;106:5825–30.

98. Doi M, Takahashi Y, Komatsu R, et al. Salt-sensitive hypertension in circadian clock-deficient Cry-null mice involves dysregulated adrenal Hsd3b6. Nat Med 2010;16:67–74.

99. Davies LA, Hu C, Guagliardo NA, et al. TASK channel deletion in mice causes primary hyperaldosteronism. Proc Natl Acad Sci U S A 2008;105: 2203–8.

100. Bhandaru M, Kempe DS, Rotte A, et al. Hyperaldosteronism, hypervolemia, and increased blood pressure in mice expressing defective APC. Am J Physiol Regul Integr Comp Physiol 2009;297:R571–5.

101. Makhanova N, Hagaman J, Kim HS, et al. Salt-sensitive blood pressure in mice with increased expression of aldosterone synthase. Hypertension 2008;51:134–40.

102. Paver WK, Pauline GJ. Hypertension and hyperpotassaemia without renal disease in a young male. Med J Aust 1964;2:305–6.

103. Arnold JE, Healy JK. Hyperkalemia, hypertension and systemic acidosis without renal failure associated with a tubular defect in potassium excretion. Am J Med 1969;47:461–72.

104. Gordon RD, Geddes RA, Pawsey CG, et al. Hypertension and severe hyperkalaemia associated with suppression of renin and aldosterone and completely reversed by dietary sodium restriction. Australas Ann Med 1970;4:287–94.

105. Barrter FC, Pronove P, Gill JR, et al. Hyperplasia of the juxtaglomerular complex with hyperaldosteronism and hypokalemic alkalosis: a new syndrome. Am J Med 1962;33:811–28.

106. de Wardener HE, Mills IH, Clapham WF, et al. Studies on the efferent mechanism of the sodium diuresis which follows the administration of intravenous saline in the dog. Clin Sci 1961;21:249–58.

107. de Wardener HE. Selective defects of tubular function. In: The kidney: an outline of normal and abnormal structure and function. 4th edition. London: Churchill Livingstone; 1973. p. 230–43.

108. DeBold AJ, Borenstein HB, Veress AT, et al. A rapid and potent natriuretic response to intravenous injection of atrial myocardial extracts in rats. Life Sci 1981;28:89–94.

109. Tunny TJ, Gordon RD. Plasma atrial natriuretic peptide in primary aldosteronism (before and after treatment) and in Bartter's and Gordon's syndromes. Lancet 1986;1:272–3.

110. Tunny TJ, Higgins BA, Gordon RD. Plasma levels of atrial natriuretic peptide in man in primary aldosteronism, in Gordon's syndrome and in Bartter's syndrome. Clin Exp Pharmacol Physiol 1986;13:341–5.

111. Gordon RD, Tunny TJ, Klemm SA. Indomethacin and atrial natriuretic peptide in Barrter's syndrome. N Engl J Med 1986;315:459.

112. Valimaki M, Pelkonen R, Tikkanen I, et al. A deficient response of atrial natriuretic peptide to volume overload in Gordon's syndrome. Acta Endocrinol (Copenh) 1989;120:331–6.

113. Gordon RD, Ravenscroft PJ, Klemm SA, et al. A new Australian kindred with the syndrome of hypertension and hyperkalemia has dysregulation of atrial natriuretic factor. J Hypertens 1988;8(Suppl 4):s323–6.

114. Ader JL, Waeber B, Suc JM, et al. [Arterial hypertension with hyperkalemia, tubular acidosis and normal renal function: Gordon syndrome and/or pseudohypoaldosteronism type II?] Arch Mal Coeur Vaiss 1988;81(Spec No):193–7 [in French].

115. Semmekrot B, Monnens L, Theelen BG, et al. The syndrome of hypertension and hyperkalaemia with normal glomerular function (Gordon's syndrome). A pathophysiological study. Pediatr Nephrol 1987;1:473–8.

116. Tormey WP, Morgan DB. Etiological considerations in Gordon's syndrome: possible role of prostaglandins. Prostaglandins Med 1980;4:107–12.

117. Stiefel P, Garcia-Morillo S, Miranda ML, et al. Gordon's syndrome: increased maximal rate of the Na-K-Cl cotransport and erythrocyte membrane replacement of sphingomyelin by phosphatidylethanolamine. J Hypertens 2000;18: 1327–30.

118. Farfel Z, Iaina A, Rosenthal T, et al. Familial hyperpotassemia and hypertension accompanied by normal plasma aldosterone levels: possible cell membrane defect. Arch Intern Med 1978;138:1828–32.

119. Disse-Nicodeme S, Desitter I, Fiquet-Kempf B, et al. Genetic heterogeneity of familial hyperkalaemic hypertension. J Hypertens 2001;19:1957–64.

120. Gordon RD, Klemm SA, Tunny TJ. Gordon's syndrome and Liddle's syndrome. In: Birkenhager WJ, Reid JL, editors. Handbook of hypertension, vol. 15 (Robertson JIS, editor. Clinical hypertension.). Amsterdam: Elsevier; 1992. p. 461–93.

121. Gordon RD. Syndrome of hypertension and hyperkalemia with normal glomerular filtration rate. Hypertension 1986;8:93–102.

122. Gordon RD, Tunny TJ, Klemm SA, et al. The syndrome of hypertension with hyperkalemia and normal glomerular filtration rate. A rare form of hypertension. In: Laragh JH, Brenner BM, editors. Hypertension: pathophysiology, diagnosis and management. New York: Raven Press; 1990. p. 1625–38.

123. Gordon RD, Klemm SA, Tunny TJ, et al. Gordon's syndrome: a sodium-volume-dependent form of hypertension with a genetic basis. In: Laragh JH, Brenner BM, editors. Hypertension: pathophysiology, diagnosis and treatment. 2nd edition. New York: Raven Press; 1995. p. 2111–23.

124. Sanjad SA, Mansour FM, Hernandez RH, et al. Severe hypertension, hyperkalemia and renal tubular acidosis responding to dietary sodium restriction. Pediatrics 1982;69:317–24.

125. Klemm SA, Gordon RD, Tunny TJ, et al. Biochemical correction in the syndrome of hypertension and hyperkalaemia by severe dietary salt restriction suggests renin-aldosterone suppression critical in pathophysiology. Clin Exp Pharmacol Physiol 1990;17:191–5.

126. Schambelan M, Sebastian A, Rector FC Jr. Mineralocorticoid-resistant renal hyperkalemia without salt wasting (type II pseudohypoaldosteronism): role of increased renal chloride reabsorption. Kidney Int 1981;19:716–27.

127. Mayan H, Mouallem M, Sharharabany M, et al. Resolution of hypertension during pregnancy in familial hyperkalemia and hypertension with the WNK4Q565E mutation. Am J Obstet Gynecol 2005;192:598–603.

128. Mansfield TA, Simon DB, Farfel Z, et al. Multilocus linkage of familial hyperkalae-mia and hypertension, pseudohypoaldosteronism type II, to chromosomes 1q31-42 and 17p11-q21. Nat Genet 1997;16:202–5.

129. O'Shaughnessy KM, Fu B, Johnson A, et al. Linkage of Gordon's syndrome to the long arm of chromosome 17 in a region recently linked to familial essential hypertension. J Hum Hypertens 1998;12:675–8.

130. Disse-Nicodeme S, Achard JM, Desitter I, et al. A new locus on chromosome 12p13.3 for pseudohypoaldosteronism type II, an autosomal dominant form of hypertension. Am J Hum Genet 2000;67:302–10.

131. Wilson FH, Disse-Nicodeme S, Choate KA, et al. Human hypertension caused by mutations in WNK kinases. Science 2001;293:1107–12.

132. Hadchouel J, Delaloy C, Faure S, et al. Familial hyperkalemic hypertension. J Am Soc Nephrol 2006;17:208–17.

133. Simon DB, Nelson-Williams C, Bia MJ, et al. Gitelman's variant of Barrter's syndrome, inherited hypokalemic alkalosis, is caused by mutations in the thiazide-sensitive Na-Cl cotransporter. Nat Genet 1996;12:24–30.

134. Mayan H, Vered I, Mouallem M, et al. Pseudohypoaldosteronism type II: marked sensitivity to thiazides, hypercalciuria, normomagnesemia, and low bone mineral density. J Clin Endocrinol Metab 2002;87:3248–54.

135. Mayan H, Melnikov S, Novikov I, et al. Familial hyperkalemia and hypertension: pathogenetic insights based on lithium clearance. J Clin Endocrinol Metab 2009;94:3010–6.

136. Weinstein SF, Allen DM, Mendoza SA. Hypertension, acidosis, and short stature associated with a defect in renal potassium excretion. J Pediatr 1974;85:353–8.

137. Rodriguez-Soriano J, Vallo A, Dominguez MJ. "Chloride-shunt" syndrome: an overlooked cause of renal hypercalciuria. Pediatr Nephrol 1989;3:113–21.

138. Klemm SA, Gordon RD, Tunny TJ, et al. The syndrome of hypertension and hy-perkalemia with normal GFR (Gordon's syndrome): is there increased proximal sodium reabsorption? Clin Invest Med 1991;14:551–8.

139. Thomsen K, Shirley DG. A hypothesis linking sodium and lithium reabsorption in the distal nephron. Nephrol Dial Transplant 2006;21:869–80.

140. Mayan H, Attar-Hertzberg D, Sharharabany M, et al. Increased urinary Na-Cl cotransporter protein in familial hyperkalemia and hypertension. Nephrol Dial Transplant 2008;23:492–6.

141. Choate KA, Kahle KT, Wilson FH, et al. WNK1, a kinase mutated in inherited hypertension with hyperkalemia, localizes to diverse Cl- -transporting epithelia. Proc Natl Acad Sci U S A 2003;100:663–8.

142. Kahle KT, Gimenez I, Hassan H, et al. WNK4 regulates apical and basolateral Cl- flux in extrarenal epithelia. Proc Natl Acad Sci U S A 2004;101:2064–9.

143. Farfel Z, Mayan H, Yaacov Y, et al. WNK4 regulates airway Na+ transport: study of familial hyperkalaemia and hypertension. Eur J Clin Invest 2005;35:410–5.

144. Kerem E, Bistritzer T, Hanukoglu A, et al. Pulmonary epithelial sodium-channel dysfunction and excess airway liquid in pseudohypoaldosteronism. N Engl J Med 1999;341:156–62.

145. Delaloy C, Hadchouel J, Imbert-Teboul M, et al. Cardiovascular expression of the mouse WNK1 gene during development and adulthood revealed by a BAC reporter assay. Am J Pathol 2006;169:105–18.

146. Levy D, DeStefano AL, Larson MG, et al. Evidence for a gene influencing blood pressure on chromosome 17. Genome scan linkage results for longitudinal blood pressure phenotypes in subjects from the Framingham Heart Study. Hypertension 2000;36:477–83.

147. Zhang H, Staessen JA. Association of blood pressure with genetic variation in WNK kinases in a white European population. Circulation 2005;112: 3371–2.
148. Glover M, Zuber AM, O'Shaughnessy KM. Hypertension, dietary salt intake, and the role of the thiazide-sensitive sodium chloride transporter NCCT. Cardiovasc Ther 2011;29(1):68–76.

Low-Renin Hypertension of Childhood

Alan A. Parsa, MD, Maria I. New, MD*

KEYWORDS

- Low-renin hypertension • Childhood • Adrenal synthetic defect
- Mineralocorticoid excess

Low-renin hypertension occurs in children as a result of several genetic mutations that cause mineralocorticoid excess or excess stimulation of the mineralocorticoid receptor.[1] The genetic disorders that cause low-renin hypertension are categorized as shown in **Box 1**.

ADRENAL SYNTHETIC DEFECTS
11β-Hydroxylase Deficiency

Congenital adrenal hyperplasia (CAH) owing to 11β-hydroxylase deficiency is the second most frequent form of CAH and represents up to 11% of all cases of CAH. The incidence of CAH is 1:100,000 births, with the highest number of cases in Moroccan Jews (1:5000–1:7000). CAH owing to 11β-hydroxylase deficiency occurs more frequently in the Sephardi Jewish population than in the Ashkenazi Jewish population. This genetic defect occurs in 2 forms: classic and nonclassic. The classic form causes a defect in the adrenal enzyme, 11β-hydroxylase as a result of the mutations encoding the enzyme **Fig. 1**.

Classic 11β-hydroxylase deficiency
Pathophysiology As a result of the enzyme defect of 11β-hydroxylase, deoxycorticosterone (DOC), a precursor of cortisol and corticosterone, accumulates.[2,3] DOC acts as a mineralocorticoid causing sodium retention (unlike the more frequent 21 hydroxylase deficiency), plasma volume expansion, and renin suppression. Because of the renin suppression, aldosterone secretion is substantially reduced. When dexamethasone is administered, the DOC level decreases, sodium retention decreases, plasma renin level increases, and the increased plasma renin stimulates the adrenal glomerulosa to

Department of Pediatrics, Mount Sinai School of Medicine, One Gustave L. Levy Place, Box 1198, New York, NY 10029, USA
* Corresponding author.
E-mail address: MARIA.NEW@MSSM.EDU

Endocrinol Metab Clin N Am 40 (2011) 369–377
doi:10.1016/j.ecl.2011.01.004

Box 1
Genetic causes of low-renin hypertension

1. Adrenal synthetic defects

   11β-Hydroxylase deficiency

   17α-Hydroxylase deficiency

2. Dexamethasone-suppressible hyperaldosteronism

3. Apparent mineralocorticoid excess

4. Primary hyperaldosteronism

   Adrenal hyperplasia

   Adrenal tumor (rare in childhood)

---

secrete aldosterone. As the DOC level decreases, the blood pressure of the patient also decreases. When the aldosterone level increases after glucocorticoid administration, it does not rise sufficiently for the hypertension to recur.

Phenotype As a result of the cortisol deficiency owing to the 11β-hydroxylase enzyme deficiency, adrenocorticotropic hormone (ACTH) level increases via the negative feedback mechanism, which then stimulates the adrenal fasciculata to oversecrete precursor hormones that are then shunted into the androgen pathway. The androgens, which are secreted by the fetal adrenal gland during fetal life, cause the affected female newborns to be born with ambiguous genitalia. Postnatally, these patients develop other hyperandrogenic symptoms, such as hirsutism, acne, hyperpigmentation, irregular menses, and impaired fertility, unless treated with glucocorticoids. Although hypokalemia should be a logical outcome of the excessive mineralocorticoid (ie, DOC), it is infrequently observed.

Genetics CAH owing to 11β-hydroxylase deficiency is caused by a mutation in the CYP11B1 gene. This gene is mapped to chromosome 8q22 and contains 9 exons. More than 40 mutations have been described in the CYP11B1 gene, which causes a decrease in cortisol secretion from the adrenal fasciculata.

Treatment The purpose of treatment is to suppress DOC secretion, reduce the blood pressure, and reduce adrenal androgens to minimize the hyperandrogenic symptoms and signs. Postnatally, the child should be treated with oral hydrocortisone (15 mg/m^2/d) rather than dexamethasone to avoid negative effects on growth. The serum hormone concentrations that are to be monitored for the adequacy of treatment are DOC, aldosterone, plasma renin concentration, Δ^4-androstenedione, and cortisol concentrations. Serum electrolyte levels (Na$^+$ and K$^+$) should be monitored along with blood pressure measurements every 3 months to assure proper clinical response to medication.

Nonclassic 11β-hydroxylase deficiency
Nonclassic 11β-hydroxylase deficiency presents with mild symptoms of hyperandrogenemia and mineralocorticoid excess.[3,4] But the signs and symptoms are variable. Plasma renin activity and renin concentrations are also variable. Genital ambiguity is either absent or mild in female newborns. In male newborns, evidence of puberty may occur precociously with an advanced bone age. Hormone levels typically

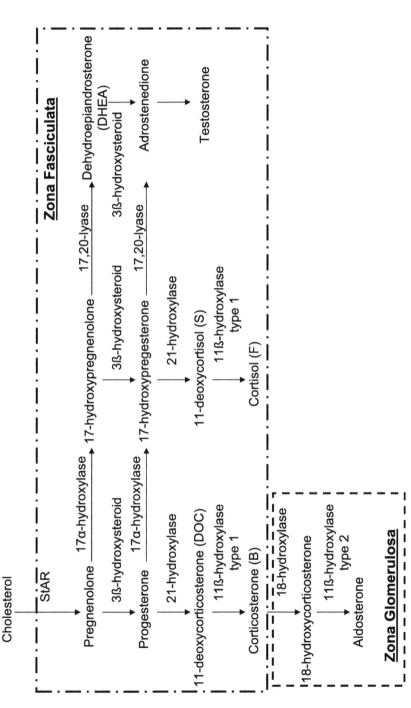

Fig. 1. Steroidogenesis in the adrenal cortex. StAR, steroidogenic acute regulatory protein.

demonstrate normal levels of cortisol, 17-hydroxyprogesterone, whereas DOC levels a somewhat elevated, but never to the extent observed in the classic form. In women, the clinical presentation may resemble polycystic ovarian syndrome. Although the frequency of nonclassic 11β-hydroxylase is unknown, it seems that it is less frequent than the classic form. White[3] observed 3 patients and reported mutations in the CYP11B1 gene in 2 patients but not in the third. In 2010, Rumsby and colleagues[4] described 7 novel mutations. The investigators reported a distinct difference between the classic (3 patients) and the nonclassic (2 patients) mutations. Further, there were 3 heterozygous carriers of nonclassic mutation who manifested the phenotype of the nonclassic form. All the genes were mapped to 8q22. This rare syndrome primarily described phenotypically and hormonally can now benefit from genetic analysis for the differences in genotype.[4]

17α-Hydroxylase Deficiency

Pathophysiology

As a result of the defective 17α-hydroxylase enzyme early in steroid synthesis (see **Fig. 1**), the 17-desoxy pathway is stimulated and the serum concentration of the 17-desoxy steroids, including DOC and corticosterone, are elevated.[5,6] Because desoxycorticosterone is a mineralocorticoid causing sodium retention, the same pathophysiology as that of 11β-hydroxylase deficiency (described earlier) applies to 17α-hydroxylase as well. Thus, renin is suppressed, aldosterone levels are very low, and hypertension is present. When dexamethasone is administered and the DOC levels decrease, the hypertension is ameliorated and the plasma renin level increases, stimulating the glomerulosa to secrete aldosterone.

Phenotype

The most prominent phenotypic evidence of 17α-hydroxylase deficiency in the 46,XY patient is the impaired virilization in utero, resulting in genital ambiguity.[7] These patients also fail to demonstrate secondary male sexual characteristics. Because of unknown reasons, breast development is a prominent feature in the 46,XY patient during puberty, whereas it is not seen in the 46,XX patient. Some of these 46,XY patients are raised as women. In 46,XX individuals, there is no genital ambiguity, but there is sexual infantilism at puberty with no breast development as evidence of estrogen insufficiency. Since the first report by Biglieri in 1966,[5] when he described the first 17α-hydroxylase deficiency in a woman with sexual infantilism, subsequent 46,XX female patients have demonstrated the inability to undergo secondary sexual characteristics at puberty.

Genotype

The gene for 17α-hydroxylase deficiency has been mapped to chromosome 10. Several mutations in the structural gene have been described. Despite its rarity, 17α-hydroxylase deficiency is prominent in Dutch Mennonites because of a founder effect resulting from immigrants from Spain and Portugal.[8] More than 46 mutations have been described to date. The frequency of 17α-hydroxylase deficiency is less than 1% of the total cases of CAH.

Treatment

Girls require estrogen to encourage puberty, whereas boys require testosterone treatment. Boys, depending on the degree of breast development, may need to undergo mammoplasty and need to continue dexamethasone treatment to maintain blood pressure control.

DEXAMETHASONE SUPPRESSIBLE HYPERALDOSTERONISM/GLUCOCORTICOID REMEDIABLE HYPERALDOSTERONISM/FAMILIAL HYPERALDOSTERONISM TYPE I

Please refer to the article by Halperin and Dluhy elsewhere in this issue.

APPARENT MINERALOCORTICOID EXCESS

Apparent mineralocorticoid excess (AME) has been regarded as prismatic because it changed the knowledge of receptor biology.[9–12] The syndrome is described in **Box 2**. Hormonal evaluation demonstrates low secretion of all adrenal hormones. The disorder was first described biochemically by New[11] in a 3-year old Zuni Indian child who survived cardiac catheterization without steroids being administered despite the very low to unmeasurable levels of adrenal steroids. The child's blood pressure was found to be markedly elevated with a very low serum potassium level. After intensive investigation, the pathophysiology of the disorder was elucidated.

Pathophysiology

In humans, protection from excess cortisol secretion occurs from the conversion of cortisol to cortisone by the enzyme 11β-hydroxysteroid type 2 (11βHSD2) in the distal convoluted tubules of the kidney. Cortisone unlike cortisol does not bind to the mineralocorticoid or glucocorticoid receptor. In AME, the 11βHSD2 enzyme is deficient as a result of a genetic defect in the 11βHSD2 gene. Cortisol secreted from the adrenal glands normally gets converted to the bioinactive form cortisone in the distal tubules of the kidney. In the patient with AME who has an 11βHSD2 deficiency, this conversion does not occur and all the cortisol secreted by the adrenals remains bioactive. Because cortisol is secreted in milligram amounts, whereas aldosterone is secreted in microgram amounts, cortisol overwhelms the mineralocorticoid receptor excluding aldosterone from binding (**Fig. 2**). Thus, the mineralocorticoid receptor of the renal distal tubule is activated by cortisol, causing hypertension and hypokalemia, suppressing renin, and causing the aldosterone secretion from the zona glomerulosa to be reduced to undetectable. Further, the bioactive cortisol enters the glucocorticoid receptor of the pituitary, causing ACTH to be severely reduced and all adrenal hormones from the fasciculata to be barely detectable.

Box 2
AME syndrome

1. Low-renin hypertension aggravated by ACTH and glucocorticoids

2. Hypokalemia aggravated by ACTH and glucocorticoids

3. Low to undetectable adrenal steroid urinary excretion

4. Low secretion rates of all adrenal steroids

5. Capacity to survive serious stress without glucocorticoid treatment

6. Remission of hypertension by salt deprivation and diuretics

7. Remission of hypertension and hypokalemia with spironolactone administration

8. Long serum half-life of cortisol

Data from New MI, Wilson RC. Steroid disorders in children: congenital adrenal hyperplasia and apparent mineralocorticoid excess. Proc Natl Acad Sci USA 1999;96:12790–7; and Cerame BI, New MI. Hormonal hypertension in children: 11beta-hydroxylase deficiency and apparent mineralocorticoid excess. J Pediatr Endocrinol Metab 2000;13:1537–47.

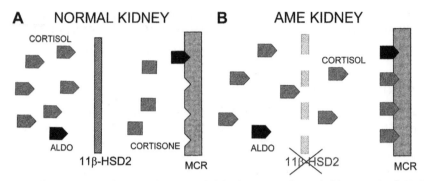

Fig. 2. (*A*) The action of 11β-hydroysteroid dehydrogenase (encoded by 11βHSD2) in the normal kidney where cortisol is converted to cortisone by 11β-hydroxysteroid dehydrogenase. Cortisone does not enter the mineralocorticoid receptor. (*B*) Absence of 11β-hydroxysteroid dehydrogenase in the AME kidney, which results in decreased conversion of cortisol to cortisone. Cortisol binds to the mineralocorticoid receptor and overwhelms it.

Genetics

The HSD11B2 gene has been mapped to chromosome 16q22.[13] Many mutations have been described (**Fig. 3**). The disorder is transmitted as an autosomal recessive trait and is more frequent in consanguineous and endogamous populations (**Fig. 4**).

Treatment

AME is potentially fatal. Patients have been reported to die from hypertensive stroke and cardiac arrest. Complications of severe hypertension and hypokalemia are common. Calcium/phosphorous disturbances occur with nephrocalcinosis. A few

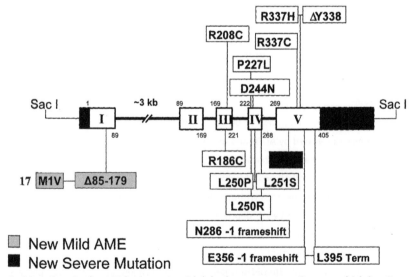

Fig. 3. Mutations in the 11β-hydroxysteroid dehydrogenase type 2 gene, which has 5 exons. The mutations in the mild as well as the severe form of AME are shown. (*Adapted from* Wilson RC, Nimkarn S, New MI. Apparent mineralocorticoid excess. Trends Endocrinol Metab 2001;12:104–11; with permission.)

AME FAMILIES – ETHNIC GROUP – NATIVE AMERICANS

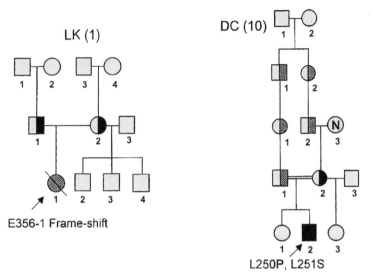

Fig. 4. Pedigree of 2 families with members with AME demonstrating consanguinity and endogamy. (*From* Wilson RC, Harbison MD, Krozowski ZS, et al. Several homozygous mutations in the gene for 11 beta-hydroxysteroid dehydrogenase type 2 in patients with apparent mineralocorticoid excess. J Clin Endocrinol Metab 1995;80:3145–50; with permission.)

cases have demonstrated rickets.[14] The syndrome has been mimicked by glycyrrhetinic acid (licorice) and carbenoxolone. The most effective treatment is spironolactone in doses from 50 to 200 mg daily. Other diuretics may be added if necessary. Renal transplantation has been reported to be a cure in a Sardinian woman with AME.[15]

MILD AME IN AN INBRED MENNONITE FAMILY

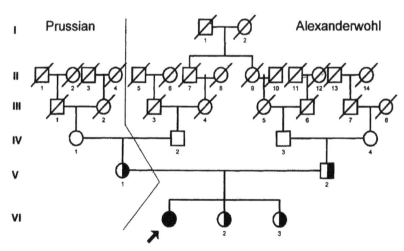

Fig. 5. Pedigree of a consanguineous Mennonite family. (*Adapted from* Wilson RC, Nimkarn S, New MI. Apparent mineralocorticoid excess. Trends Endocrinol Metab 2001;12:104–11; with permission.)

Mild Forms of AME

A Mennonite child from Kansas was diagnosed locally with low-renin hypertension, and AME was suspected.[16,17] The diagnosis, however, was unclear because the patient, a 12-year-old girl, did not have hypokalemia, low birth weight, or severe hypertension. The patient presented with low renin levels, mild hypertension, and low aldosterone concentrations. Consanguinity was prominent in the pedigree (**Fig. 5**). The final proof of the diagnosis for AME was in the DNA analysis, which demonstrated a new and specific mutation of the mild form of AME (see **Fig. 3**).

PRIMARY HYPERALDOSTERONISM

Primary hyperaldosteronism in childhood is extremely rare. In childhood, it is most frequently the result of adrenal hyperplasia. Treatment of this disorder is very controversial and no treatment has resulted in great success in lowering aldosterone and blood pressure. Primary aldosteronism as a result of an aldosterone-secreting adrenal adenoma (Conn syndrome), which is a frequent cause of hyperaldosteronism in adults, is almost never seen in childhood. If primary aldosteronism occurs, it responds to the removal of the tumor.

REFERENCES

1. New MI, Geller DS, Fallo F. Monogenic low renin hypertension [review]. Trends Endocrinol Metab 2005;16(3):92–7.
2. Bhangoo A, Wilson R, New MI, et al. Donor splice mutation in the 11β-hydroxylase (CYP11B1) gene resulting in sex reversal: a case report and review of the literature. J Pediatr Endocrinol Metab 2006;19:1267–82.
3. White PC, Schmitt K, Kofler R, et al. CYP11B1 mutations causing non-classic adrenal hyperplasia due to 11 beta-hydroxylase deficiency. Hum Mol Genet 1997;6:1829–34.
4. Rumsby G, Arlt W, Krone N, et al. Functional consequences of seven novel mutations in the CYP11B1 gene: four mutations associated with nonclassic and three mutations causing classic 11 beta-hydroxylase deficiency. J Clin Endocrinol Metab 2010;95:779–88.
5. Biglieri EG. 17-Hydroxylation deficiency in man. J Clin Invest 1966;45:1946–54.
6. Miller WL. Steroid 17 α-hydroxylase deficiency—not rare everywhere. J Clin Endocrinol Metab 2004;89(1):40–2.
7. New MI (with the technical assistance of Suvannakul L). Male pseudohermaphroditism due to 17α hydroxylase deficiency. J Clin Invest 1970;49:1930–41.
8. Imai T, Yanase T, Waterman MR, et al. Canadian Mennonites and individuals residing in the Friesland region of the Netherlands share the same molecular basis of 17α hydroxylase deficiency. Hum Genet 1992;89:95–6.
9. Ulick S, Ramirez LC, New MI. An abnormality in steroid reductive metabolism in a hypertensive syndrome. J Clin Endocrinol Metab 1977;44:799–802.
10. Morineau G, Sulmont V, Salomon R, et al. Apparent mineralocorticoid excess: report of six new cases and extensive personal experience. J Am Soc Nephrol 2006;17(11):3176–84.
11. New MI, Levine LS, Biglieri EG, et al. Evidence for an unidentified steroid in a child with apparent mineralocorticoid hypertension. J Clin Endocrinol Metab 1977;44:924–33.
12. Wilson RC, Harbison MD, Krozowski ZS, et al. Several homozygous mutations in the gene for 11 beta-hydroxysteroid dehydrogenase type 2 in patients with

apparent mineralocorticoid excess. J Clin Endocrinol Metab 1995;80(11): 3145–50.

13. Krozowski Z, Baker E, Obeyesekere V, et al. Localization of the gene for human 11 beta-hydroxysteroid dehydrogenase type 2 (HSD11B2) to chromosome band 16q22. Cytogenet Cell Genet 1995;71(2):124–5.

14. Mendonça BB, Batista MC, Kater CE. Spironolactone-reversible rickets associated with 11β-hydroxysteroid dehydrogenase deficiency syndrome. J Pediatr 1986;109(6):989–93.

15. Palermo M, Delitala G, Sorba G, et al. Does kidney transplantation normalize cortisol metabolism in apparent mineralocorticoid excess syndrome? J Endocrinol Invest 2000;23(7):457–62.

16. Lavery GG, Ronconi V, Draper N, et al. Late-onset apparent mineralocorticoid excess caused by novel compound heterozygous mutations in the HSD11B2 gene. Hypertension 2003;42:123–9.

17. Ugrasbul F, Wiens T, Rubinstein P, et al. Prevalence of mild apparent mineralocorticoid excess in Mennonites. J Clin Endocrinol Metab 1999;84:4735–8.

Cushing's Syndrome: All Variants, Detection, and Treatment

Susmeeta T. Sharma, MBBS, Lynnette K. Nieman, MD*

KEYWORDS

- Cushing's syndrome • Hypertension • Glucocorticoids
- Ectopic ACTH secretion
- 11 Beta-hydroxysteroid dehydrogenase • Hypercortisolemia

Cushing's syndrome is a rare disorder that results from prolonged and pathologic exposure to excess glucocorticoids. The incidence of Cushing's syndrome varies depending on the population studied, anywhere from 2 to 3 cases per million population per year.[1–3] More recent data suggests that this is probably an underestimate and Cushing's syndrome may be more common than previously thought.[4,5] Iatrogenic Cushing's syndrome caused by the administration of supraphysiologic doses of glucocorticoids is probably much more common (although underreported) than endogenous causes.

The clinical presentation of Cushing's syndrome varies widely. Although the diagnosis is straightforward in full-blown cases, establishing the diagnosis can be difficult in mild hypercortisolism especially because none of the signs or symptoms is pathognomonic of the syndrome (**Box 1**). However, some of the signs that have been reported to better distinguish Cushing's syndrome from simple obesity include proximal muscle weakness, easy bruising, violaceous striae greater than 1 cm, and hypertension.[6,7] The clinical presentation differs in children, in whom weight gain and growth retardation are more prominent.[8]

Biochemical confirmation of hypercortisolism is necessary when the clinical presentation suggests Cushing's syndrome. According to the 2008 Endocrine Society

---

This work was supported by the intramural program of the *Eunice Kennedy Shriver* National Institute of Child Health and Human Development, National Institutes of Health.

On part of the NIH, Dr Nieman participates in a Cooperative Research and Development Agreement (CRADA) with HRA-Pharma to evaluate mifepristone treatment of ectopic ACTH secretion. Dr Sharma has nothing to disclose.

Program on Reproductive and Adult Endocrinology, *Eunice Kennedy Shriver* National Institute of Child Health and Human Development, National Institutes of Health, Building 10, CRC, 1East, Room 3140, 10 Center Drive, Bethesda, MD 20892-1109, USA

* Corresponding author.

E-mail address: niemanl@nih.gov

Endocrinol Metab Clin N Am 40 (2011) 379–391

doi:10.1016/j.ecl.2011.01.006

0889-8529/11/$ – see front matter. Published by Elsevier Inc.

endo.theclinics.com

Box 1
Signs and symptoms of Cushing's syndrome

Hypertension

Adipose

    Weight gain

    Increased centripetal, supraclavicular, temporal, or dorsocervical fat

Skin

    Hirsutism

    Striae (especially if >1-cm diameter and purple)

    Easy bruising

    Plethora

Reproductive system

    Menstrual irregularity

    Amenorrhea

    Decreased libido

Psychiatric and cognitive

    Depression

    Emotional lability

    Irritability

    Decreased memory

    Decreased concentration

Skeleton and muscle

    Proximal muscle weakness

    Reduced bone mineral density

    Fractures

Metabolism

    Impaired glucose tolerance

    Diabetes

---

guidelines, any of the following tests can be used for the initial diagnosis of Cushing's syndrome: 24-hour urinary free cortisol, late-night salivary cortisol, or a dexamethasone suppression test (DST, either as a 1-mg overnight test or the longer low-dose test using 2 mg/d over 48 hours).[9]

After 2 different abnormal tests establish the diagnosis, the cause of Cushing's syndrome must be determined. Endogenous Cushing's syndrome can be divided into adrenocorticotropin (ACTH)-dependent and independent forms. ACTH-independent Cushing's syndrome (15%) results from increased autonomous production of cortisol from adrenal tumors (adenoma or carcinoma) or hyperplasia. Corticotropin-dependent causes of Cushing's syndrome include ACTH production from pituitary (Cushing's disease, 70%) or other tumors (ectopic Cushing's syndrome, 15%) and, rarely, corticotropin-releasing hormone (CRH)–producing tumors.[10,11]

Measurement of plasma ACTH level is the first step in the differential diagnosis strategy. A low normal or undetectable value reflects suppression of the normal corticotropes by excess cortisol and points to an adrenal source of hypercortisolemia. In these so-called ACTH-independent forms, imaging of the adrenal glands with computerized tomography or magnetic resonance imaging (MRI) should be performed to identify the sites of abnormality.

Conversely, an elevated or inappropriately normal ACTH level reflects a pituitary or an ectopic source of ACTH as a cause of excessive cortisol (as the normal corticotropes are suppressed). Differentiating between these two etiologies can be challenging. Pituitary MRI should be obtained first. If a pituitary mass larger than 6 mm is found, and biochemical testing with CRH stimulation test and high-dose 8-mg DST are consistent with Cushing's disease, no further testing is necessary. If the biochemical testing is discordant and the pituitary MRI is normal or equivocal (mass <6 mm), bilateral inferior petrosal sinus sampling (IPSS) should be strongly considered. Alternatively, IPSS may be obtained without additional biochemical testing because it has the highest diagnostic accuracy. A significant central-to-peripheral ACTH gradient during IPSS (more than 2 before, and more than 3 after CRH administration) indicates Cushing's disease. In the absence of a gradient, a search for an ectopic source should be performed using various imaging modalities.[3,10]

HYPERTENSION IN CUSHING'S SYNDROME

The increased mortality of Cushing's syndrome is caused in part by an increased risk of vascular disease up to 5 times the population average.[2,12] In one prospective study, ultrasound identified atherosclerotic plaques in both carotid arteries in 8 of 25 subjects with active Cushing's disease and 2 of 32 age-, sex-, and body mass index-matched controls.[13]

Hypertension, impaired glucose tolerance, diabetes, dyslipidemia, and visceral obesity are common cardiovascular risk factors in patients with Cushing's syndrome. Hypertension, although not invariable, is a frequent feature of endogenous Cushing's syndrome with a prevalence of approximately 80% in adults. It is even more common (95%) in ectopic Cushing's syndrome[14]; whereas, in children and adolescents, it is less common (about 47%).[15] By contrast, hypertension is present in only about 20% of patients with iatrogenic Cushing's syndrome, where it correlates with the daily dose of glucocorticoid.[16,17]

Studies have clearly shown that in the general population, the chance of myocardial infarction, heart failure, stroke, and kidney disease increases as blood pressure increases.[18] In a meta-analysis of 61 prospective studies of individuals aged 40 to 69 years, Lewington and colleagues[19] reported that for every 20-mm Hg systolic or 10-mm Hg diastolic increase in blood pressure, there is a 2-fold increase in mortality from ischemic heart disease and stroke.

Because of the potential impact of hypertension on morbidity and mortality, it is important to understand its causes and to treat it. The purpose of this article is to review the various possible mechanisms leading to hypertension in Cushing's syndrome and its treatment.

Physiology of Blood Pressure in Cushing's Syndrome

Healthy adults have a diurnal variation in blood pressure, with a decrease in blood pressure during sleep. This decrease parallels that of cortisol, and may reflect decreased sensitivity to catecholamines. The absence of sleep-related decrease in blood pressure is found in several pathologic conditions, including glucocorticoid-induced hypertension.[20,21]

In 2004, Zacharieva and colleagues[22] performed 24-hour ambulatory blood pressure monitoring in 100 subjects with Cushing's syndrome (80 with Cushing's disease and 20 with adrenal causes) and 40 subjects with essential hypertension. They found that the nighttime decrease in blood pressure in subjects with each type of Cushing's syndrome was significantly reduced compared with subjects with essential hypertension. However, the nocturnal fall in heart rate was preserved in both groups of subjects. The blunted decrease in nighttime blood pressure improved with treatment of Cushing's syndrome and the degree of improvement was negatively correlated with the duration of hypercortisolism. Administration of supraphysiologic doses of exogenous glucocorticoids leads to a similar loss of the nocturnal fall in blood pressure.[23]

Pathogenesis of Hypertension in Cushing's Syndrome

Glucocorticoids play an important role in blood pressure regulation. Several mechanisms have been postulated to explain how hypercortisolism leads to hypertension in Cushing's syndrome. These mechanisms include mineralocorticoid effects of cortisol, activation of the renin angiotensin system (RAS), and the action of cortisol on peripheral and systemic vasculature.[17,24]

Mineralocorticoid Effects of Cortisol: Role of 11 Beta-hydroxysteroid Dehydrogenase

Cortisol binds to both type 1 (mineralocorticoid) and type 2 (glucocorticoid) receptors. It is likely that glucocorticoid-induced hypertension is mediated through effects of cortisol on both receptors. At the cellular level, cortisol availability is modulated by the 2 isoforms of the enzyme 11 beta-hydroxysteroid dehydrogenase (11βHSD).[25]

11βHSD1 is a nicotinamide adenine dinucleotide phosphate (NADPH)-dependent enzyme that is most abundantly expressed in liver and adipose tissue. It has bidirectional activity and catalyzes both dehydrogenation (conversion of cortisol to cortisone) and reduction (conversion of cortisone to cortisol) reactions. In vivo, it predominantly functions as a reductase, converting inactive cortisone to active cortisol. This reductase activity relies on high NADPH concentrations, which in turn are dependent on the activity of hexose-6-phosphate dehydrogenase within the endoplasmic reticulum.

11βHSD2 is an NADPH-dependent enzyme and predominantly acts as a dehydrogenase to convert cortisol into inactive cortisone. It is abundantly expressed in the classical mineralocorticoid target tissues, including the renal cortex, colon, and salivary glands.[17,25] Both 11βHSD1 and 11βHSD2 are present in vascular endothelial cells, coronary artery cells, and vascular smooth muscles, thereby modulating local access of cortisol to the vasculature.[26,27]

In vitro, the mineralocorticoid receptor has similar binding affinity for both cortisol and aldosterone. However, the circulating levels of cortisol in healthy individuals are about 100- to 1000-times higher than aldosterone levels. The in vivo selectivity of the renal mineralocorticoid receptor for aldosterone requires conversion of cortisol to cortisone by 11βHSD2, rendering it unable to bind to the mineralocorticoid receptor.[28,29]

The global activity of 11βHSD can be assessed by measurement of urinary steroid metabolites. Both cortisol and cortisone undergo A-ring reduction by 5 α- and 5 β-reductases and 3 α-hydroxysteroid dehydrogenase, yielding 5 β-tetrahydrocortisol (THF), 5 α-tetrahydrocortisol (allo-THF) and 5 β-tetrahydrocortisone (THE). The overall 11βHSD1 and 11βHSD2 activity in the body is reflected in the ratio of urinary cortisol and cortisone metabolites (THF + allo-THF/THE). Alternatively, urine cortisol-to-cortisone ratio or plasma cortisol-to-cortisone ratio can also help in the evaluation.[25,30]

One potential etiology for hypertension in Cushing's syndrome is decreased renal conversion of cortisol to cortisone, which would increase mineralocorticoid action.

In Cushing's syndrome, the urinary THF + allo-THF/THE ratio is elevated, especially in patients with the highest urine free cortisol. These findings suggest that high cortisol levels can overwhelm the 11βHSD2 enzyme because of substrate saturation leading to spillover of cortisol to the mineralocorticoid receptor. This result may cause a functional mineralocorticoid excess state with hypokalemia, increased renal tubular sodium reabsorption, intravascular volume expansion, and hypertension.[14,31] These findings are similar to those in patients with inactivating mutations of 11βHSD2 who have a syndrome of apparent mineralocorticoid excess (SAME).[25] However, in SAME, the aldosterone and renin levels are suppressed in comparison to those seen in Cushing's syndrome.

Other studies suggest that cortisol-induced hypertension is not primarily mediated via sodium retention. Connell and colleagues[32] gave ACTH (1 mg/d) to healthy volunteers on a sodium-restricted diet (15 mmol/d). They noted that systolic blood pressure rose significantly from a mean value of 116 mm Hg to 125 mm Hg and plasma volume rose from a mean of 2.8 L to 3.6 L. The level of increase in blood pressure was less than that seen in previous studies in which ACTH was given to subjects on a normal-sodium diet, suggesting that dietary sodium restriction lessens but does not prevent the rise in blood pressure with hypercortisolemia. Williamson and colleagues[33] demonstrated that mineralocorticoid blockade with spironolactone (400 mg/d) did not affect the increased blood pressure seen in subjects given cortisol (80 and 200 mg/d), even though it completely blocked salt and water retention. In another study, Whitworth and colleagues[34] showed that administration of synthetic glucocorticoids with little or no mineralocorticoid activity increased blood pressure without salt and water retention. Finally, the glucocorticoid antagonist mifepristone can normalize blood pressure in Cushing's syndrome but does not bind to the mineralocorticoid receptor.[35] These findings indicate that a functional mineralocorticoid excess state is not the sole pathogenic mechanism, and the glucocorticoid receptor is involved in the development of hypertension in Cushing's syndrome.

GLUCOCORTICOID EFFECTS ON VASCULATURE
Enhanced Action of the Renin Angiotensin System

In rodent models, glucocorticoids increase angiotensinogen production.[36] Despite this potential increase in substrate, plasma angiotensin II levels and renin activity are usually normal or suppressed in patients with Cushing's syndrome. However, animal studies have shown that glucocorticoids increase angiotensin II receptor type 1 concentration in brain and peripheral tissue. They also enhance angiotensin II-stimulated inositol phosphate-3 production in vascular smooth muscle cells[37,38] and its central pressor effects.[39] Patients with Cushing's syndrome show an increased pressor response to angiotensin II, suggesting increased sensitivity to the agent. These data support the concept that the renin angiotensin system may play a role in the pathophysiology of glucocorticoid-induced hypertension through upregulation of central and peripheral angiotensin II receptors.

Inhibition of Vasodilators

In addition to enhancing RAS activity, glucocorticoids impair vasodilation.[40] Although circulating levels of the vasodilator atrial natriuretic peptide (ANP) are increased in experimental and clinical conditions of glucocorticoid excess, in vitro studies show that glucocorticoids decrease its biologic activity.[41] Sala and colleagues[40] administered physiologic doses of ANP to normotensive healthy volunteers, and subjects with

Cushing's disease or essential hypertension. Despite a 4-fold increase in ANP levels in all groups, the biologic response, increase in plasma and urine cGMP, was much lower in subjects with Cushing's disease.

Glucocorticoids also decrease production of nitric oxide synthase, which is responsible for the synthesis of another vasodilator, nitric oxide.[42] Glucocorticoids also inhibit production of other potent vasodilators, such as prostacyclin, prostaglandin E2, and kallikrein.[43,44] This inhibition may increase blood pressure by decreasing peripheral vasodilation.

Enhanced Vascular Reactivity to Vasopressors

Glucocorticoids increase the vascular sensitivity to the effects of catecholamines. Studies in healthy volunteers demonstrate that glucocorticoids increase the sensitivity to infusions of phenylephrine, angiotensin II, and norepinephrine resulting in an increase in peripheral vascular resistance and mean arterial blood pressure.[44–46] Although plasma concentrations of various vasopressor hormones are normal in patients with Cushing's syndrome, an increase in beta-adrenergic receptor sensitivity has been documented.[45]

Endothelin-1 (ET-1) is a potent vasoconstrictor produced by vascular smooth muscle cells and endothelial cells. Plasma levels of ET-1 are significantly elevated in patients with Cushing's syndrome.[47] However, studies looking at the role of ET-1 in glucocorticoid-induced hypertension have conflicting results. On one hand, dexamethasone decreases endothelin receptors in the kidney and the nonselective endothelin antagonist bosentan has no effect on ACTH-induced hypertension in rats. On the other hand, in animal studies, chronic use of endothelin type-A receptor antagonist normalizes blood pressure in 11βHSD inhibitor-induced hypertension.[48] Therefore, the contribution of the endothelin-1 pathway to glucocorticoid-induced hypertension requires further study.

Glucocorticoids also appear to downregulate the expression of the sodium-calcium exchanger in vascular smooth muscle cells, which in turn increases the cytoplasmic concentration of calcium, and leads to vasoconstriction.[49] Plasma levels of erythropoietin, another vasoconstrictor, have also been shown to increase with glucocorticoids and may play a role in glucocorticoid induced hypertension.[50]

Other Indirect Factors

Obstructive sleep apnea (OSA) has been reported in patients with Cushing's syndrome.[51] This finding represents an additional etiology because OSA is associated with hypertension. Moreover, obesity-associated hypertension may occur regardless of cortisol levels and may also contribute to hypertension in Cushing's syndrome.

MANAGEMENT OF HYPERTENSION IN CUSHING'S SYNDROME

Because excess cortisol levels in Cushing's syndrome mediate hypertension, the therapeutic goal is to find and surgically remove the cause of excess glucocorticoids. Although this may lead to resolution or improvement of hypertension, in some cases complete normalization is not achieved. In patients with occult ACTH-secreting tumors, as well as in those awaiting surgery, antihypertensive agents and antiglucocorticoid agents are useful adjunctive therapies.

MEDICAL MANAGEMENT

Although the optimal therapy for Cushing's syndrome is surgical, medical treatment of hypercortisolism is often required while awaiting surgery and also when surgery is contraindicated or a tumor cannot be found. Medical agents include compounds that modulate ACTH release (dopamine and somatostatin agonists), inhibit steroidogenesis (metyrapone, ketoconazole, and mitotane), or block glucocorticoid action at its receptor (mifepristone). Normalization of cortisol is generally associated with improved blood pressure, although metyrapone may exacerbate hypertension by increasing mineralocorticoid production.

The steroidogenesis inhibitors metyrapone and ketoconazole have a rapid onset of action. However, because of an escape phenomenon where ACTH secretion overrides control of hypercortisolemia, these drugs are usually not effective as the sole long-term treatment for Cushing's disease. They are usually used as adjunctive agents after surgery or radiotherapy, or in preparation for surgery. The escape phenomenon is less likely with high doses of mitotane, presumably because of its adrenolytic effects. The choice of agent is individualized depending on the side-effect profile and other factors (**Table 1**). One of the main concerns with all medical agents is overtreatment that can render patients adrenally insufficient. Therefore, all patients receiving such treatment should be educated in the use of glucocorticoids in an emergency.

Agents evaluated for inhibition of pituitary tumoral ACTH secretion include bromocriptine, cabergoline, octreotide, and the investigational somatostatin-dopamine chimeric drug SOM230.[52] Successful normalization or control of hypercortisolemia leads to better control of hypertension. However, these agents are not uniformly effective and their role in treatment of ACTH-dependent Cushing's syndrome is not defined. Despite early promise, peroxisome proliferator activated receptor γ agonists are not effective.[53,54]

In addition to antiglucocorticoid agents, antihypertensive agents should be used. Patients usually require more than 1 agent to reach the target blood pressure levels

Table 1
Steroidogenesis inhibitors and glucocorticoid antagonist for treatment of hypercortisolism

Name	Mechanism of Action	Time to Onset of Action	Side Effects	Other Concerns
Metyrapone	Inhibits CYP11B1	Days	Hirsutism, hypertension, gastrointestinal effects	In United States, available only from the manufacturer as of 2010
Ketoconazole	Inhibits CYP11B1 and CYP11A1	Days	Gastrointestinal, gynecomastia, rarely hepatic dyscrasia	Enzyme inhibition leads to decreased testosterone; requires gastric acidity for bioavailability
Mitotane	Adrenolytic; inhibits CYP11B1 and CYP11A1; possibly other actions	Months	Gastrointestinal (common); central nervous system (lethargy, dizziness)	Hepatic enzyme inducer; teratogenic; fat soluble
Mifepristone	Reversible blockade of glucocorticoid receptor	Days	Risk of adrenal insufficiency	Also antagonizes androgen and progesterone receptor

recommended by JNC 7. Because the upregulation of RAS may be involved in glucocorticoid-induced hypertension, angiotensin-converting enzyme inhibitors (ACEI) and angiotensin II receptor blockers (ARB) are recommended. ACEIs and ARBs ameliorate hypertension in almost 50% of patients who are hypertensive with Cushing's disease.[55–57] Although adrenergic blockade and calcium channel blockers may be ineffective alone, they may be useful in combination therapy.[58]

Hypertension can be difficult to control with antihypertensive agents without normalization of hypercortisolemia. Fallo and colleagues[59] conducted a retrospective study of 40 subjects with hypertension in Cushing syndrome; 28 had received conventional antihypertensive therapy and 12 were treated with ketoconazole. Blood pressure normalized in only 4 of the 28 subjects on conventional treatment. A total of 12 of the remaining 24 subjects were placed on ketoconazole, with normalization of blood pressure in all but 1 subject. In the second group, 11 of the 12 subjects achieved normal blood pressure with ketoconazole alone. Whether this reflects bias in allocation to either treatment or suboptimal use of antihypertensive medications is not known. Specific treatment of hypertension and normalization of cortisol levels is essential in Cushing 's syndrome.

SURGICAL TREATMENT OF CUSHING'S SYNDROME

Surgical excision of cortisol or ACTH-producing tumors remains the optimal treatment of Cushing's syndrome. Worldwide, transsphenoidal resection of pituitary adenoma for Cushing's disease has immediate postoperative cure rates of 78% to 97%, with best results with microadenomas and experienced neurosurgeons. Unilateral or bilateral adrenalectomy is used for primary adrenal disease, depending on its location. Localization and surgical excision of nonmetastatic ectopic ACTH-secreting tumors leads to cure. Bilateral adrenalectomy can be considered when a tumor cannot be localized or other treatments have failed.[10]

Not all patients become normotensive, even after curative surgery for Cushing's syndrome. Studies have shown that about one-third of adult patients continue to have hypertension after surgery.[60–62] Persistent hypertension after surgery correlates with the duration, but not the severity, of preoperative hypertension. These findings are similar to rates of persistent hypertension after treatment of other forms of secondary hypertension in adults, and probably reflect irreparable damage or remodeling of the vasculature from long-standing hypertension. By contrast, children and adolescents show complete resolution of hypertension within 1 year after surgical cure.[15] The exact reason for this is not known but it may be related to the shorter duration of hypercortisolemia or vascular protective factors in younger patients.

SUMMARY

Cushing's syndrome results from chronic pathologic exposure to glucocorticoids. Hypertension is present in almost 80% of patients with Cushing's syndrome and if left uncontrolled can lead to an increased cardiovascular risk and mortality. Although the exact pathophysiology leading to hypertension in Cushing's syndrome is still not known, several possible mechanisms have been proposed (**Fig. 1**). These mechanisms include the presence of a functional mineralocorticoid excess state secondary to substrate saturation of the 11βHSD2 enzyme, upregulation of the renin angiotensin system, inhibition of vasodilators, and an enhanced vasoreactivity to vasopressors. Control of hypercortisolemia is important for blood pressure control. Normalization of hypercortisolemia via surgical resection of the source of excess glucocorticoids (adrenal pathology, pituitary adenoma, or an ectopic tumor) remains the therapeutic

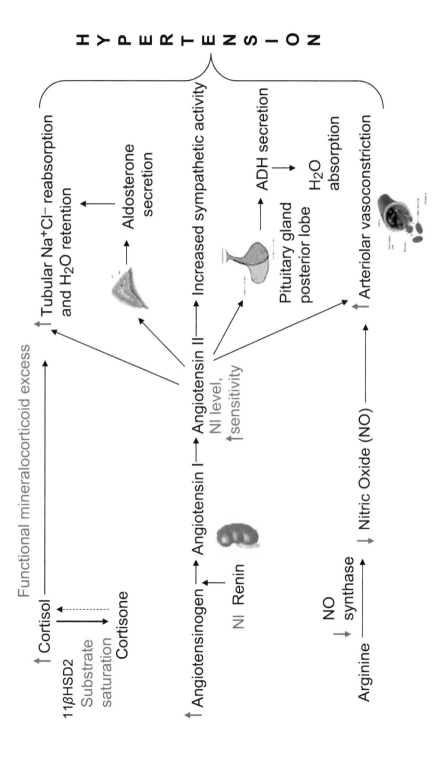

Fig. 1. Pathogenesis of hypertension in Cushing's syndrome. Text and arrows in red show the effect of excess glucocorticoids on the renin-angiotensin system and other pathways involved. ↑, increased; ↓, decreased; Nl, normal.

goal. Antiglucocorticoid drugs and antihypertensive agents should be used as adjunctive modes of treatment to normalize blood pressure.

REFERENCES

1. Lindholm J, Juul S, Jorgenson JO, et al. Incidence and late prognosis of Cushing's syndrome: a population based study. J Clin Endocrinol Metab 2001;86:117–23.
2. Etxabe J, Vazquez JA. Morbidity and mortality in Cushing's disease: an epidemiological approach. Clin Endocrinol (Oxf) 1994;40:479–84.
3. Newell-Price J, Bertagna X, Grossman AB, et al. Cushing's syndrome. Lancet 2006;367:1605–17.
4. Catargi B, Rigalleau V, Poussin A, et al. Occult Cushing's syndrome in type-2 diabetes. J Clin Endocrinol Metab 2003;88:5808–13.
5. Leibowitz G, Tsur A, Chayen SD, et al. Pre-clinical Cushing's syndrome: an unexpected frequent cause of poor glycaemic control in obese diabetic patients. Clin Endocrinol (Oxf) 1996;44:717–22.
6. Nugent CA, Warner HR, Dunn JT, et al. Probability theory in the diagnosis of Cushing's syndrome. J Clin Endocrinol Metab 1964;24:621–7.
7. Ross EJ, Linch DC. Cushing's syndrome-killing disease: discriminatory value of signs and symptoms aiding early diagnosis. Lancet 1982;2(8299):646–9.
8. Magiakou MA, Mastorakos G, Oldfield EH, et al. Cushing's syndrome in children and adolescents: presentation, diagnosis, and therapy. N Engl J Med 1994;331:629–36.
9. Nieman LK, Biller BM, Findling JW, et al. The diagnosis of Cushing's syndrome: an endocrine society clinical practice guideline. J Clin Endocrinol Metab 2008;93(5):1526–40.
10. Nieman LK, Ilias I. Evaluation and treatment of Cushing's syndrome. Am J Med 2005;118:134–46.
11. Ilias I, Torpy DJ, Pacak K, et al. Cushing's syndrome due to ectopic corticotrophin secretion: twenty years experience at National Institutes of Health. J Clin Endocrinol Metab 2005;90:4955–62.
12. Torpy DJ, Mullen N, Ilias I, et al. Association of hypertension and hypokalemia with Cushing's syndrome caused by ectopic ACTH secretion. Ann N Y Acad Sci 2002;970:134–44.
13. Faggiano A, Pivonello R, Spiezia S, et al. Cardiovascular risk factors and common carotid artery caliber and stiffness in patients with Cushing's disease during active disease and 1 year after disease remission. J Clin Endocrinol Metab 2003;88:2527–33.
14. Stewart PM, Walker BR, Holder F. II beta-hydroxysteroid dehydrogenase activity in Cushing's syndrome: explaining the mineralocorticoid excess state of the ectopic adrenocorticotropin syndrome. J Clin Endocrinol Metab 1995;80:3617–20.
15. Magiakou MA, Mastorakos G, Zachman K, et al. Blood pressure in children and adolescents with Cushing's syndrome before and after surgical cure. J Clin Endocrinol Metab 1997;82:1734–8.
16. Treadwell BLJ, Sever ED, Savage O, et al. Side-effects of long-term treatment with corticosteroids and corticotrophin. Lancet 1964;1(7343):1121–3.
17. Fraser R, Davies DL, Connell JM. Hormones and hypertension. Clin Endocrinol 1989;31:701–46.
18. Chobanian AV, Bakris GL, Black HR, et al. The seventh report of the Joint National Committee on prevention, detection, evaluation and treatment of high blood pressure. Hypertension 2003;42:1206–52.

19. Lewington S, Clarke R, Qizilbash N, et al. Age-specific relevance of usual blood pressure to vascular mortality: a meta-analysis of individual data for one million adults in 61 prospective studies. Lancet 2002;360(9349):1903–13.

20. Speiker C, Barenbrock M, Rahn KH, et al. Circadian blood pressure variations in endocrine disorders. Blood Press 1993;2:35–9.

21. Imai Y, Abe S, Sasaki S, et al. Altered circadian blood pressure rhythm in patients with Cushing's syndrome. Hypertension 1988;12:11–9.

22. Zacharieva S, Orbetzova M, Stoynev A, et al. Circadian blood pressure profile in patients with Cushing's syndrome before and after treatment. J Endocrinol Invest 2004;27:924–30.

23. Imai Y, Abe S, Sasaki S, et al. Exogenous glucocorticoid eliminates or reverses circadian blood pressure variations. J Hypertens 1989;7:113–20.

24. Magiakou MA, Smyrnaki P, Chrousos GP. Hypertension in Cushing's syndrome. Best Pract Res Clin Endocrinol Metab 2006 Sep;20(3):467–82.

25. Quinkler M, Stewart PM. Hypertension and the Cortisol-Cortisone shuttle. J Clin Endocrinol Metab 2003;88(6):2384–92.

26. Hatakeyama H, Inaba S, Miyamori I. 11 beta hydroxysteroid dehydrogenase in cultured human vascular cells: possible role in development of hypertension. Hypertension 1999;33:1179–84.

27. Brem A, Bina R, King T, et al. Localization of 2 11-betahydroxysteroid dehydrogenase isoforms in aortic endothelial cells. Hypertension 1998;31:459–62.

28. Edwards CR, Stewart PM, Burt D, et al. Localization of 11-beta hydroxysteroid dehydrogenase – tissue specific protector of the mineralocorticoid receptor. Lancet 1988;2(8618):986–9.

29. Funder JW, Pearce PT, Smith R, et al. Mineralocorticoid action: target tissue specificity is enzyme, not receptor, mediated. Science 1988;242:583–5.

30. Dotsch J, Dorr HG, Stall GK, et al. Effect of glucocorticoid excess on cortisol/cortisone ratio. Steroids 2001;66:817–20.

31. Ulick S, Wang JZ, Blumenfeld JD, et al. Cortisol inactivation overload: a mechanism of mineralocorticoid hypertension in the ectopic adrenocorticotropin syndrome. J Clin Endocrinol Metab 1992;74:963–7.

32. Connell JM, Whitworth JA, Davies DL, et al. Hemodynamic, hormonal, and renal effects of adrenocorticotrophic hormone in sodium-restricted man. J Hypertens 1988;6(1):17–23.

33. Williamson PM, Kelly JJ, Whitworth JA. Dose-response and mineralocorticoid activity in cortisol-induced hypertension in humans. J Hypertens Suppl 1996; 14(5):S37–41.

34. Whitworth JA, Gordon D, Andrews J, et al. The hypertensive effect of synthetic glucocorticoids in man: role of sodium and volume. J Hypertens 1989;7: 537–49.

35. Nieman LK, Chrousos GP, Kellner C, et al. Successful treatment of Cushing's syndrome with the glucocorticoid antagonist RU 486. J Clin Endocrinol Metab 1985;61:536–40.

36. Klett C, Ganten D, Hellmann W, et al. Regulation of hepatic angiotensinogen synthesis and secretion by steroid hormones. Endocrinology 1992;130: 3660–8.

37. Sato A, Suzuki H, Murakami M, et al. Glucocorticoid increases angiotensin II type 1 receptor and its gene expression. Hypertension 1994;23:25–30.

38. Shelat SG, King JL, Flanagan-Cato LM, et al. Mineralocorticoids and glucocorticoids cooperatively increase salt intake and angiotensin II receptor binding in rat brain. Neuroendocrinology 1999;69:339–51.

39. Scheuer DA, Bechtold AG. Glucocorticoids potentiate central actions of angiotensin to increase arterial blood pressure. Am J Physiol Regul Integr Comp Physiol 2001;280:R1719–26.

40. Sala C, Ambrosi B, Morganti A. Blunted vascular and renal effects of exogenous atrial natriuretic peptide in patients with Cushing's disease. J Clin Endocrinol Metab 2001;86:1957–61.

41. Yasunari K, Kohno M, Murakawa K, et al. Glucocorticoids and atrial natriuretic factor receptors on vascular smooth muscle. Hypertension 1990;16:581–6.

42. Kelm M. The L-arginine-nitric oxide pathway in hypertension. Curr Hypertens Rep 2003;5:80–6.

43. Axelrod L. Inhibition of prostacyclin production mediates permissive effect of glucocorticoids on vascular tone. Perturbations of this mechanism contribute to pathogenesis of Cushing's syndrome and Addison's disease. Lancet 1983;23: 904–6.

44. Handa M, Kondo K, Suzuki H, et al. Role of prostaglandins and pressure sensitivity to norepinephrine. Hypertension 1984;6(2):236–41.

45. McKnight JA, Rooney DP, Whitehead H, et al. Blood pressure responses to phenylephrine infusions in subjects with Cushing's syndrome. J Hum Hypertens 1995; 9:855–8.

46. Pirpiris M, Sudhir K, Yeung S, et al. Pressor responsiveness in corticosteroid-induced hypertension in humans. Hypertension 1992;19(6):567–74.

47. Kirilov G, Tomova A, Dakovska L, et al. Elevated plasma endothelin as an additional cardiovascular risk factor in patients with Cushing's syndrome. Eur J Endocrinol 2003;149:549–53.

48. Ruschitzka F, Quaschning T, Noll G, et al. Endothelin-1 type A receptor antagonism prevents vascular dysfunction and hypertension induced by 11 beta hydroxysteroid dehydrogenase inhibition: role of nitric oxide. Circulation 2001; 103(25):3129–35.

49. Smith L, Smith JB. Regulation of sodium-calcium exchanger by glucocorticoids and growth factors in vascular smooth muscle. J Biol Chem 1994;269(44): 27527–31.

50. Kelly JJ, Martin A, Whitworth JA. Role of erythropoietin in cortisol-induced hypertension. J Hum Hypertens 2000;14(3):195–8.

51. Shipley JE, Schteingart DE, Tandon R, et al. Sleep architecture and sleep apnoea in patients with Cushing's disease. Sleep 1992;15:514–8.

52. Nieman LK. Medical therapy of Cushing's disease. Pituitary 2002;5:77–82.

53. Suri D, Weiss RE. Effect of pioglitazone on adrenocorticotropic hormone and cortisol secretion in Cushing's disease. J Clin Endocrinol Metab 2005;90(3): 1340–6.

54. Kreutzer J, Jeske I, Hofmann B, et al. No effect of the PPAR-gamma agonist rosiglitazone on ACTH or cortisol secretion in Nelson's syndrome or Cushing's disease in vitro and in vivo. Clin Neuropathol 2009;28(6):430–9.

55. Zacharieva S, Orbetzova M, Natchev E, et al. Losartan in Cushing's syndrome. Methods Find Exp Clin Pharmacol 1998;20:163–8.

56. Dalakos TG, Elias AN, Anderson GH Jr, et al. Evidence for an angiotensinogenic mechanism of the hypertension of Cushing's syndrome. J Clin Endocrinol Metab 1978;46:114–8.

57. Zacharieva S, Torbova S, Orbetzova M, et al. Trandolapril in Cushing's disease: short-term trandolapril treatment in patients with Cushing's disease and essential hypertension. Methods Find Exp Clin Pharmacol 1988;20:433–8.

58. Baid S, Nieman LK. Glucocorticoid excess and hypertension. Curr Hypertens Rep 2004;6(6):493–9.
59. Fallo F, Paoletta A, Tona F, et al. Response of hypertension to conventional anti-hypertensive treatment and/or steroidogenesis inhibitors in Cushing's syndrome. J Intern Med 1993;234:595–8.
60. Fallo F, Sonino N, Barzon L, et al. Effect of surgical treatment on hypertension in Cushing's syndrome. Am J Hypertens 1996;9:77–80.
61. Colao A, Pivonello R, Spiezia S, et al. Persistence of increased cardiovascular risk in patients with Cushing's disease after five years of successful cure. J Clin Endocrinol Metab 1999;84:2664–72.
62. Mishra AK, Agarwal A, Gupta S, et al. Outcome of adrenalectomy for Cushing's syndrome: experience from a tertiary care center. World J Surg 2007;31(7): 1425–32.

How Do Glucocorticoids Cause Hypertension: Role of Nitric Oxide Deficiency, Oxidative Stress, and Eicosanoids

Sharon L.H. Ong, BSc(Med), MBBS, FRACP[a,b,]*,
Judith A. Whitworth, AC, MBBS, DSc, MD, PhD, FRACP[c]

KEYWORDS

- Glucocorticoid • Hypertension • Nitric oxide • Oxidative stress
- Prostanoids • 20-hydroxyeicosatetranoic acid

The discovery of the anti-inflammatory effects of corticosteroid hormones by Philip Hench and colleagues in 1929 revolutionized the treatments of various inflammatory conditions. Today, glucocorticoids are widely used in inflammatory conditions and in chemotherapeutic and immunosuppressive regimens for the treatment of both cancer and solid organ transplantation. Unfortunately, chronic usage of systemic glucocorticoids at supraphysiological doses, sometimes inevitable for certain medical conditions, often leads to iatrogenic Cushing syndrome, which is more common than its endogenous counterpart. Cushing syndrome, both endogenous and iatrogenic, is associated with several cardiovascular and metabolic side effects. Approximately 80% of patients with Cushing syndrome have hypertension.[1] Around 20% of patients receiving exogenous glucocorticoids have been reported to have hypertension, which can be severe in some cases.[2,3]

Adrenocorticotropic hormone (ACTH) is another cause of Cushing syndrome. Endogenous ACTH excess due to pituitary ACTH overproduction (Cushing disease), such as in pituitary adenoma or ectopic ACTH release, can be associated with hypertension. The use of synthetic ACTH is currently limited to some neurologic conditions such as infantile spasms and diagnosis of certain endocrine conditions

The authors have nothing to disclose.

[a] Department of Nephrology, St George Hospital, 50 Montgomery Street, Kogarah, Sydney, NSW 2217, Australia

[b] St George Hospital Clinical School, Faculty of Medicine, University of New South Wales, Sydney, NSW 2052, Australia

[c] John Curtin School of Medical Research, Australian National University, Building 131, Garran Road, Acton, Canberra, ACT 0200, Australia

* Corresponding author.

E-mail address: s.ong@unsw.edu.au

Endocrinol Metab Clin N Am 40 (2011) 393–407
doi:10.1016/j.ecl.2011.01.010
0889-8529/11/$ – see front matter. Crown Copyright © 2011 Published by Elsevier Inc. All rights reserved.

endo.theclinics.com

but, even acutely in endocrine diagnosis, has been associated with hypertension. ACTH-induced hypertension is explicable in terms of effects of cortisol in humans and corticosterone in rodents.[4] There are major similarities between ACTH-induced and glucocorticoid-induced hypertension in terms of their rate of onset, requirement for salt loading and volume expansion, role in nitric oxide–redox imbalance, and their responses to tetrahydrobiopterin and antioxidants, as is discussed in this review (**Table 1**). Similarly, subtle differences between ACTH-induced and glucocorticoid-induced hypertension have also been identified (**Table 2**), although the exact reasons for these differences remain unclear.

HEMODYNAMIC FEATURES OF GLUCOCORTICOID-INDUCED HYPERTENSION

Glucocorticoid administration produces highly significant elevations in systolic blood pressure and, to a lesser extent, diastolic blood pressure, in man and animals.[5,6] These effects become evident rapidly. In humans, hypertension is observed within 24 hours of oral cortisol administration, reaching a peak in 4 to 5 days.[6,7] Dexamethasone-induced hypertension in rats,[8–10] dogs,[11,12] and humans[13] develops within 1 to 2 days of dexamethasone administration. Similarly, ACTH treatment induces hypertension rapidly in sheep,[14] rats,[15] and humans.[6,16]

Several experimental studies have been performed to evaluate the hemodynamic profiles of glucocorticoid-induced hypertension. Dexamethasone-induced hypertension in humans, induced by 1 mg oral dexamethasone given thrice daily for 7 days, was associated with a significant increase in calculated total peripheral resistance without any significant difference in the measured cardiac output and heart rate compared with their normotensive counterparts.[13] In rats, dexamethasone-induced hypertension (10 μg/rat/d, given subcutaneously) was also associated with increases in total peripheral resistance but not cardiac output, heart rate and stroke volume.[17] The increase in total peripheral resistance was not attributed to increases in resistances in the renal, mesenteric, or hindquarter vascular beds, although it may reflect cumulative changes from several vascular beds.[17] Pretreatment with minoxidil in dexamethasone-hypertensive rats failed to prevent hypertension despite significant reduction in total peripheral resistance in these rats.[17] At a higher dose, dexamethasone-induced hypertension in dogs (0.5 mg/kg/d, given orally) was accompanied by a reduction in cardiac output and elevated calculated total peripheral resistance.[11,12]

Table 1
Similarities of ACTH-induced and glucocorticoid-induced hypertension

Characteristics	ACTH-HT and GC-HT	Glucocorticoid	References
Onset	Rapid	Cortisol, DEX	6–8,14,15,24,63
Requirement for salt loading	No	Cortisol, DEX	22,24,25,84–86
Associated with nitric oxide deficiency	Yes	Corticosterone, cortisol, DEX	4,7,34,46,54,59,87,88
Associated with oxidative stress	Yes	DEX	9,54,57,60
Response to antioxidants (tempol, apocynin, folic acid, NAC)	Yes	DEX	8–10,54,57,58,60
Response to BH$_4$ supplementation	No	DEX	53,54
Response to allopurinol	No	DEX	60,63
Response to minoxidil	No	DEX	17,20

Abbreviations: ACTH-HT, adrenocorticotropic hormone–induced hypertension; BH$_4$, tetrahydrobiopterin; DEX, dexamethasone; GC-HT, glucocorticoid-induced hypertension; NAC, N-acetylcysteine.

Table 2
Differences of ACTH-induced and glucocorticoid-induced hypertension

BP Response to the Following:	ACTH-HT	GC-HT	Glucocorticoid	References
L-Arginine	↓	↔	DEX	8,34,39,40
GC antagonist (DHEA)	↔	↓	DEX	89,90
Vasopressin antagonist	↔	↓	DEX	31,91
Aspirin	↓	↔	DEX	61
20-HETE inhibitor (HET0016)	↓	↔	DEX	36
Characteristics:				
Total peripheral resistance	↔	↑	DEX	17,19
Renal vascular resistance	↑	↔	DEX	17,19
Cardiac output	↑	↔	DEX	17,19
Urinary 20-HETE excretion	↑	↔	DEX	73

Abbreviations: 20-HETE, 20-hydroxyeicosatetraenoic acid; DHEA, dehydroepiandrosterone.

Hypertension caused by hydrocortisone (cortisol) in humans (200 mg/d, orally) was associated with increased cardiac output[5] and renal vascular resistance,[6] but not with changes in total peripheral resistance or heart rate.[5] Reduction in cardiac output by the β-adrenergic blocker atenolol was unsuccessful in preventing hypertension due to hydrocortisone in humans,[5] suggesting that the increase in cardiac output (which may be due to concomitant increase in plasma volume) is not essential for the development of hydrocortisone-induced hypertension.[6] The calcium channel receptor blocker felodipine, which reduces total peripheral resistance, had no effect on hypertension caused by cortisol administration in humans.[18]

ACTH-induced hypertension in rats (0.5 mg/kg subcutaneous corticotropin per day) was also characterized by increased cardiac output and renal vascular resistance but with no change in total peripheral resistance.[19] The hemodynamic mechanisms of ACTH hypertension in rats were tested using atenolol (to reduce cardiac output) and ramipril at a dose that effectively reduces renal vascular resistance only.[20] Although atenolol successfully prevented the increase in cardiac output due to ACTH, it did not prevent the development of ACTH hypertension in rats.[20] Ramipril, on the other hand, effectively prevented both increases in renal vascular resistance and hypertension in rats.

Thus, hypertension due to synthetic glucocorticoids with predominant glucocorticoid activity is associated with raised total peripheral resistance, but this hemodynamic alteration is not essential for dexamethasone-induced blood pressure increase. On the other hand, hypertension due to endogenous glucocorticoids such as cortisol is characterized by the increase in cardiac output and renal vascular resistance, although the former is not crucial for the development of hypertension.

MECHANISMS OF GLUCOCORTICOID-INDUCED HYPERTENSION

Sodium and water retention is still accepted by many as a mechanism of glucocorticoid-induced hypertension. This view is based on the notion that cortisol causes both hypertension and water retention by means of glucocorticoid activation of the mineralocorticoid receptors. Nevertheless, a causal relationship between cortisol-induced water retention and hypertension is lacking. Inhibition of the mineralocorticoid receptors using spironolactone failed to prevent either cortisol-induced hypertension in humans[21,22] or ACTH-induced hypertension in rats.[23] ACTH has been shown to result in hypertension despite dietary salt restriction to 15 mmol/L, although dietary salt loading potentiated the hypertensive response to ACTH.[24,25] Evaluations of a range of synthetic glucocorticoids including prednisolone, methyl-prednisolone, dexamethasone, and triamcinolone showed induction of hypertension without evidence of plasma volume expansion and urinary sodium retention.[25] These data demonstrated that sodium and water retention are not essential for the development of glucocorticoid-induced hypertension.

Several other common pathophysiological mechanisms of hypertension have been tested in glucocorticoid-induced hypertension models. Currently available data suggest that sympathetic nerve stimulation is not a candidate mechanism in glucocorticoid-induced hypertension. Using microneurographic recordings of the common peroneal nerves, cortisol-induced and dexamethasone-induced hypertensive subjects were shown to have suppression of muscle sympathetic activity.[26] Furthermore, there were no significant differences between plasma neuropeptide Y concentration in normotensive and hypertensive patients with Cushing syndrome.[27] Neuropeptide Y immunoreactivity was also unchanged with cortisol.

Some vasopressor hormones such as angiotensin II, arginine vasopressin, and endothelins have been implicated in glucocorticoid-induced hypertension. In normal human subjects, cortisol treatment for 5 days resulted in a nonsignificant increase in urinary endothelin excretion.[28] However, a 50% increase in plasma endothelin-1 level has been reported in human subjects on reducing doses of prednisolone over 5 days.[29] Rats treated with dexamethasone (2 mg/kg/d for 12 days) also had raised plasma endothelin levels.[30] Arginine vasopressin, another vasopressor hormone, has been evaluated in glucocorticoid-induced hypertension. Ijima and Malik[31] showed that treatment with an arginine vasopressin V_1 receptor antagonist successfully reduced mean arterial pressure in dexamethasone-induced hypertensive but not control rats. In humans, cortisol treatment did not alter plasma arginine vasopressin, but it has been suggested that glucocorticoid-induced hypertension is mediated by increased expression of the V_{1a} arginine vasopressor receptor via increased mRNA stability[32] and not by increased plasma arginine vasopressin concentration.[11] It is likely that arginine vasopressin may play a role in the genesis of glucocorticoid-induced hypertension, but the role of endothelins remains unclear. Further assessments using endothelin antagonist in vitro in a glucocorticoid-induced hypertensive model is necessary. The role of angiotensin II is discussed by Krakoff elsewhere in this issue, and is beyond the scope of this review.

Current interest focuses on the role of nitric oxide, oxidative stress, and their interactions with arachidonic acid metabolism.

THE NITRIC OXIDE SYSTEM AND GLUCOCORTICOID-INDUCED HYPERTENSION

The notion that nitric oxide plays a role in the development of glucocorticoid-induced hypertension stemmed from the observation of reduced urinary nitrate and nitrite concentrations (metabolites of nitric oxide) in a patient with Cushing syndrome before and after the administration of the nitric oxide precursor L-arginine.[33] Cortisol treatment (80 mg/d given orally) in healthy male subjects on restricted nitrate diet resulted in significant reduction in plasma nitrate and nitrite concentration without evidence of increase nitrate clearance, reduction of L-arginine availability, or increased asymmetric dimethyl arginine (an endogenous nitric oxide synthase inhibitor) concentrations.[7] ACTH-induced[34] and dexamethasone-induced hypertension[35,36] in rats were also associated with decreased plasma nitrate and nitrite concentrations. Furthermore, the nitric oxide donor isosorbide dinitrate prevented hypertension due to ACTH in the rat.[37] Oral cortisol increased blood pressure and threshold for a depressor response to the nitric oxide donor glyceryl trinitrate in man, implicating the presence of decreased nitric oxide availability in cortisol-induced hypertension in humans.[38] These data implicate nitric oxide deficiency in the genesis of glucocorticoid-induced hypertension. Results from manipulations of the nitric oxide system at different levels (reviewed below; **Fig. 1**) had also provided greater insight into how the nitric oxide system is altered in glucocorticoid-induced hypertension.

L-Arginine Availability and Delivery

L-Arginine is a specific precursor of nitric oxide synthesis. Aberrations in its utilization by nitric oxide synthase can potentially lead to a state of nitric oxide deficiency. L-Arginine supplementation (0.6% in food), as a way to overcome any deficit in L-arginine availability, prevents ACTH-induced hypertension in rats.[39] L-Arginine, however, did not prevent dexamethasone-induced hypertension in rats[40] or cortisol-induced hypertension in humans.[41] Thus, decreased L-arginine availability is a feature of ACTH hypertension in rats, but not dexamethasone hypertension in rats and cortisol hypertension in humans. The reason for these different outcomes remains unclear, although these studies highlight the differences in the mechanism of ACTH and dexamethasone-induced hypertension, as well as showing that nitric oxide deficiency in glucocorticoid-induced hypertension is not simply the result of insufficient L-arginine. The fact that the nitric oxide synthase inhibitor N-nitro-L-arginine successfully

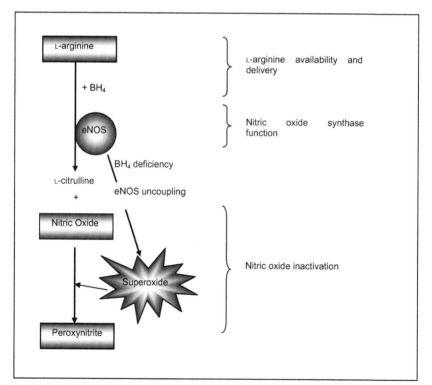

Fig. 1. The L-arginine–nitric oxide pathway. BH_4, tetrahydrobiopterin; eNOS, endothelial nitric oxide synthase.

inhibited the preventative effect of L-arginine on ACTH hypertension in rats indicates that the L-arginine effect is mediated through nitric oxide synthesis.[42]

Defective L-arginine transport could also result in a state of relative intracellular deficiency. This mechanism was tested in cortisol-induced hypertension human subjects on a nitrate-restricted diet. This study showed that cellular L-arginine transport in peripheral blood mononuclear cells (in vitro) and in forearm vasculature (in vivo) was not affected by orally administered cortisol (250 mg over 24 hours).[43] Whether this translates to dexamethasone-induced hypertension is unclear and is yet to be determined.

Nitric Oxide Synthase Function

Nitric oxide synthase inhibition
One of the ways to investigate whether the state of nitric oxide deficiency in glucocorticoid-induced hypertension is a consequence of the inhibition of nitric oxide biosynthesis is to examine the effect of direct inhibition of nitric oxide synthase. The nitric oxide synthase inhibitor N-nitro-L-arginine (approximately 17–30 mg/kg/d orally) not only induced hypertension in control rats but also resulted in an additive hypertensive response in ACTH-hypertensive and dexamethasone-hypertensive rats.[44,45] This response suggested that glucocorticoid-induced hypertension is not entirely attributable to nitric oxide inhibition because if this were the case, a further increase in blood pressure should not be apparent in the treated rats.

Nitric oxide synthase mRNA downregulation
At the molecular level, Wallerath and colleagues[35] have demonstrated in vitro that dexamethasone treatment resulted in a considerable downregulation of endothelial nitric oxide synthase (eNOS) mRNA and protein in cultured human and bovine endothelial cells, as well as in aorta, kidney, and liver of dexamethasone-induced hypertensive rats. This process seemed to involve mRNA destabilization and a decrease in transcription in the eNOS gene.[35] These investigators subsequently demonstrated that dexamethasone significantly increased blood pressure in wild-type eNOS$^{+/+}$ mice but did not further increase the blood pressure in the already-hypertensive eNOS$^{-/-}$ mice.[46] Suppression of inducible NOS and eNOS mRNA and encoded protein expression in the kidney have also been demonstrated in ACTH-induced hypertensive rats.[47] These data further confirmed the notion that glucocorticoid impairs nitric oxide production by downregulating the expression and limiting the activity of nitric oxide synthase.

Uncoupling of endothelial nitric oxide synthase
For any of the NOS isoforms to effectively catalyze the production of nitric oxide, a sufficient amount of the cofactor tetrahydrobiopterin (BH_4) is essential.[48] When BH_4 is limiting, whether due to decreased synthesis or increased oxidation, eNOS uncoupling impairs the L-arginine catalytic process, resulting in the formation of superoxide instead of nitric oxide.[49]

Guanosine triphosphate (GTP) cyclohydrolase 1 is the rate-limiting enzyme responsible for the de novo production of BH_4. In vitro treatment of cultured rat cardiac microvascular endothelial cells with dexamethasone has been shown to suppress GTP cyclohydrolase gene expression and thus decrease nitric oxide production in this cell line.[50] Johns and colleagues[51] demonstrated a blunted endothelium-dependent vasorelaxation to A23187 in aortic rings of dexamethasone-induced hypertensive rats. These investigators proposed that this effect was a consequence of diminution in BH_4-mediated eNOS activity, based on their in vitro experiments demonstrating reductions in GTP cyclohydrolase mRNA levels in dexamethasone-incubated rat aortic rings.[51] In another study, ex vivo analysis of the aorta of dexamethasone-induced hypertensive rats showed a time-dependent decrease in maximal relaxation in response to acetylcholine as well as a decrease in GTP cyclohydrolase 1 mRNA expression.[52] Based on these findings, nitric oxide deficiency due to decreased BH_4 availability has been proposed in glucocorticoid-induced hypertension.

The authors have evaluated the role of BH_4 and sepiapterin supplementation in both ACTH-hypertensive and dexamethasone-induced hypertensive rats.[45,53,54] Daily treatment with BH_4, at a dose (10 mg/kg, intraperitoneally) known to increase plasma BH_4, while partially preventing the onset of hypertension in spontaneously hypertensive rats,[55] failed to prevent ACTH-induced hypertension. BH_4 treatment also did not prevent dexamethasone-induced hypertension in rats despite detectable levels of plasma BH_4 concentrations.[54] The BH_4 donor sepiapterin, at a dose that effectively increased plasma BH_4, was unable to prevent ACTH-induced and dexamethasone-induced hypertension in the rat.[45] This evidence clearly indicates that eNOS uncoupling consequent on BH_4 deficiency is not a candidate mechanism of nitric oxide deficiency in these models.

Increased Inactivation

Nitric oxide deficiency may also be caused by oxidative inactivation by superoxide anion and other reactive oxygen species. Its interaction with superoxide, which forms the powerful oxidant peroxynitrite, is significantly faster than dismutation of superoxide by superoxide dismutase. Iuchi and colleagues[56] reported raised vascular production of peroxynitrite in a hypertensive patient with Cushing syndrome. These investigators also observed increased immunostaining of nitrotyrosine residue, a biomarker of nitric oxide radical–derived oxidant, in skeletal muscle vasculature.[56] Thus, oxidative stress and nitric oxide–redox imbalance are implicated in the pathogenesis of glucocorticoid-induced hypertension.

OXIDATIVE STRESS AND GLUCOCORTICOID HYPERTENSION

There is now a body of evidence implicating oxidative stress in the causation of glucocorticoid-induced hypertension. Aortic lucigenin-enhanced chemiluminescence,[57–59] a biomarker of tissue oxidative stress, and plasma F_2-isoprostane concentration[9,36,54,57,60] is increased in ACTH-induced and dexamethasone-induced hypertensive rats.

The response of glucocorticoid-induced hypertension to antioxidants further illustrates the significance of oxidative stress in this form of hypertension. The superoxide scavenger tempol prevented and reversed glucocorticoid-induced hypertension in the rat, most likely by intracellular reactive oxygen species reduction without significant alterations in plasma F_2-isoprostane concentrations.[9,57] Drugs without any specific antihypertensive action such as aspirin,[61] folate,[54] atorvastatin,[59] and N-acetylcysteine[10,58] were also effective in preventing glucocorticoid hypertension in the rat, presumably because of their antioxidative properties.

Factors influencing the availability of reactive oxygen species such as increased production by the different superoxide generating systems and impaired removal in the vasculature may contribute to the state of oxidative stress in glucocorticoid-induced hypertensive models.

Increased Reactive Oxygen Species Production

Of the numerous reactive oxygen species–producing systems, the nicotinamide adenine dinucleotide phosphate (NAD(P)H) oxidase, xanthine oxidase, and eNOS in its uncoupled state are the best studied in glucocorticoid-induced hypertension.

The authors have demonstrated that the NAD(P)H oxidase pathway is the main source of superoxide in glucocorticoid-induced hypertension in the rat. Whether this translates to glucocorticoid-induced hypertension in humans is unclear. In rats, the NAD(P)H oxidase inhibitor apocynin successfully prevented hypertension and attenuated the raised plasma F_2-isoprostane concentrations induced by ACTH.[60] Dexamethasone-induced hypertension in rats was also prevented by apocynin.[8] Angiotensin II–induced stimulation of the NAD(P)H oxidase pathway contributes to oxidative stress in gluococorticoid-induced hypertension. Blockade of angiotensin II receptors using losartan prevented ACTH-induced hypertension and ACTH-induced increase in plasma F_2-isoprostane concentration.[62] By contrast, losartan prevented and reversed dexamethasone-induced hypertension without altering F_2-isoprostane concentration.[62] The angiotensin-converting enzyme inhibitor ramipril prevented ACTH hypertension in rats, although its effect on biomarkers of oxidative stress has not been demonstrated.[20] The effect of renin-angiotensin system inhibition in glucocorticoid-induced hypertension is partly due to oxidative stress reduction, although not exclusively. The other effects of the renin-angiotensin system in glucocorticoid-induced hypertension are reviewed by Krakoff and colleagues elsewhere in this issue.

Although the xanthine oxidase system is an important source of superoxide, it was shown not to play a major role in the generation of nitric oxide imbalance in glucocorticoid-induced hypertension. Treatment with allopurinol was unsuccessful in preventing both ACTH-induced and dexamethasone-induced hypertension.[60,63] Endothelial NOS, in its uncoupled form, is another source of vascular superoxide. However, this is unlikely to be a major contributor of oxidative stress in the glucocorticoid-induced hypertensive model, as attempts to prevent its uncoupling by BH_4 or sepiapterin supplementation were unsuccessful in preventing glucocorticoid-induced hypertension.

Impaired Reactive Oxygen Species Degradation

Endogenous antioxidants such as superoxide dismutase, catalase, glutathione-S-transferase, and glutathione peroxidase provide cells with defense against toxic reactive oxygen species. The imbalance resulting from an increase in reactive oxygen species production and the availability of endogenous antioxidants can potentially result in tissue injury. Rajashree and Puvanakrishnan[64] have demonstrated that dexamethasone-induced hypertensive rats had increased thiobarbituric acid reactants (a marker of tissue lipid peroxidation), decreased levels of catalase and superoxide dismutase in the heart but not in the kidney, and a decrease followed by a subsequent increase in glutathione-S-transferase and glutathione peroxidase activity in both the heart and kidney. In another study, dexamethasone-induced oxidative stress in veal calves was associated with increased serum glutathione peroxidase activity.[65] These changes may, in part, be attributable to compensatory induction of endogenous antioxidant enzymes in response to oxidative stress, although a direct effect of glucocorticoids on naturally occurring antioxidants cannot be discounted.[66] Even though dysregulation of endogenous antioxidants is a feature of glucocorticoid-induced hypertension, it remains unclear as to whether it plays an important role in its pathogenesis.

EICOSANOIDS

Eicosanoids, which are products of metabolism of arachidonic acid, consist of several vasoactive substances such as prostaglandin E_2, prostacyclin, thromboxane A_2, and 20-hydroxyeicosatetraenoic acid (20-HETE). The roles of the vasodilator prostanoids (prostaglandin I_2 [prostacyclin] and prostaglandin E_2) and 20-HETE have been evaluated in glucocorticoid-induced hypertension.

Glucocorticoid Inhibition of Vasodilator Prostanoid Production

It was initially proposed that glucocorticoid inhibition of phospholipase would inhibit prostacyclin synthesis, increase vascular tone, and thus contribute to hypertension.[67] This proposal was supported by in vitro studies demonstrating dexamethasone-induced inhibition of prostaglandin synthesis via the inhibition of phospholipase A_2 activity,[68–70] resulting in the reduction of arachidonic acid.

Falardeau and Martineau[71] reported that dexamethasone-induced hypertensive rats (dexamethasone dose: 3 mg/L, drinking water, approximately 146–160 μg/d, 7 days) had reduced urinary excretion of PGI-M, a marker of prostacyclin biosynthesis. Prostaglandin E_2 was significantly lower in dexamethasone-treated rats (dexamethasone dose: 2.5×10^7 mol dexamethasone/rat/d or 0.1 mg/rat/d orally), just before the development of hypertension.[72] At a significantly lower dexamethasone dose (20 μg/kg/d, approximately 4 μg/rat/d), urinary prostacyclin was not significantly altered compared with control rats.[73] In humans, urinary prostanoid excretion after cortisol administration (200 mg/d for 5 days) was raised or not significantly altered.[28] Whether these differences were caused by the different glucocorticoids, different doses, and/or different species remains unclear. Furthermore, it is questionable whether urinary prostaglandins correlate with circulating or tissue prostaglandin levels.

Administration of the cyclooxygenase inhibitor indomethacin to cortisol-treated individuals resulted in increased pressor responsiveness and threshold to phenylephrine but not to angiotensin II.[74] Although this study did not specifically determine whether glucocorticoid-induced hypertension is mediated by a decrease in vasodilator prostanoids, the finding that cyclooxygenase inhibition with indomethacin did not further potentiate glucocorticoid-induced hypertension suggested that prostaglandin depletion may have a role.

Glucocorticoid-Induced Hypertension and 20-Hydroxyeicosatetranoic Acid

20-HETE is a potent vasoconstrictor that can potentiate vascular smooth muscle response to vasoconstrictor and myogenic stimuli.[75] It also plays an important role in regulating renal tubular sodium reabsorption, resulting in natriuretic and diuretic properties.[75]

The interactions of nitric oxide and 20-HETE have been recognized (**Fig. 2**). The catalytic activity of cytochrome P450 enzymes can be inhibited by nitric oxide or nitric oxide donors.[76] 20-HETE can be inhibited directly and functionally by nitric oxide.[77–79] In addition, 20-HETE has the ability to reduce eNOS activation[80] and accelerate degradation of nitric oxide by increasing NAD(P)H oxidase–related superoxide overproduction,[81] which may further decrease the availability of nitric oxide and exacerbate hypertension. Therefore, 20-HETE production is likely to be increased in the presence of nitric oxide deficiency.

ACTH-induced, but not dexamethasone-induced hypertensive rats increased urinary 20-HETE excretion[73] and renal microsomal 20-HETE formation.[36] Inhibition of 20-HETE synthesis with HET0016 effectively prevented and reversed ACTH-induced hypertension but not dexamethasone-induced hypertension in rats.[36] These studies demonstrated that 20-HETE may play a role in the development of ACTH-induced hypertension. The presence of oxidative stress and nitric oxide deficiency in this model may be implicated in increased 20-HETE formation in this model.

The absence of a response to HET0016, however, does not completely eliminate the possibility of a role of renal 20-HETE in dexamethasone-induced (10 μg/rat/d)

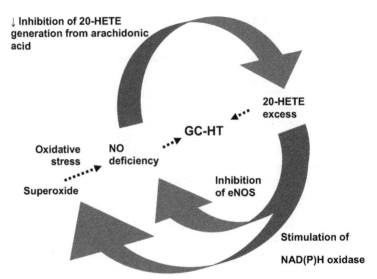

Fig. 2. Proposed mechanism of glucocorticoid-induced hypertension involving 20-HETE. 20-HETE, 20-hydroxyeicosatetraenoic acid; eNOS, endothelial nitric oxide synthase; GC-HT, glucocorticoid-induced hypertension; NAD(P)H, nicotinamide adenine dinucleotide phosphate; NO, nitric oxide.

hypertension, as higher dexamethasone doses in rats (0.3–1 mg/kg/d) have been reported to result in increased renal 20-HETE production.[82,83] It is also possible that the dexamethasone-induced hypertensive model has a higher threshold for the effects of 20-HETE. Thus, dexamethasone at higher doses could influence 20-HETE production, and the likely effect on blood pressure regulation warrants further investigations in future studies.

CLINICAL PERSPECTIVES: FROM BENCH TO BEDSIDE

Prolonged glucocorticoid administration, sometimes at supraphysiological doses, frequently leads to hypertension. Although the range of antihypertensive drugs can be tried to treat this complication, currently available evidence points to the use of nitric oxide donors and angiotensin-converting enzyme inhibitors (by limiting the angiotensin II effect on the NAD(P)H oxidase pathway) as therapeutic strategy. Diuretics and salt restriction are indicated for glucocorticoids with significant mineralocorticoid activity.

Lowering the renal vascular resistance with an angiotensin-converting enzyme inhibitor is logical in cortisol-induced, hydrocortisone-induced, and ACTH-induced hypertension. In ACTH-induced hypertension in rats, the angiotensin-converting enzyme inhibitor ramipril prevented the increase in blood pressure at a dose that also effectively reduced renal vascular resistance.[20] Although an increase in total peripheral resistance is a feature of dexamethasone-induced hypertension, the utility of a vasodilator such as minoxidil is limited, based on evidence in rats.[17] The efficacy of minoxidil in human glucocorticoid hypertension remains questionable.

β-Adrenergic receptor blockers,[5,20] calcium channel blockers,[18] and the xanthine oxidase inhibitor allopurinol[60,63] have been shown to be ineffective in this form of hypertension. Although 20-HETE inhibition is effective in ACTH-induced hypertension in rats,[36] it is not available for use in the clinical setting.

REFERENCES

1. Ross EJ, Linch DC. Cushing's syndrome-killing disease: discriminatory value of signs and symptoms aiding early diagnosis. Lancet 1982;320:646–9.
2. Treadwell BL, Sever ED, Savage O, et al. Side-effects of long-term treatment with corticosteroids and corticotrophin. Lancet 1964;283:1121–3.
3. Savage O, Copeman WS, Chapman L, et al. Pituitary and adrenal hormones in rheumatoid arthritis. Lancet 1962;279:232–5.
4. Mangos GJ, Turner SW, Fraser TB, et al. The role of corticosterone in corticotrophin (ACTH)-induced hypertension in the rat. J Hypertens 2000;18:1849–55.
5. Pirpiris M, Yeung S, Dewar E, et al. Hydrocortisone-induced hypertension in men. The role of cardiac output. Am J Hypertens 1993;6:287–94.
6. Connell JM, Whitworth JA, Davies DL, et al. Effects of ACTH and cortisol administration on blood pressure, electrolyte metabolism, atrial natriuretic peptide and renal function in normal man. J Hypertens 1987;5:425–33.
7. Kelly JJ, Tam SH, Williamson PM, et al. The nitric oxide system and cortisol-induced hypertension in humans. Clin Exp Pharmacol Physiol 1998;25:945–6.
8. Hu L, Zhang Y, Lim PS, et al. Apocynin but not L-arginine prevents and reverses dexamethasone-induced hypertension in the rat. Am J Hypertens 2006;19:413–8.
9. Zhang Y, Croft KD, Mori TA, et al. The antioxidant tempol prevents and partially reverses dexamethasone-induced hypertension in the rat. Am J Hypertens 2004;17:260–5.
10. Krug S, Zhang Y, Mori TA, et al. N-Acetylcysteine prevents but does not reverse dexamethasone-induced hypertension. Clin Exp Pharmacol Physiol 2008;35:979–81.
11. Nakamoto H, Suzuki H, Kageyama Y, et al. Characterization of alterations of hemodynamics and neuroendocrine hormones in dexamethasone induced hypertension in dogs. Clin Exp Hypertens A 1991;13:587–606.
12. Nakamoto H, Suzuki H, Kageyama Y, et al. Depressor systems contribute to hypertension induced by glucocorticoid excess in dogs. J Hypertens 1992;10:561–9.
13. Pirpiris M, Sudhir K, Yeung S, et al. Pressor responsiveness in corticosteroid-induced hypertension in humans. Hypertension 1992;19:567–74.
14. Scoggins BA, Allen KJ, Coghlan JP, et al. Haemodynamics of ACTH-induced hypertension in sheep. Clin Sci (Lond) 1979;57(Suppl 5):333s–6s.
15. Turner SW, Wen C, Li M, et al. Adrenocorticotrophin dose-response relationships in the rat: haemodynamic, metabolic and hormonal effects. J Hypertens 1998;16:593–600.
16. Whitworth JA. Adrenocorticotrophin and steroid-induced hypertension in humans. Kidney Int Suppl 1992;37:S34–7.
17. Ong SL, Zhang Y, Sutton M, et al. Hemodynamics of dexamethasone-induced hypertension in the rat. Hypertens Res 2009;32:889–94.
18. Whitworth JA, Williamson PM, Ramsey D. Haemodynamic response to cortisol in man: effects of felodipine. Hypertens Res 1994;17:137–42.
19. Wen C, Fraser T, Li M, et al. Hemodynamic profile of corticotropin-induced hypertension in the rat. J Hypertens 1998;16:187–94.
20. Wen C, Fraser T, Li M, et al. Haemodynamic mechanisms of corticotropin (ACTH)-induced hypertension in the rat. J Hypertens 1999;17:1715–23.
21. Montrella-Waybill M, Clore JN, Schoolwerth AC, et al. Evidence that high dose cortisol-induced Na+ retention in man is not mediated by the mineralocorticoid receptor. J Clin Endocrinol Metab 1991;72:1060–6.

22. Williamson PM, Kelly JJ, Whitworth JA. Dose-response relationships and mineralocorticoid activity in cortisol-induced hypertension in humans. J Hypertens 1996; Suppl 14:S37–41.

23. Li M, Wen C, Fraser T, et al. Adrenocorticotrophin-induced hypertension: effects of mineralocorticoid and glucocorticoid receptor antagonism. J Hypertens 1999; 17:419–26.

24. Whitworth JA, Saines D, Scoggins BA. Potentiation of ACTH hypertension in man with salt loading. Clin Exp Pharmacol Physiol 1985;12:239–43.

25. Connell JM, Whitworth JA, Davies DL, et al. Haemodynamic, hormonal and renal effects of adrenocorticotrophic hormone in sodium-restricted man. J Hypertens 1988;6:17–23.

26. Macefield VG, Williamson PM, Wilson LR, et al. Muscle sympathetic vasoconstrictor activity in hydrocortisone-induced hypertension in humans. Blood Press 1998;7:215–22.

27. Tabarin A, Minot AP, Dallochio M, et al. Plasma concentration of neuropeptide Y in patients with adrenal hypertension. Regul Pept 1992;42:51–61.

28. Whitworth JA, Williamson PM, Mangos G, et al. Cardiovascular consequences of cortisol excess. Vasc Health Risk Manag 2005;1:291–9.

29. Borcsok I, Schairer HU, Sommer U, et al. Glucocorticoids regulate the expression of the human osteoblastic endothelin A receptor gene. J Exp Med 1998;188: 1563–73.

30. Takahashi K, Suda K, Lam HC, et al. Endothelin-like immunoreactivity in rat models of diabetes mellitus. J Endocrinol 1991;130:123–7.

31. Iijima F, Malik KU. Contribution of vasopressin in dexamethasone-induced hypertension in rats. Hypertension 1988;11:I42–6.

32. Murasawa S, Matsubara H, Kizima K, et al. Glucocorticoids regulate V1a vasopressin receptor expression by increasing mRNA stability in vascular smooth muscle cells. Hypertension 1995;26:665–9.

33. Saruta T. Mechanism of glucocorticoid-induced hypertension. Hypertens Res 1996;19:1–8.

34. Wen C, Li M, Fraser T, et al. L-Arginine partially reverses established adrenocorticotrophin-induced hypertension and nitric oxide deficiency in the rat. Blood Press 2000;9:298–304.

35. Wallerath T, Witte K, Schafer SC, et al. Down-regulation of the expression of endothelial NO synthase is likely to contribute to glucocorticoid-mediated hypertension. Proc Natl Acad Sci U S A 1999;96:13357–62.

36. Zhang Y, Wu JH, Vickers JJ, et al. The role of 20-hydroxyeicosatetraenoic acid in glucocorticoid-induced hypertension. J Hypertens 2009;27:1609–16.

37. Andrews MC, Schyvens CG, Zhang Y, et al. Nitric oxide donation lowers blood pressure in adrenocorticotrophic hormone-induced hypertensive rats. Clin Exp Hypertens 2004;26:499–509.

38. Kelly JJ, Tam SH, Williamson PM, et al. Decreased threshold for the nitric oxide donor glyceryl trinitrate in cortisol-induced hypertension in humans. Clin Exp Pharmacol Physiol 2007;34:1317–8.

39. Turner SW, Wen C, Li M, et al. L-Arginine prevents corticotropin-induced increases in blood pressure in the rat. Hypertension 1996;27:184–9.

40. Li M, Fraser T, Wang J, et al. Dexamethasone-induced hypertension in the rat: effects of L-arginine. Clin Exp Pharmacol Physiol 1997;24:730–2.

41. Kelly JJ, Williamson P, Martin A, et al. Effects of oral L-arginine on plasma nitrate and blood pressure in cortisol-treated humans. J Hypertens 2001;19: 263–8.

42. Wen C, Li M, Whitworth JA. Role of nitric oxide in adrenocorticotrophin-induced hypertension: L-arginine effects reversed by N-nitro-L-arginine. Clin Exp Pharmacol Physiol 2000;27:887–90.
43. Chin-Dusting JP, Ahlers BA, Kaye DM, et al. L-Arginine transport in humans with cortisol-induced hypertension. Hypertension 2003;41:1336–40.
44. Li M, Dusting GJ, Whitworth JA. Inhibition of NO synthesis has an additive effect on hypertension induced by ACTH in conscious rats. Clin Exp Pharmacol Physiol 1992;19:675–81.
45. Thida M, Earl J, Zhao Y, et al. Effects of sepiapterin supplementation and NOS inhibition on glucocorticoid-induced hypertension. Am J Hypertens 2010;23: 569–74.
46. Wallerath T, Godecke A, Molojavyi A, et al. Dexamethasone lacks effect on blood pressure in mice with a disrupted endothelial NO synthase gene. Nitric Oxide 2004;10:36–41.
47. Lou Yk, Wen C, Li M, et al. Decreased renal expression of nitric oxide synthase isoforms in adrenocorticotropin-induced and corticosterone-induced hypertension. Hypertension 2001;37:1164–70.
48. Schmidt K, Werner ER, Mayer B, et al. Tetrahydrobiopterin-dependent formation of endothelium-derived relaxing factor (nitric oxide) in aortic endothelial cells. Biochem J 1992;281(Pt 2):297–300.
49. Alp NJ, Channon KM. Regulation of endothelial nitric oxide synthase by tetrahydrobiopterin in vascular disease. Arterioscler Thromb Vasc Biol 2004;24: 413–20.
50. Simmons WW, Ungureanu-Longrois D, Smith GK, et al. Glucocorticoids regulate inducible nitric oxide synthase by inhibiting tetrahydrobiopterin synthesis and L-arginine transport. J Biol Chem 1996;271:23928–37.
51. Johns DG, Dorrance AM, Tramontini NL, et al. Glucocorticoids inhibit tetrahydrobiopterin-dependent endothelial function. Exp Biol Med 2001;226: 27–31.
52. Mitchell BM, Dorrance AM, Webb RC. GTP cyclohydrolase 1 downregulation contributes to glucocorticoid hypertension in rats. Hypertension 2003;41: 669–74.
53. Zhang Y, Pang T, Earl J, et al. Role of tetrahydrobiopterin in adrenocorticotropic hormone-induced hypertension in the rat. Clin Exp Hypertens 2004;26:231–41.
54. Miao Y, Zhang Y, Lim PS, et al. Folic acid prevents and partially reverses glucocorticoid-induced hypertension in the rat. Am J Hypertens 2007;20:304–10.
55. Hong H-J, Hsiao G, Cheng TH, et al. Supplementation with tetrahydrobiopterin suppresses the development of hypertension in spontaneously hypertensive rats. Hypertension 2001;38:1044–8.
56. Iuchi T, Akaike M, Mitsui T, et al. Glucocorticoid excess induces superoxide production in vascular endothelial cells and elicits vascular endothelial dysfunction. Circ Res 2003;92:81–7.
57. Zhang Y, Jang R, Mori TA, et al. The anti-oxidant tempol reverses and partially prevents adrenocorticotrophic hormone-induced hypertension in the rat. J Hypertens 2003;21:1513–8.
58. Mondo CK, Zhang Y, Possamai V, et al. N-Acetylcysteine antagonizes the development but does not reverse ACTH-induced hypertension in the rat. Clin Exp Hypertens 2006;28:73–84.
59. Mondo CK, Yang WS, Zhang N, et al. Anti-oxidant effects of atorvastatin in dexamethasone-induced hypertension in the rat. Clin Exp Pharmacol Physiol 2006;33:1029–34.

60. Zhang Y, Chan MM, Andrews MC, et al. Apocynin but not allopurinol prevents and reverses adrenocorticotropic hormone-induced hypertension in the rat. Am J Hypertens 2005;18:910–6.
61. Zhang Y, Miao Y, Whitworth JA. Aspirin prevents and partially reverses adreno-corticotropic hormone-induced hypertension in the rat. Am J Hypertens 2007; 20:1222–8.
62. He Y, Zhang Y, Whitworth JA. Losartan prevents and reverses glucocorticoid-induced hypertension. Hypertension 2009;53:043.
63. Ong SL, Vickers JJ, Zhang Y, et al. Role of xanthine oxidase in dexamethasone-induced hypertension in rats. Clin Exp Pharmacol Physiol 2007;34:517–9.
64. Rajashree S, Puvanakrishnan R. Dexamethasone induced alterations in the levels of proteases involved in blood pressure homeostasis and blood coagulation in rats. Mol Cell Biochem 1999;197:203–8.
65. Carletti M, Cantiello M, Giantin M, et al. Serum antioxidant enzyme activities and oxidative stress parameters as possible biomarkers of exposure in veal calves illegally treated with dexamethasone. Toxicol In Vitro 2007;21:277–83.
66. Crawford DR, Davies KJ. Adaptive response and oxidative stress. Environ Health Perspect 1994;102(Suppl 10):25–8.
67. Axelrod L. Inhibition of prostacyclin production mediates permissive effect of glucocorticoids on vascular tone. Perturbations of this mechanism contribute to pathogenesis of Cushing's syndrome and Addison's disease. Lancet 1983;1: 904–6.
68. Flower RJ, Blackwell GJ. Anti-inflammatory steroids induce biosynthesis of a phospholipase A2 inhibitor which prevents prostaglandin generation. Nature 1979;278:456–9.
69. Hirata F, Schiffmann E, Venkatasubramanian K, et al. A phospholipase A2 inhibitory protein in rabbit neutrophils induced by glucocorticoids. Proc Natl Acad Sci U S A 1980;77:2533–6.
70. Russo-Marie F, Duval D. Dexamethasone-induced inhibition of prostaglandin production dose not result from a direct action on phospholipase activities but is mediated through a steroid-inducible factor. Biochim Biophys Acta 1982;712: 177–85.
71. Falardeau P, Martineau A. Prostaglandin I2 and glucocorticoid-induced rise in arterial pressure in the rat. J Hypertens 1989;7:625–32.
72. Handa M, Kondo K, Suzuki H, et al. Urinary prostaglandin E2 and kallikrein excretion in glucocorticoid hypertension in rats. Clin Sci (Lond) 1983;65:37–42.
73. Zhang Y, Hu L, Mori TA, et al. Arachidonic acid metabolism in glucocorticoid-induced hypertension. Clin Exp Pharmacol Physiol 2008;35:557–62.
74. Whitworth JA, Connell JM, Gordon D, et al. Effects of indomethacin on steroid-induced changes in pressor responsiveness in man. Clin Exp Pharmacol Physiol 1988;15:305–10.
75. Miyata N, Roman RJ. Role of 20-hydroxyeicosatetraenoic acid (20-HETE) in vascular system. J Smooth Muscle Res 2005;41:175–93.
76. Morgan ET, Ullrich V, Daiber A, et al. Cytochromes P450 and flavin monooxygenases—targets and sources of nitric oxide. Drug Metab Dispos 2001;29:1366–76.
77. Alonso-Galicia M, Drummond HA, Reddy KK, et al. Inhibition of 20-HETE production contributes to the vascular responses to nitric oxide. Hypertension 1997;29: 320–5.
78. Oyekan AO, Youseff T, Fulton D, et al. Renal cytochrome P450 omega-hydroxylase and epoxygenase activity are differentially modified by nitric oxide and sodium chloride. J Clin Invest 1999;104:1131–7.

79. Sun CW, Alonso-Galicia M, Taheri MR, et al. Nitric oxide-20-hydroxyeicosatetrae-noic acid interaction in the regulation of K$^+$ channel activity and vascular tone in renal arterioles. Circ Res 1998;83:1069–79.
80. Cheng J, Ou JS, Singh H, et al. 20-Hydroxyeicosatetraenoic acid causes endo-thelial dysfunction via eNOS uncoupling. Am J Physiol Heart Circ Physiol 2008; 294:H1018–26.
81. Wang JS, Singh H, Zhang F, et al. Endothelial dysfunction and hypertension in rats transduced with CYP4A2 adenovirus. Circ Res 2006;98:962–9.
82. Lin F, Abraham NG, Schwartzman ML. Cytochrome P450 arachidonic acid omega-hydroxylation in the proximal tubule of the rat kidney. Ann N Y Acad Sci 1994;744:11–24.
83. Sanchez-Mendoza A, Lopez-Sanchez P, Vazquez-Cruz B, et al. Angiotensin II modulates ion transport in rat proximal tubules through CYP metabolites. Biochem Biophys Res Commun 2000;272:423–30.
84. Whitworth JA, Gordon D, Andrews J, et al. The hypertensive effect of synthetic glucocorticoids in man: role of sodium and volume. J Hypertens 1989;7:537–49.
85. Humphrey TJ, Fan JS, Coghlan JP, et al. Inter-relationships between sodium and potassium intake and the blood pressure effects of ACTH in sheep. J Hypertens 1983;1:19–26.
86. Mills EH, Coghlan JP, Denton DA, et al. The effect of sodium depletion and potassium loading on cortisol induced hypertension in sheep. Acta Endocrinol (Copenh) 1986;113:298–304.
87. Mondo CK, Yang WS, Su JZ, et al. Atorvastatin prevented and reversed dexamethasone-induced hypertension in the rat. Clin Exp Hypertens 2006;28: 499–509.
88. Turner SW, Mangos GJ, Whitworth JA. Nitric oxide synthase activity in adrenocorticotrophin-induced hypertension in the rat. Clin Exp Pharmacol Physiol 2001;28:881–3.
89. Shafagoj Y, Opoku J, Qureshi D, et al. Dehydroepiandrosterone prevents dexamethasone-induced hypertension in rats. Am J Physiol Endocrinol Metab 1992;263:E210–3.
90. Li M, Wen C, Martin A, et al. Dehydroepiandrosterone does not prevent adrenocorticotrophin-induced hypertension in conscious rats. Clin Exp Pharma-col Physiol 1996;23:435–7.
91. Fraser TB, Turner SW, Wen C, et al. Vasopressin V1a receptor antagonism does not reverse adrenocorticotrophin-induced hypertension in the rat. Clin Exp Phar-macol Physiol 2000;27:866–70.

Glucocorticoids and Cardiovascular Risk Factors

Erika A. Strohmayer, MD[a],*, Lawrence R. Krakoff, MD[b]

KEYWORDS

- Glucocorticoids • Diabetes • Glucose metabolism
- Dyslipidemia • Hypertension • Cardiovascular risk
- C-reactive protein

Almost from the first extensive clinical descriptions of Cushing's syndrome, experts have recognized that excess exposure to the human glucocorticoid cortisol or the various synthetic glucocorticoids leads to hypertension, diabetes, and a high occurrence of atherosclerotic cardiovascular disease, stroke, and cardiac artery disease.[1] One might conclude that atherosclerosis is a variant of the complications of glucocorticoid excess. The resultant degree of cardiovascular disease caused by glucocorticoid therapy is best explained not by hypertension alone, but rather by the metabolic effects of prolonged glucocorticoid treatment on other pathways, particularly impaired glucose tolerance, including overt diabetes, and disturbances in serum lipids. The original enthusiasm toward glucocorticoids for treatment of various diseases has been tempered by recognition of its risks. Therefore, steroid-sparing regimens in the development of disease-modifying therapeutics have reduced exposure to glucocorticoids. This article explores the potential mechanisms of glucocorticoid-induced hyperglycemia and dyslipidemia. Interactions between glucocorticoids and other potential cardiovascular risk factors are also reviewed.

GLUCOCORTICOIDS, GLUCOSE METABOLISM, AND DIABETES

In patients treated with glucocorticoids, the odds ratio for development of new-onset diabetes mellitus has been reported to be 1.36 to 2.31.[2] The prevalence of abnormal

Financial Disclosures: The authors have nothing to disclose.
[a] Division of Endocrinology and Diabetes and Bone Disease, Mount Sinai School of Medicine, One Gustave L. Levy Place, New York, NY 10029, USA
[b] Mount Sinai School of Medicine, One Gustave L Levy Place, Box 1030, New York, NY 10029-6574, USA
* Corresponding author.
E-mail address: Erika.strohmayer@mountsinai.org

Endocrinol Metab Clin N Am 40 (2011) 409–417
doi:10.1016/j.ecl.2011.01.011
0889-8529/11/$ – see front matter © 2011 Elsevier Inc. All rights reserved.

endo.theclinics.com

glucose metabolism in postrenal transplant patients taking glucocorticoids has been reported to be 17% to 32%.[3,4] Smaller studies in patients treated with glucocorticoids for various neurologic diseases[5] and rheumatoid arthritis[6] have reported even greater prevalence. The risk of impaired glucose tolerance is probably not a sole consequence of the underlying disorder, because abnormal glucose metabolism has been observed in experimental studies of healthy subjects who were given glucocorticoids for a brief duration.[7–9]

Glucocorticoid-induced diabetes is similar to type 2 diabetes because glucocorticoids impair glucose metabolism mainly through increased insulin resistance. This mechanism is in contrast to type 1 diabetes, which results from autoimmune destruction of pancreatic islet cells, rendering patients insulin-dependent. To investigate the mechanism of glucocorticoid-induced hyperglycemia, Pagano and colleagues[7] evaluated prednisolone administration for 7 days in healthy volunteers. A 50% reduction in insulin sensitivity was shown using insulin clamp methods.[7] Subsequent studies[9,10] support these findings. The increased insulin resistance occurs in the liver, resulting in increased basal glucose production, and the periphery (adipose and skeletal tissues) where glucose use is impaired.

Insulin stimulates peripheral glucose uptake through binding to its receptor, stimulating glucose transport 4 (GLUT4) to the cell surface, and activating a signaling cascade that promotes use of glucose within the cell, including glycogen synthesis. By interfering with this signaling cascade, glucocorticoids impair glucose use through postreceptor defects, such as diminished GLUT4 expression and migration[11] and decreased glycogen synthesis.[12,13] Human studies are limited but support the notion of glucocorticoid-induced postreceptor defects. Reduction of glycogen synthase activity after glucocorticoid administration has been shown in muscle biopsies from healthy controls[14] and renal transplant patients.[15] Some experts have proposed that glucocorticoids may indirectly reduce insulin signaling through increased protein catabolism and intracellular lipid accumulation[16]; however, studies supporting these indirect mechanisms are lacking.

Glucocorticoids also increase insulin resistance in the liver, thus enhancing hepatic endogenous glucose production. This effect was shown by Rizza and colleagues,[8] who performed euglycemic hyperinsulinemic clamp studies on healthy volunteers after infusion of either cortisol or saline. Cortisol increased fasting glucose production, and more insulin was required to reduce this glucose production after cortisol infusion than after saline.[8] Because endogenous hepatic glucose production is accomplished through gluconeogenesis and glycogenolysis, experts believe that glucocorticoids promote these processes. Animal studies[17] show that glucocorticoids induce expression of key enzymes of gluconeogenesis. Glucocorticoid augmentation of counterregulatory hormones (ie, glucagon) has also been implicated.[18]

In response to decreased insulin sensitivity, the pancreatic beta cell normally increases insulin secretion to maintain normal glucose homeostasis. Type 2 diabetes results from progressive loss of beta cell function, diminishing this compensation and resulting in hyperglycemia.[19] Glucocorticoids have been suggested to cause beta cell dysfunction, but human studies reporting on glucocorticoid effect on insulin secretion are mixed. Both enhancement[20] and inhibition[21] of insulin secretion after exposure to glucocorticoids has been shown. Moreover, insulin secretion may not increase enough to compensate for the amplified insulin resistance.[22]

Glucocorticoids seem to have differential effects depending on dosage and duration of exposure, degree of glucose level achieved, measurement of insulin secretion (ie, hyperglycemic clamp versus oral glucose tolerance test), and vulnerability of the population studied. Studies[23,24] using higher doses for up to 3 days in healthy subjects show enhanced secretion of insulin, whereas those in susceptible individuals (ie, obese subjects) are more consistent with inadequate insulin secretion.[22]

The effect of long-term glucocorticoid exposure on insulin secretion in healthy humans has not been prospectively evaluated, and observational data from patients on glucocorticoid therapy may be confounded by the effect of inflammation on beta cell function, although this effect is not well described. Dessein and Joffe[25] attempted to discern the effects of inflammation by looking at inflammatory markers, diseased activity, and a homeostatic model of beta cell function in 94 patients with rheumatoid arthritis. Elevated highly sensitive C-reactive protein (CRP) correlated with reduced beta cell function, but this relationship lost significance when adjusted for abdominal waist circumference. Therefore, inflammatory disease states may induce beta cell dysfunction through indirect mechanisms.

Glucocorticoids are believed to interfere with the signaling pathways of various insulin secretagogues, including glucose. The exact mechanisms are unknown but several have been supported by in vitro studies, including reduced glucose uptake and oxidation,[26,27] and upregulation of potassium-gated ion channels, impairing depolarization and leading to decreased calcium influx; a stimulus for insulin granule release.[28] Increased beta cell death after incubation with dexamethasone has also been shown.[29]

Understanding of the mechanisms of glucocorticoid-induced diabetes will lead to the development of novel therapeutic agents for anti-inflammatory drugs. Glucocorticoid receptor agonists that have anti-inflammatory properties without metabolic side effects are already being investigated.[16] Currently, the significant increased risks for diabetes and subsequent cardiovascular disease associated with glucocorticoids are important to understand so that patients can be monitored and treated appropriately.

GLUCOCORTICOIDS AND LIPIDS

Glucocorticoid administration is a known, reversible cause of dyslipidemia. The prevalence of dyslipidemia among transplant recipients taking glucocorticoids is more than 80% for heart, 60% to 70% for renal, and 45% for liver.[30] These results may be confounded by concurrent use of other immunosuppressant agents. However, patients treated with glucocorticoid monotherapy for inflammatory diseases such as sarcoidosis, uveitis,[31] systemic lupus erythematosus,[32] and asthma[33] also show increased rates of dyslipidemia. Duration and cumulative glucocorticoid dose are important determinants of glucocorticoid-induced dyslipidemia. Studies evaluating steroid-sparing regimens or alternate-day dosing of prednisone show reduced rates of dyslipidemia after cardiac[34] and renal transplant.[35] Underlying inflammation probably contributes to dyslipidemia in these populations. Still, alterations in lipid metabolism have been shown in investigations of glucocorticoids in healthy human subjects.[36,37]

Glucocorticoids have a differential effect on lipid profiles in normal subjects versus those with underlying disease. Increased high-density lipoprotein (HDL), variable increases in total cholesterol (TC) and triglycerides (TG), and unchanged low-density lipoprotein (LDL) have been reported in small, short-term prospective studies in healthy subjects,[36–38] whereas observational studies of patients treated with glucocorticoids for asthma, cardiac or renal transplants, and rheumatoid arthritis have shown elevations of TC, TG, and LDL, and variable changes in HDL.[39]

The reasons behind the observed differences between healthy subjects and patients are multifactorial. Chronic inflammation promotes dyslipidemia. Cytokines involved in the inflammatory cascade lead to decreases in HDL and increases in very-low-density lipoprotein (VLDL), LDL, and TG.[40] Chronic illness can also lead to changes in eating habits that alter lipid profiles. Studies in healthy subjects are necessarily brief and have limited effects compared with the prolonged duration of glucocorticoid treatment in patients with chronic diseases. Glucocorticoid treatment may have different short-term and long-term effects on lipids. Moreover, the variable results in HDL levels among patients are dose-related and disease-dependent. For example, increased HDL was seen in patients treated with a mean dose of prednisone, 5 mg daily, for rheumatoid arthritis,[41] whereas decreased HDL in postcardiac transplant patients is potentiated by glucocorticoid treatment.[30]

The mechanisms through which glucocorticoids induce dyslipidemia are not well elucidated. Experts have suggested that glucocorticoid-induced hepatic insulin resistance leads to increased production of VLDL and subsequent increased TG and LDL levels.[38,42] Hydrocortisone and dexamethasone have been shown in vitro to alter LDL degradation and internalization in fibroblasts and macrophages, respectively, which are important for atherosclerotic plaque formation.[43,44] In this way, glucocorticoids may exert atherogenic effects. The observed rise in HDL may be from direct hepatic production of HDL or secondary to glucocorticoid-induced lipoprotein lipase activity, which hydrolyzes VLDL to HDL.[38] However, lipoprotein lipase activity has been shown to be decreased in some rat studies.[45] Furthermore, the observed increases in lipoprotein lipase may be correlative and not causative.[37]

The metabolism of TGs has important metabolic and possible cardiovascular consequences. Lipolysis is the process of conversion of TGs to free fatty acids. Through beta-oxidation, free fatty acids are used as fuel in adipose, hepatic, and muscle tissue. In states of energy excess, lipogenesis occurs where free fatty acids are converted to TGs and used for storage or released into the circulation. Excessive lipid accumulation can lead to organ-specific consequences. For example, intramyocellular lipid accumulation promotes insulin resistance.[46] Glucocorticoids have variable effects on free fatty acid metabolism in a site-specific manner.

Glucocorticoid alteration in hepatic free fatty acid metabolism can lead to hepatic steatosis. In rats, dexamethasone administration resulted in intrahepatic TG accumulation.[47] Interruption of glucocorticoid receptor activity reverses hepatic steatosis in mice models of fatty liver.[48] Human studies are lacking. However, one study[49] showed that 20% of patients with endogenous Cushing's syndrome met criteria for hepatic steatosis through CT evaluation. Come case reports have linked glucocorticoid therapy to hepatic steatosis.[50–53]

The effect of glucocorticoid on adipose and intravascular lipid metabolism was recently reviewed elsewhere.[54] Most in vitro and some in vivo reports support increased whole-body lipolysis after glucocorticoid administration.[54] Glucocorticoids may have differential effects on subcutaneous and visceral fat metabolism, which may explain the body fat redistribution exhibited by patients with endogenous Cushing's syndrome, in whom subcutaneous fat decreases and visceral fat increases.[55,56] Clinical studies of exogenous glucocorticoid administration are less prevalent. One study[57] examining patients with temporal arteritis treated with prednisolone found that truncal fat increased more than peripheral fat in a dose-dependent manner. Increased central adiposity is a key feature of the metabolic syndrome, which is associated with systemic inflammation and increased cardiovascular morbidity and mortality.[58] The underlying mechanisms through which excess glucocorticoids modulate body fat content and distribution are being explored. These mechanisms may provide insight for future therapeutic strategies to reduce visceral adiposity and subsequent cardiovascular risk.

GLUCOCORTICOIDS AND OTHER RISK FACTORS

The diverse actions of glucocorticoids on other systems may also contribute to increased cardiovascular risk. Elsewhere in this issue, Ong and Whitworth summarize recent advances in understanding of how glucocorticoid treatment causes hypertension. The renin–angiotensin system may contribute to increased cardiovascular disease even when hypertension is not present.[59] Unlike mineralocorticoid excess, which suppresses the renin system, glucocorticoid therapy tends to increase plasma renin activity, partly through increased levels of angiotensinogen.[60] Drugs that block the renin–angiotensin system, angiotensin-converting enzyme inhibitors, or angiotensin receptor blockers may be effective for glucocorticoid therapy–related hypertension, but may also prevent cardiovascular pathology through alternate mechanisms.

Inflammation is now recognized as an important component of atherosclerotic cardiovascular disease, as reflected in the relationship between CRP and pathology.[61] Glucocorticoids have a powerful anti-inflammatory effect, suggesting that glucocorticoid therapy would retard rather than promote atherosclerotic disease. CRP is reduced after glucocorticoid treatment for certain inflammatory disorders, including giant cell arterits,[62] polymyalgia rheumatic,[63] and periodontitis.[64] Brotman and colleagues[36] showed a significant reduction in CRP in healthy subjects treated with dexamethasone for 5 days. Dernellis and Panaretou[65] showed that patients with persistent atrial fibrillation converted to sinus rhythm who were treated with methylprednisone for 5 months had lower CRP values and less recurrence of atrial fibrillation. How reduction in CRP correlates with other cardiovascular risks remains to be determined. Further studies are needed to address this issue. Glucocorticoid therapy may have a beneficial anti-inflammatory effect in preventing atherosclerosis that is masked by the hypertension, impaired glucose tolerance, and induced dyslipidemia associated with long-term treatment.

SUMMARY

Glucocorticoids remain a valuable and necessary component of therapy for many diseases. Nonetheless, sustained glucocorticoid treatment increases potential for future cardiovascular disease through multiple pathways, resulting in a tradeoff between benefit and harm. This article, and one by Ong and Whitworth elsewhere in this issue, summarize these pathways. Safe, alternate strategies for minimizing the need for glucocorticoids are urgently needed.

REFERENCES

1. Plotz CM, Knowlton AI, Ragan C. The natural history of Cushing's syndrome. Am J Med 1952;13(5):597–614.
2. Clore JN, Thurby-Hay L. Glucocorticoid-induced hyperglycemia. Endocr Pract 2009;15(5):469–74.
3. Chan HW, Cheung CY, Liu YL, et al. Prevalence of abnormal glucose metabolism in Chinese renal transplant recipients: a single centre study. Nephrol Dial Transplant 2008;23(10):3337–42.
4. Bonato V, Barni R, Cataldo D, et al. Analysis of posttransplant diabetes mellitus prevalence in a population of kidney transplant recipients. Transplant Proc 2008;40(6):1888–90.
5. Iwamoto T, Kagawa Y, Naito Y, et al. Steroid-induced diabetes mellitus and related risk factors in patients with neurologic diseases. Pharmacotherapy 2004;24(4):508–14.

6. Panthakalam S, Bhatnagar D, Klimink P. The prevalence and management of hyperglycaemia in patients with rheumatoid arthritis on corticosteroid therapy. Scott Med J 2004;49(4):139–41.

7. Pagano G, Cavalloperin P, Cassader M, et al. An in vivo and in vitro study of the mechanism of prednisone-induced insulin resistance in healthy subjects. J Clin Invest 1983;72(5):1814–20.

8. Rizza RA, Mandarino LJ, Gerich JE. Cortisol-induced insulin resistance in man: impaired suppression of glucose-production and stimulation of glucose-utilization due to a postreceptor defect of insulin action. J Clin Endocrinol Metab 1982;54(1):131–8.

9. Abdelmannan D, Tahboub R, Genuth S, et al. Effect of dexamethasone on oral glucose tolerance in normal individuals. Endocr Pract 2010;16(5):770–7.

10. Nicod N, Giusti V, Besse C, et al. Metabolic adaptations to dexamethasone-induced insulin resistance in healthy volunteers. Obes Res 2003;11(5):625–31.

11. Weinstein SP, Wilson CM, Pritsker A, et al. Dexamethasone inhibits insulin-stimulated recruitment of GLUT4 to the cell surface in rat skeletal muscle. Metabolism 1998;47(1):3–6.

12. Ruzzin J, Wagman AS, Jensen J. Glucocorticoid-induced insulin resistance in skeletal muscles: defects in insulin signalling and the effects of a selective glycogen synthase kinase-3 inhibitor. Diabetologia 2005;48(10):2119–30.

13. Buren J, Lai YC, Lundgren M, et al. Insulin action and signalling in fat and muscle from dexamethasone-treated rats. Arch Biochem Biophys 2008; 474(1):91–101.

14. Henriksen JE, Alford F, Vaag A, et al. Intracellular skeletal muscle glucose metabolism is differentially altered by dexamethasone treatment of normoglycemic relatives of type 2 diabetic patients. Metabolism 1999;48(9):1128–35.

15. Ekstrand A, Schalin Jantti C, Lofman M, et al. The effect of (steroid) immunosuppression on skeletal muscle glycogen metabolism in patients after kidney transplantation. Transplantation 1996;61(6):889–93.

16. van Raalte DH, Ouwens DM, Diamant M. Novel insights into glucocorticoid-mediated diabetogenic effects: towards expansion of therapeutic options? Eur J Clin Invest 2009;39(2):81–93.

17. Jin JY, DuBois DC, Almon RR, et al. Receptor/gene-mediated pharmacodynamic effects of methylprednisolone on phosphoenolpyruvate carboxykinase regulation in rat liver. J Pharmacol Exp Ther 2004;309(1):328–39.

18. Dirlewanger M, Schneiter P, Paquot N, et al. Effects of glucocorticoids on hepatic sensitivity to insulin and glucagon in man. Clin Nutr 2000;19(1):29–34.

19. Stumvoll M, Goldstein BJ, van Haeften TW. Type 2 diabetes: principles of pathogenesis and therapy. Lancet 2005;365(9467):1333–46.

20. Vila G, Krebs M, Riedl M, et al. Acute effects of hydrocortisone on the metabolic response to a glucose load: increase in first-phase insulin secretion. Eur J Endocrinol 2010;163(2):225–31.

21. Kalhan SC, Adam PA. Inhibitory effect of prednisone on insulin-secretion in man: model for duplication of blood-glucose concentration. J Clin Endocrinol Metab 1975;41(3):600–10.

22. Besse C, Nicod N, Tappy L. Changes in insulin secretion and glucose metabolism induced by dexamethasone in lean and obese females. Obes Res 2005; 13(2):306–11.

23. Matsumoto K, Yamasaki H, Akazawa S, et al. High-dose but not low-dose dexamethasone impairs glucose tolerance by inducing compensatory failure of pancreatic beta-cells in normal men. J Clin Endocrinol Metab 1996;81:2621–6.

24. Beard JC, Halter JB, Best JD, et al. Dexamethasone-induced insulin resistance enhances b-cell responsiveness to glucose level in normal men. Am J Physiol 1984;247(5):E592–6.
25. Dessein PH, Joffe BI. Insulin resistance and impaired beta cell function in rheumatoid arthritis. Arthritis Rheum 2006;54(9):2765–75.
26. Gremlich S, Roduit R, Thorens B. Dexamethasone induces posttranslational degradation of GLUT2 and inhibition of insulin secretion in isolated pancreatic beta cells. Comparison with the effects of fatty acids. J Biol Chem 1997;272(6): 3216–22.
27. Khan A, Ostenson CG, Berggren PO, et al. Glucocorticoid increases glucose cycling and inhibits insulin release in pancreatic-islets of ob/ob mice. Am J Physiol 1992;263(4):E663–6.
28. Ullrich S, Berchtold S, Ranta F, et al. Serum- and glucocorticoid-inducible kinase 1 (SGK1) mediates glucocorticoid-induced inhibition of insulin secretion. Diabetes 2005;54(4):1090–9.
29. Ranta F, Avram D, Berchtold S, et al. Dexamethasone induces cell death in insulin-secreting cells, an effect reversed by exendin-4. Diabetes 2006;55(5): 1380–90.
30. Miller LW. Cardiovascular toxicities of immunosuppressive agents. Am J Transplant 2002;2(9):807–18.
31. Zimmerman J, Fainaru M, Eisenberg S. The effects of prednisone therapy on plasma lipoproteins and apolipoproteins: a prospective study. Metabolism 1984;33(6):521–6.
32. Ettinger WH, Goldberg AP, Applebaum-Bowden D, et al. Dyslipoproteinemia in systemic lupus erythematosus. Effect of corticosteroids. Am J Med 1987;83(3): 503–8.
33. el-Shaboury AH, Hayes TM. Hyperlipidaemia in asthmatic patients receiving long-term steroid therapy. Br Med J 1973;2(5858):85–6.
34. Keogh A, Macdonald P, Harvison A, et al. Initial steroid-free versus steroid-based maintenance therapy and steroid withdrawal after heart transplantation: two views of the steroid question. J Heart Lung Transplant 1992;11(2 Pt 2):421–7.
35. Curtis JJ, Galla JH, Woodford SY, et al. Effect of alternate-day prednisone on plasma lipids in renal transplant recipients. Kidney Int 1982;22(1):42–7.
36. Brotman DJ, Girod JP, Garcia MJ, et al. Effects of short-term glucocorticoids on cardiovascular biomarkers. J Clin Endocrinol Metab 2005;90(6):3202–8.
37. Taskinen MR, Kuusi T, Yki-Jarvinen H, et al. Short-term effects of prednisone on serum lipids and high density lipoprotein subfractions in normolipidemic healthy men. J Clin Endocrinol Metab 1988;67(2):291–9.
38. Ettinger WH Jr, Hazzard WR. Elevated apolipoprotein-B levels in corticosteroid-treated patients with systemic lupus erythematosus. J Clin Endocrinol Metab 1988;67(3):425–8.
39. Sholter DE, Armstrong PW. Adverse effects of corticosteroids on the cardiovascular system. Can J Cardiol 2000;16(4):505–11.
40. Esteve E, Ricart W, Fernandez-Real JM. Dyslipidemia and inflammation: an evolutionary conserved mechanism. Clin Nutr 2005;24(1):16–31.
41. Garcia-Gomez C, Nolla JM, Valverde J, et al. High HDL-cholesterol in women with rheumatoid arthritis on low-dose glucocorticoid therapy. Eur J Clin Invest 2008;38(9):686–92.
42. Stern MP, Kolterman OG, Fries JF, et al. Adrenocortical steroid treatment of rheumatic diseases. Effects on lipid metabolism. Arch Intern Med 1973;132(1): 97–101.

43. Henze K, Chait A, Albers JJ, et al. Hydrocortisone decreases the internalization of low density lipoprotein in cultured human fibroblasts and arterial smooth muscle cells. Eur J Clin Invest 1983;13(2):171–7.
44. Hirsch LJ, Mazzone T. Dexamethasone modulates lipoprotein metabolism in cultured human monocyte-derived macrophages. Stimulation of scavenger receptor activity. J Clin Invest 1986;77(2):485–90.
45. Bagdade JD, Yee E, Albers J, et al. Glucocorticoids and triglyceride transport: effects on triglyceride secretion rates, lipoprotein lipase, and plasma lipoproteins in the rat. Metabolism 1976;25(5):533–42.
46. Boden G, Shulman GI. Free fatty acids in obesity and type 2 diabetes: defining their role in the development of insulin resistance and beta-cell dysfunction. Eur J Clin Invest 2002;32(Suppl 3):14–23.
47. Cole TG, Wilcox HG, Heimberg M. Effects of adrenalectomy and dexamethasone on hepatic lipid metabolism. J Lipid Res 1982;23(1):81–91.
48. Lemke U, Krones-Herzig A, Berriel Diaz M, et al. The glucocorticoid receptor controls hepatic dyslipidemia through Hes1. Cell Metab 2008;8(3):212–23.
49. Rockall AG, Sohaib SA, Evans D, et al. Hepatic steatosis in Cushing's syndrome: a radiological assessment using computed tomography. Eur J Endocrinol 2003; 149(6):543–8.
50. Dourakis SP, Sevastianos VA, Kaliopi P. Acute severe steatohepatitis related to prednisolone therapy. Am J Gastroenterol 2002;97(4):1074–5.
51. Itoh S, Igarashi M, Tsukada Y, et al. Nonalcoholic fatty liver with alcoholic hyalin after long-term glucocorticoid therapy. Acta Hepatogastroenterol (Stuttg) 1977; 24(6):415–8.
52. Kitahara A, Saga K, Koide S, et al. Iatrogenic hyperadrenocorticism and steato-hepatitis caused by unapproved medicine. Intern Med 2008;47(13):1231–6.
53. Nanki T, Koike R, Miyasaka N. Subacute severe steatohepatitis during predniso-lone therapy for systemic lupus erythematosis. Am J Gastroenterol 1999;94(11): 3379.
54. Macfarlane DP, Forbes S, Walker BR. Glucocorticoids and fatty acid metabolism in humans: fuelling fat redistribution in the metabolic syndrome. J Endocrinol 2008;197(2):189–204.
55. Rockall AG, Sohaib SA, Evans D, et al. Computed tomography assessment of fat distribution in male and female patients with Cushing's syndrome. Eur J Endocri-nol 2003;149(6):561–7.
56. Rebuffe-Scrive M, Krotkiewski M, Elfverson J, et al. Muscle and adipose tissue morphology and metabolism in Cushing's syndrome. J Clin Endocrinol Metab 1988;67(6):1122–8.
57. Nordborg E, Schaufelberger C, Bosaeus I. The effect of glucocorticoids on fat and lean tissue masses in giant cell arteritis. Scand J Rheumatol 1998;27(2): 106–11.
58. Isomaa B, Almgren P, Tuomi T, et al. Cardiovascular morbidity and mortality asso-ciated with the metabolic syndrome. Diabetes Care 2001;24(4):683–9.
59. Yusuf S, Sleight P, Pogue J, et al. Effects of an angiotensin-converting-enzyme inhibitor, ramipril, on cardiovascular events in high-risk patients. The Heart Outcomes Prevention Evaluation Study Investigators. N Engl J Med 2000; 342(3):145–53.
60. Krakoff LR, Elijovich F. Cushing's syndrome and exogenous glucocorticoid hyper-tension. Clin Endocrinol Metab 1981;10(3):479–88.
61. Ridker PM, Morrow DA. C-reactive protein, inflammation, and coronary risk. Car-diol Clin 2003;21(3):315–25.

62. Andersson R, Malmvall BE, Bengtsson BA. Acute phase reactants in the initial phase of giant cell arteritis. Acta Med Scand 1986;220(4):365–7.
63. Mallya RK, Hind CR, Berry H, et al. Serum C-reactive protein in polymyalgia rheumatica. A prospective serial study. Arthritis Rheum 1985;28(4):383–7.
64. Renvert S, Lindahl C, Roos-Jansaker AM, et al. Short-term effects of an anti-inflammatory treatment on clinical parameters and serum levels of C-reactive protein and proinflammatory cytokines in subjects with periodontitis. J Periodontol 2009;80(6):892–900.
65. Dernellis J, Panaretou M. Relationship between C-reactive protein concentrations during glucocorticoid therapy and recurrent atrial fibrillation. Eur Heart J 2004; 25(13):1100–7.

Blood Pressure Effects of the Oral Contraceptive and Postmenopausal Hormone Therapies

Angela Boldo, MD[a], William B. White, MD[b],*

KEYWORDS

• Blood pressure monitoring • Hormone therapy • Menopause
• Oral contraceptives • Postmenopausal

ORAL CONTRACEPTIVE USE IN CLINICAL PRACTICE

In North America, oral contraceptive pills (OCPs) are among the most commonly prescribed birth-control methods, used by 19% of women in general and by approximately 80% of women at some time during their life.[1] Contraceptive hormones were first introduced in the 1960s and contained 2 to 5 times as much estrogen and 5 to 10 times as much progestin as presently used combination agents. OCPs are classified in generations (first to fourth) depending on their timing of introduction into the market as well as by the dose of estrogen and type of progestin used. First-generation OCPs contained 150 μg of ethinyl estradiol compared with 50 μg in the second-generation pills and 20 to 35 μg in the currently available preparations. Some OCPs contain mestranol as the estrogen. These estrogens are combined with different types of progestin that use the same dose throughout the cycle (monophasic) or at increasing weekly doses to mimic the natural hormonal cycle (biphasic or triphasic).

The first-generation oral contraceptive progestins (norethindrone and ethynodiol diacetate) were replaced by more potent second-generation progestins (levonorgestrel and norgestrel) that allowed for lower dosages to be used. The third-generation oral contraceptive progestins (desogestrel, norgestimate, and gestodene) and the fourth-generation progestins (chlormadinone acetate and drospirenone) have fewer androgenic and metabolic side effects. Drospirenone is also an aldosterone

---

[a] Division of Endocrinology, Dartmouth-Hitchcock Medical Center, Lebanon, NH, USA
[b] Division of Hypertension and Clinical Pharmacology, Pat and Jim Calhoun Cardiology Center, University of Connecticut School of Medicine, 263 Farmington Avenue Farmington, CT 06032-3940, USA
* Corresponding author.
E-mail address: wwhite@nso1.uchc.edu

Endocrinol Metab Clin N Am 40 (2011) 419–432
doi:10.1016/j.ecl.2011.01.008
0889-8529/11/$ – see front matter © 2011 Elsevier Inc. All rights reserved.

endo.theclinics.com

antagonist with both androgenic and diuretic effects. Most OCPs are taken for 21 days out of a 28-day cycle but new low-dose formulations exist that when taken daily produce only 0 to 4 menses per year. Contraceptive hormones also can be delivered by transdermal patches or via a vaginal ring. Progestin-only contraceptives are available through oral route, injection, implant, or intrauterine devices (**Table 1**).[2]

ORAL CONTRACEPTIVE AND THE DEVELOPMENT OF HYPERTENSION

Many studies have shown that OCPs can induce significant increases in blood pressure (BP) with chronic use.[3–6] In a prospective cohort study of 68,297 normotensive women, there was a 1.8 relative increase in the risk of developing hypertension in 4 years (the absolute incidence rates ranged from 0.5% to 1.9% depending on the age of the women). Increased BPs decreased quickly with cessation of oral contraceptives.[7] In women with stage 1 hypertension, an average increase of 8 mm Hg in the systolic BP has been observed between the users of a low-dose OCP and controls.[8] In hypertensive women,[9] a decrease in the systolic pressure of 15 mm Hg has been observed after discontinuation of OCPs.[10] The dose and type of progestin might influence the incidence rates of hypertension[3] but women taking progesterone-only preparations show few increases in BP.[3,4] Increases in BP nearly always seem to be reversible after 4 weeks of discontinuation of the OCP; in contrast during the 7-day pill-free period of the 21/28 cycles of most preparations, BP does not become lower versus the active treatment period.[6]

Hypertension has been reported even with the newer low-estrogen-dose monophasic pills.[5,6] In a study using 24-hour BP monitoring, an increase of systolic BP by 8 mm Hg was observed in normotensive women after 6 to 9 months of low-dose (30 µg estrogen) oral contraceptive use.[11] Meade and colleagues[5] reported larger BP effects of estrogen doses of 50 µg versus 30 µg OCPs; part of the hypertensive effect was attributed to the progesterone used (norgestrel).

A newer progestin, drospirenone, has antimineralocorticoid diuretic effects, which seem to produce lower BPs when combined with OCP estrogen doses. Eighty women were randomized into 4 groups of drospirenone 3 mg and 3 doses of ethinyl estradiol (30 µg, 20 µg, and 15 µg) and a control group administered 30 µg of ethinyl estradiol and 150 µg of levonorgestrel. Systolic and diastolic BPs decreased by 1 to 4 mm Hg in the 3 drospirenone groups and increased by 1 to 2 mm Hg in the levonorgestrel group. Women treated with drospirenone also had a significant loss of weight ranging from 0.8 to 1.7 kg (**Fig. 1**). This study also reported increased plasma renin activity and aldosterone in the drospirenone groups, presumably from sodium loss and feedback from the blockade of mineralocorticoid receptors.[12]

Regarding progestogen-only preparations, a cross-sectional survey in England found increased BP in patients on oral contraceptives containing estrogen and progesterone but not in patients taking a progestin-only pill.[4]

PATHOPHYSIOLOGY OF ORAL CONTRACEPTIVE USE AND THE DEVELOPMENT OF HYPERTENSION

Causes of BP increase in women taking oral contraceptives are multifactorial and complex. Activation of the renin-angiotensin system (RAS) is involved in increasing BP in oral contraceptive users. A study in rats showed that the promoter region in the angiotensinogen gene is responsive to estrogen, and exogenous estrogen administration increased the concentration of angiotensinogen[13] and consequently has the potential to increase plasma concentration of angiotensin II. In humans, increased levels of plasma renin activity, angiotensinogen, and angiotensin II have been observed in OCP users, and the increase in renal vascular resistance is at least partially abolished by angiotensin II blockade with losartan (**Fig. 2**).[14] Conversely, OCP users show a higher activation of nitric oxide (NO) activation, modulating the hemodynamic effects of RAS activation by enhancing endothelial-dependent vasodilatation.[15]

Although in healthy women an increase in angiotensin II as discussed earlier induces a reduction in renin release, women who become hypertensive on oral contraceptives seem to have an incomplete negative feedback response for renin production, leading to activation of the RAS with a subsequent increase in BP.[16] The synthetic progestins are unable to mitigate the salt-retaining and water-retaining effects of estrogen because unlike natural progesterone, which induces mineralocorticoid receptor antagonism, they lack this effect.

The antimineralocorticoid effect of drospirenone is similar to natural progesterone. This compound is a derivative of 17-α-spironolactone that inhibits ovulation and leads to a mild natriuresis which slightly activates the RAS.[17] Drospirenone attenuates the vascular effects of estrogen; this characteristic was shown in aldosterone salt-treated rats, in which the beneficial effect of 17-β-estradiol (natural estrogen) on vascular function was abolished by medroxyprogesterone but not by drospirenone. In addition, drospirenone has shown protective effects on cardiac hypertrophy and endothelial function in rats.[18]

PHENOTYPE AND BP EFFECTS OF ORAL CONTRACEPTIVE

Women who generally have higher BPs have been hypothesized to be more susceptible to the hypertensive effects of OCPs. However, there has been no obvious influence of age, family history, ethnicity, or body mass index (calculated as weight in kilograms divided by the square of height in meters) in either a prospective study of normotensive women[7] or a cross-sectional study that evaluated BP responses to oral contraceptives according to race and ethnicity.[19] The latter study did show increased BP with oral contraceptive use in those women who had family history of hypertension or history of hypertension during pregnancy.[19]

TREATMENT OF EXOGENOUS OCP-INDUCED HYPERTENSION

Stopping OCP in patients with hypertension has been shown to reduce systolic BP and is clearly a first-line consideration in OCP-induced hypertension.[10] The challenge is when no alternate form of contraception is feasible or acceptable. Because the RAS is involved in the mechanism of OCP-induced hypertension, the use of angiotensin II blockade becomes a rational consideration for treatment. Despite higher levels of plasma renin activity in OCP users compared with patients with essential hypertension, captopril induced similar changes in BP and renal hemodynamics in both groups, supporting the use of angiotensin-converting enzyme (ACE) inhibitors in the treatment of patients with OCP-induced hypertension.[20] The BP increase and increase in renal vascular resistance with OCPs were also partially reversed with an angiotensin II receptor blocker (see **Fig. 2**).[14] The change in oral contraception in premenopausal women who developed hypertension on estrogen-containing OCPs to progestin-only preparation or to formulations shown to have antimineralocorticoid effect with lowering BP (drospirenone) are options, but no studies evaluating this strategy have been performed. In postmenopausal women, the addition of hormonal replacement therapy (HRT) with drospirenone to hypertensive postmenopausal women on enalapril decreased BP by a mean of 9/5 mm Hg, suggesting an additive BP effect of drospirenone in hypertensive patients on ACE inhibitors.[21] Drospirenone-based hormone

Table 1
Overview of hormonal contraception formulations available in the United States

	Dose	Brand/Trade Name
Oral Triphasic Formulation		
Estrogen/progestin[a]		
Ethinyl estradiol/desogestrel	25 µg/0.1, 0.125, 0.15 mg	Cyclessa
Ethinyl estradiol/ levonorgestrel	30 µg/0.05 mg, 40 µg/0.075 mg, 30 µg/0.125 mg	Enpresse, Trivora
Ethinyl estradiol/ norgestimate	25 µg/0.18, 0.215, 0.25 mg	Ortho Tri-Cyclen Lo
	35 µg/0.18, 0.215, 0.25 mg	Ortho Tri-Cyclen, Tri-Previfem, Tri-Sprintec, TriNessa
Ethinyl estradiol/ norethindrone	35 µg/0.5, 0.75, 1 mg	Necon 7/7/7, Ortho-Novum 7/7/7
	35 µg/0.5, 1, 0.5 mg	Aranelle, Tri-Norinyl[b]
Oral Monophasic Formulation		
Estrogen/progestin[c]		
Ethinyl Estradiol/levonorgestrel	20 µg/0.09 mg	Lybrel
	20 µg/0.1 mg	Alesse, Aviane, Lutera
	30 µg/0.15 mg	Jolessa, Levora, Nordette, Protia, Quasense, Seasonale[c]
	30 µg/0.15 mg, 10 µg/0 mg	Seasonique[d]
Ethinyl estradiol/desogestrel	30 µg/0.15 mg	Apri, Desogen, Reclipsen
Ethinyl Estradiol/ norethindrone	20 µg/1 mg[e]	Junel 21 1/20, Loestrin 21 1/20
	30 µg/1.5 mg	Loestrin 24 Fe 1/20,[e] Microgestin 1/20, Microgestin Fe 1/20
	35 µg/0.4 mg	Junel 21 1.5/30, Loestrin 21 1.5/30
	35 µg/0.5 mg	Loestrin Fe 1.5/30, Microgestin 1.5/30, Microgestin FE 1.5/30
	35 µg/1 mg	Balziva, Femcom Fe, Ovcon 35
	50 µg/1 mg	Brevicon, Medicon, Necon 0.5/35
		Necon 1/35, Norinyl 1/35, Ortho-Novum 1/35
		Necon 1/50, Ovcon 50
Ethinyl estradiol/norgestrel	30 µg/0.3 mg	Cryselle, Lo/Ovral, Low-Ogestrel
Ethinyl estradiol/ norgestimate	35 µg/0.25 mg	MonoNessa, Ortho-Cyclen, Previfem, Sprintec
Mestranol/norethindrone	50 µg/1 mg	Norinyl 1/50
Ethinyl estradiol/ drospirenone	20 µg/3 mg[e]	Yaz
	30 µg/3 mg	Ocella, Yasmin
Ethinyl estrodiol/ethynodiol	35 µg/1 mg	Kelnor, Zovia 1/35
	50 µg/1 mg	Zovia 1/50

(continued on next page)

Table 1 *(continued)*		
	Dose	**Brand/Trade Name**
Ethinyl estradiol/desogestrel	30 μg/0.15 mg	Ortho-Cept
Nonoral Combined Formulations		
Transdermal estrogen/ progestin		
Ethinyl estradiol/ norelgestromin	20 μg/0.15 mg/d patch	Ortho Evra
Vaginal ring estrogen/ progestin		
Ethinyl estradiol/ etonogestrel vaginal	15 μg/0.12 mg/d vaginal ring	NuvaRing
Progestin Only		
Oral progestin only		
Norethindrone	0.35 mg	Camilla, Errin, Jolivette, Nor-QD, OrthoMicronor, Ovrette
Progestin Injection		
Medroxyprogesterone acetate	150 mg, intramuscular, every 3 months	Depo-Provera
	104 mg, subcutaneous, every 3 months	Depo-SubQ Provera
Progestin-releasing IUD		
Levonorgestrel	52 mg intrauterine device, daily release 20 μg	Mirena

[a] 21 active tablets and 7 placebo, active tablets divided into 7 tablet doses as indicated.
[b] Active pills are divided into 7 tablet doses, 9 tablet doses followed by 5 tablet doses.
[c] 21 active tablets and 7 placebo, active tablets are all same dose.
[d] 91-day extended formulation available with 84 consecutive active tablets and 7 placebo or 10 μg estradiol.
[e] 24 active tablets and 4 placebo.

therapy has also been shown to decrease BP in postmenopausal hypertensive women on hydrochlorothiazide.[22]

ORAL CONTRACEPTIVES AND OTHER CARDIOVASCULAR RISKS

Cardiovascular event rates differ significantly for middle-aged men and women, because of differences in risk factors and hormones.[23] In animal models, estrogen-deficient animals (cynomolgus monkey) not receiving exogenous hormones develop twice the level of atherosclerosis, and exposure to OCPs prevents this effect.[24] Adams and colleagues[25] found a significant inhibitory effect of ethinyl estradiol on atherosclerosis progression whereas treatment with progesterone alone had no effect on atherosclerosis prevention.

The increased risk of cardiovascular disease with OCP use in clinical studies is controversial. The Nurses' Health Study, an 8-year self-reported prospective study on the use of OCP and risk of cardiovascular disease, found no evidence of increase of the risk of cardiovascular disease in past users of oral contraceptives, even with

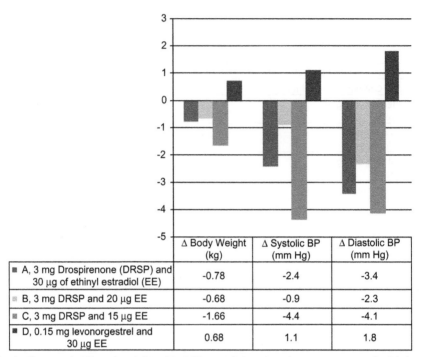

	Δ Body Weight (kg)	Δ Systolic BP (mm Hg)	Δ Diastolic BP (mm Hg)
■ A, 3 mg Drospirenone (DRSP) and 30 μg of ethinyl estradiol (EE)	-0.78	-2.4	-3.4
▨ B, 3 mg DRSP and 20 μg EE	-0.68	-0.9	-2.3
■ C, 3 mg DRSP and 15 μg EE	-1.66	-4.4	-4.1
■ D, 0.15 mg levonorgestrel and 30 μg EE	0.68	1.1	1.8

Fig. 1. Changes in BP and weight with OCP containing drospirenone compared with levo-norgestrel. Mean changes (Δ) in body weight, systolic BP, and diastolic BP at 6 months of treatment compared with baseline in the treatment groups A, B, C, and the control group D. At 6 months, weight changes in groups A, B, and C, changes in systolic BP in group C, and diastolic BP in groups A and C were significantly different from those in group D. (*Data from* Oelkers W, Foidart JM, Dombrovicz N, et al. Effects of a new oral contraceptive containing an antimineralocorticoid progestogen, drospirenone, on the reninaldosterone system, body weight, blood pressure, glucose tolerance, and lipid metabolism. J Clin Endocrinol Metab 1995;80:1816–21.)

prolonged use.[26] Among current users, there was a 2.5-fold increased relative risk of adverse cardiovascular events, believed to be associated with prothrombotic effects of estrogen.[26] In a case-control study with second-generation and third-generation OCPs, there was no association between OCP use and myocardial infarction. Smoking was an important comorbid risk factor.[27] Another case-control study by Sidney and colleagues[28] found no increase in risk of myocardial infarction with current or past use of OCP and even found no increased risk associated with age or smoking. In contrast, Tanis and colleagues[29] found an increase in risk of a first myocardial infarction in women using first-generation and second-generation OCP and did not show any increased risk with third-generation. Smoking, but not age, also increased the risk. Thus, even although OCPs might decrease atherosclerosis progression in animal models, the overall risk of cardiovascular disease seems to be the same or higher in women with current but no increase in past use of oral contraceptives. No cardiovascular data are available for the fourth-generation OCPs.

Oral contraceptives also affect the cardiovascular system indirectly by altering hemostasis and lipoproteins. The OCPs have been shown to increase risk of venous thromboembolic events, particularly in women who smoke cigarettes. In 1 study the

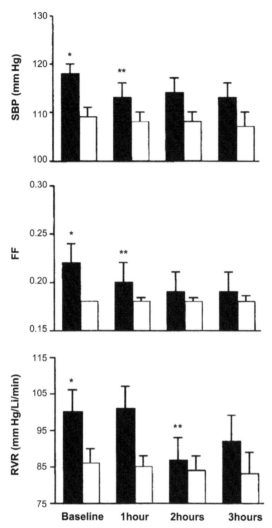

Fig. 2. Response of systolic blood pressure (SBP), filtration fraction (FF), and renal vascular resistance (RVR) to the subdepressor dose of losartan in users of oral contraceptives (OC, *solid bars*) and in nonusers of OC (*open bars*). *P<.05 versus OC nonusers baseline values. **P<.05 versus baseline. (*From* Kang AK, Duncan JA, Cattran DC, et al. Effect of oral contraceptives on the renin angiotensin system and renal function. Am J Physiol Regul Integr Comp Physiol 2001;280:R810; with permission.)

risk of venous thromboembolic events was 4 times higher with OCP with less than 50 μg of ethinyl estradiol versus nonusers, with higher risk in obese patients and those with thrombophilia.[30] Studies have shown relations among the dose of estrogen[31] in the OCP, the type of progesterone,[32] and the occurrence of venous thromboembolic events. For example, the risk of venous thromboembolism is higher in patients taking OCP containing 50 μg of estrogen compared with 30 μg of estrogen.[31] The type of progestin also alters risk and this was shown by an increased risk of nonfatal thromboembolism linked to the newer-generation progestins (desogestrel and gestodene) compared with levonorgestrel.[32] There seems to be a balanced effect of oral contraceptive on hemostasis by stimulating both coagulation and fibrinolytic activity over baseline in OCP containing 20 and 30 μg of ethinyl estradiol.[33,34]

Premenopausal women show a dose-related response of exogenous hormones on the lipid profile. In a controlled, randomized study, the effects of a reduced dose second-generation oral contraceptive formulation (20 μg of ethinyl estradiol and 100 μg of levonorgestrel) and a reference formulation (30 μg of ethinyl estradiol and 150 μg of levonorgestrel) on lipids and hemostasis showed reductions in high-density lipoprotein (HDL) levels by 26% and 40%, respectively. The low-density lipoprotein (LDL) increased by 3% and 25%, respectively, and triglycerides increased by 10% and 37%, respectively.[34] A second study found a similar effect on HDL reductions and increase in LDL and triglyceride but without statistical significance between the 20-μg and 30-μg doses of ethinyl estradiol.[35] Second-generation progestins show a clear adverse influence on lipid metabolism and this is in part because of their ability to counteract the favorable estrogen effect on HDL and LDL. In contrast, third-generation and fourth-generation OCPs seem to have beneficial effects on the lipid profile. A study evaluating low-estrogen OCP (20 μg ethinyl estradiol) containing desogestrel (third-generation OCP) and drospirenone (fourth-generation OCP) has shown that both had a similar effect on lipid levels, increasing HDL (11% and 16%, respectively) and decreasing LDL (10% and 18%, respectively).[36] Compared with the progestin levonorgestrel, drospirenone significantly increased serum triglyceride and HDL and slightly decreased LDL.[12] Whereas progestin seems to directly affect the lipid profile, progesterone-only pills (desogestrel and levonorgestrel) seem to have minimal effect on lipid profile, with no changes in LDL cholesterol.[37] In contrast, over longer periods of time in postmenopausal women, hormonal replacement in the Women's Health Initiative (WHI) trial showed an increase in HDL and triglyceride and a decrease in LDL.[38]

Platelets and platelet function play a critical role in the pathogenesis of cardiovascular events. Incubation of platelets with 17-β-estradiol inhibits adenosine-diphosphate–induced platelet aggregation in vitro.[39] In addition, 17-β-estradiol has been shown to have an important role in inhibiting platelet aggregation by affecting Ca^{++} concentration and increasing NO synthesis.[40] Certain progestins, including medroxyprogesterone, attenuate the 17-β-estradiol–induced NO production that inhibits platelet aggregation by endothelial cells, suggesting a negative effect of the progestin.[41] Clinical studies also show that platelet function is altered during the menstrual cycle. Platelet aggregation is relatively enhanced in the luteal phase compared with the follicular phase in young women not on OCPs.[42] Platelet activation was shown to peak around the time of ovulation.[43] To study the effect of OCPs on platelet function, Roell and colleagues[44] conducted a cross-sectional study comparing platelet function in women taking different types of monophasic oral contraceptives with women not taking OCP in the luteal and follicular phase. These investigators reported that progesterone plays a key role in altering platelet function compared with estrogen. The alteration of platelet function observed in second-generation and third-generation pills seems to be within the physiologic changes observed as well in the natural menstrual cycle, but the fourth-generation antiandrogen-containing progestin was associated with increased platelet aggregability. All OCPs also increased von Willebrand factor mediated by the progesterone component. On the other hand, conjugated estrogens (0.625 mg/d) inhibited platelet aggregation in postmenopausal women.[45] These studies show that whereas estrogen seems to inhibit aggregation in both in vitro and in vivo studies, progesterone may increase platelet aggregation, hence promoting thrombosis.

POSTMENOPAUSAL HORMONE THERAPY AND HYPERTENSION

Estrogen was first used as an effective treatment of menopausal vasomotor symptoms in the 1960s but its use declined after being linked to endometrial cancer until the 1980s, when the addition of progesterone was found to mitigate that effect.[46] After the reports from the WHI trial in 2002 that showed increases in the risk of coronary heart disease, breast cancer, stroke, and thromboembolism in older women, the use of postmenopausal estrogen therapy declined substantially.[38,47] The use of combined HRT in WHI increased the relative risk of coronary heart disease by 29% in women more than the age of 70 years.[47] but did not have a deleterious cardiovascular effect in the younger women in the trial. Hormone therapy also did not show a clinical benefit in the secondary prevention of cardiovascular events in the Heart and Estrogen/Progestin Replacement Study.[48]

The frequency of hot flushes and night sweats, the major indication today of HRT, is reduced in about 75% with its use.[49] HRT is commonly prescribed as conjugated estrogen/medroxyprogesterone in various dosages (0.625 mg/2.5 mg, 0.45 mg/1.5 mg, 0.3 mg/1.5 mg) or only as conjugated estrogen for patients after hysterectomy. Various oral combinations with different estrogens (estradiol, esterified estrogen, ethinyl estradiol) and progestins (medroxyprogesterone, norethindrone acetate, drosperinone) can be found as well as estradiol patches with or without progestin (norethindrome or levonorgestrel). The same dose of estrogen without progesterone might be less effective because of the independent effect of medroxyprogesterone on hot flush reduction.[50]

PATHOPHYSIOLOGY OF POSTMENOPAUSAL HYPERTENSION

The prevalence of hypertension increases with age in postmenopausal women because systolic BP increases by about 5 mm Hg per decade. Although hypertension is less common among women than men in early adulthood, the incidence of hypertension increases more rapidly in women than in men after the fifth decade of life, reaching a prevalence rate that is equal to or greater than in men during the sixth decade.[51]

Increases in BP associated with the initiation of the menopause may be mediated in part through reduction in arterial compliance and the loss of estrogen.[52] Mechanisms include increased salt sensitivity, decreased endothelial NO production, and upregulation of the angiotensin II subtype 1 receptor that causes functional activation of angiotensin II. The RAS and NO pathways play a central role in BP control and electrolyte balance. Salt-sensitive hypertension is accompanied by activation of RAS and downregulation of endothelial NO synthase, decreasing NO bioavailability. Estrogen downregulates both angiotensin II subtype 1 receptor expression and activation of NO synthase with NO release. Estrogen also causes antioxidant and vasodilatory effects through inhibition of endothelin synthesis and nicotinamide adenine dinucleotide phosphate oxidase. After menopause, estrogen deficiency results in increased salt sensitivity and hypertension, especially in genetically prone women.[15,53]

Loss of estrogen is not the only mechanism of increased BP in postmenopausal women, because conventional hormone replacement does not typically decrease BP.[54] Other possible factors may involve the relative hyperandrogenic state via activation of the RAS, increases in plasma levels of the vasoconstrictor endothelin, and increases in oxidative stress.[53,55]

It is more likely that administration of hormone therapy may increase the BP during menopause. Prelevic and colleagues[56] studied healthy postmenopausal women on hormonal therapy for at least 5 years and showed increases in systolic BP up to 9 mm Hg. Similar findings were reported from the WHI. The WHI study assessed major health benefits and risks of estrogen plus progestin component in postmenopausal women aged 50 to 79 years with an intact uterus[38,47] and estrogen alone in postmenopausal women with previous hysterectomy.[57] The estrogen plus progestin arm was terminated after an average of 5.2 years because overall risks exceeded benefits. The combined therapy showed increases in coronary heart disease events, breast cancer, stroke, pulmonary embolism, and systolic hypertension.[38,47] The estrogen-only arm showed no increase in cardiovascular risk but showed a small increase in the absolute risk of stroke.

Because the WHI reported that the frequently used combination of conjugated equine estrogens with medroxyprogesterone acetate may increase cardiovascular morbidity in older postmenopausal women,[47] interest developed for providing a new estrogen/progesterone combination with a potentially lower cardiovascular risk profile. The progestin drospirenone has the potential of reducing body weight and BP because of its mechanism of mineralocorticoid receptor blockade. A combination product containing small doses of 17-β-estradiol and drosperinone was developed for the treatment of menopausal symptoms. This progestin was evaluated in combination with 17-β-estradiol in postmenopausal women with stage 1 hypertension[58] and in stage 1 and 2 hypertension[59] and was shown to lower systolic BP without causing hyperkalemia. Randomized, double-blind clinical trials were performed to evaluate the effect on BP of drosperinone 1 mg, 2 mg, and 3 mg in combination with estradiol versus estradiol alone and placebo in postmenopausal women with stage 1 to 2 hypertension. Significant reductions in 24-hour systolic BPs were observed at doses of 2 mg and 3 mg of drosperinone in combination with 17-β-estradiol (6.1 and 4.7 mm Hg, respectively) but not by 1 mg of drosperinone with estradiol or estradiol alone (**Fig. 3**).[59] The BP-lowering effects and potassium-sparing effects of drospirenone could lead to a beneficial cardiovascular effect in this population relative to other progestins.

RALOXIFENE AND CARDIOVASCULAR RISK

Raloxifene is a selective estrogen receptor modulator that exerts estrogen-agonistic action on bone, lipids, and the cardiovascular system and has an estrogen-antagonistic

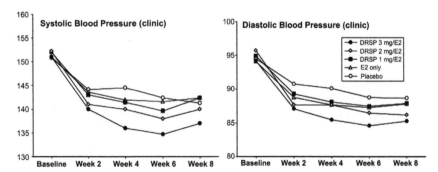

Fig. 3. Effects of drospirenone (DRSP) in combination with 17-β-estradiol (E2), estradiol alone, and placebo on systolic and diastolic BP in women with postmenopausal hypertension. (*From* White WB, Hanes V, Chauhan V, et al. Effects of a new hormone therapy, drospirenone and 17-beta-estradiol, in postmenopausal women with hypertension. Hypertension 2006;48:250; with permission.)

effect on the breast and uterus. Its positive effect on bone and osteoporosis is well established in several studies and has been the major clinical indication for raloxifene. The RUTH (Raloxifene Use for The Heart) trial showed no difference in overall mortality, cardiovascular mortality, or cardiovascular events in postmenopausal women with coronary heart disease or at increased risk for cardiovascular disease with the use of raloxifene. The drug decreased LDL and increased HDL, showing a beneficial lipid response but increased the risk for venous thromboembolism and fatal stroke.[60] Raloxifene therapy was shown not to change BP, plasma renin activity, or aldosterone plasma concentration significantly in populations of both normotensive and hypertensive postmenopausal women.[61] Raloxifene also showed beneficial effects on brachial arterial endothelial function and significant decrease in carotid wall thickness in osteoporotic women[62] and may indicate a decrease in cardiovascular risk. This study also showed a significant decrease in LDL level.[62] Raloxifene seems to have positive effects in a variety of cardiovascular risk factors, but no effect on cardiovascular morbidity or mortality.

SUMMARY

Numerous studies have shown significant increases in BP in women taking oral contraceptives. The primary mechanism for this effect seems to be related to activation of the RAS mediated by estrogen and the inability of most synthetic progestins to antagonize this effect. The exception is drospirenone, which in higher doses may decrease BP and weight.[12,58] No clear evidence of influence of age, family history, ethnicity, or body mass index has been found to predispose patients to increases in BP with the use of contraceptive pills.

Menopause is associated with BP increase and conventional hormonal replacement that can further increase morbidity and mortality from cardiovascular and thromboembolic disease, particularly in women more than 65 to 70 years of age. As seen with oral contraceptives, drospirenone if used as progestin in postmenopausal hormone also showed improvement in BP control because of its antimineralocorticoid effect.

REFERENCES

1. Chandra A, Martinez GM, Mosher WD, et al. Fertility, family planning, and reproductive health of U.S. women: data from the 2002 National Survey of Family Growth. Vital Health Stat 23 2005;(25):1–160.
2. Shufelt CL, Bairey Merz CN. Contraceptive hormone use and cardiovascular disease. J Am Coll Cardiol 2009;53:221–31.
3. Wilson ES, Cruickshank J, McMaster M, et al. A prospective controlled study of the effect on blood pressure of contraceptive preparations containing different types and dosages of progestogen. Br J Obstet Gynaecol 1984;91:1254–60.
4. Dong W, Colhoun HM, Poulter NR. Blood pressure in women using oral contraceptives: results from the Health Survey for England 1994. J Hypertens 1997; 15:1063–8.
5. Meade TW, Haines AP, North WR, et al. Haemostatic, lipid, and blood-pressure profiles of women on oral contraceptives containing 50 microgram or 30 microgram oestrogen. Lancet 1977;2:948–51.
6. Nichols M, Robinson G, Bounds W, et al. Effect of four combined oral contraceptives on blood pressure in the pill-free interval. Contraception 1993;47:367–76.
7. Chasan-Taber L, Willett WC, Manson JE, et al. Prospective study of oral contraceptives and hypertension among women in the United States. Circulation 1996;94:483–9.

8. Narkiewicz K, Graniero GR, D'Este D, et al. Ambulatory blood pressure in mild hypertensive women taking oral contraceptives. A case-control study. Am J Hypertens 1995;8:249–53.

9. Lubianca JN, Faccin CS, Fuchs FD. Oral contraceptives: a risk factor for uncontrolled blood pressure among hypertensive women. Contraception 2003;67: 19–24.

10. Lubianca JN, Moreira LB, Gus M, et al. Stopping oral contraceptives: an effective blood pressure-lowering intervention in women with hypertension. J Hum Hypertens 2005;19:451–5.

11. Cardoso F, Polonia J, Santos A, et al. Low-dose oral contraceptives and 24-hour ambulatory blood pressure. Int J Gynaecol Obstet 1997;59:237–43.

12. Oelkers W, Foidart JM, Dombrovicz N, et al. Effects of a new oral contraceptive containing an antimineralocorticoid progestogen, drospirenone, on the renin-aldosterone system, body weight, blood pressure, glucose tolerance, and lipid metabolism. J Clin Endocrinol Metab 1995;80:1816–21.

13. Gordon MS, Chin WW, Shupnik MA. Regulation of angiotensinogen gene expression by estrogen. J Hypertens 1992;10:361–6.

14. Kang AK, Duncan JA, Cattran DC, et al. Effect of oral contraceptives on the renin angiotensin system and renal function. Am J Physiol Regul Integr Comp Physiol 2001;280:R807–13.

15. Cherney DZ, Scholey JW, Cattran DC, et al. The effect of oral contraceptives on the nitric oxide system and renal function. Am J Physiol Renal Physiol 2007;293: F1539–44.

16. Saruta T, Nakamura R, Nagahama S, et al. Effects of angiotensin II analog on blood pressure, renin and aldosterone in women on oral contraceptives and toxemia. Gynecol Obstet Invest 1981;12:11–20.

17. Oelkers W. Drospirenone, a progestogen with antimineralocorticoid properties: a short review. Mol Cell Endocrinol 2004;217:255–61.

18. Arias-Loza PA, Hu K, Schafer A, et al. Medroxyprogesterone acetate but not drospirenone ablates the protective function of 17 beta-estradiol in aldosterone salt-treated rats. Hypertension 2006;48:994–1001.

19. Khaw KT, Peart WS. Blood pressure and contraceptive use. Br Med J (Clin Res Ed) 1982;285:403–7.

20. Ribstein J, Halimi JM, du Cailar G, et al. Renal characteristics and effect of angiotensin suppression in oral contraceptive users. Hypertension 1999;33: 90–5.

21. Preston RA, Alonso A, Panzitta D, et al. Additive effect of drospirenone/17-beta-estradiol in hypertensive postmenopausal women receiving enalapril. Am J Hypertens 2002;15:816–22.

22. Preston RA, Norris PM, Alonso AB, et al. Randomized, placebo-controlled trial of the effects of drospirenone-estradiol on blood pressure and potassium balance in hypertensive postmenopausal women receiving hydrochlorothiazide. Menopause 2007;14:408–14.

23. Mendelsohn ME, Karas RH. The protective effects of estrogen on the cardiovascular system. N Engl J Med 1999;340:1801–11.

24. Kaplan JR, Manuck SB, Anthony MS, et al. Premenopausal social status and hormone exposure predict postmenopausal atherosclerosis in female monkeys. Obstet Gynecol 2002;99:381–8.

25. Adams MR, Anthony MS, Manning JM, et al. Low-dose contraceptive estrogen-progestin and coronary artery atherosclerosis of monkeys. Obstet Gynecol 2000;96:250–5.

26. Stampfer MJ, Willett WC, Colditz GA, et al. A prospective study of past use of oral contraceptive agents and risk of cardiovascular diseases. N Engl J Med 1988; 319:1313–7.

27. Dunn N, Thorogood M, Faragher B, et al. Oral contraceptives and myocardial infarction: results of the MICA case-control study. BMJ 1999;318:1579–83.

28. Sidney S, Siscovick DS, Petitti DB, et al. Myocardial infarction and use of low-dose oral contraceptives: a pooled analysis of 2 US studies. Circulation 1998;98:1058–63.

29. Tanis BC, van den Bosch MA, Kemmeren JM, et al. Oral contraceptives and the risk of myocardial infarction. N Engl J Med 2001;345:1787–93.

30. Sidney S, Petitti DB, Soff GA, et al. Venous thromboembolic disease in users of low-estrogen combined estrogen-progestin oral contraceptives. Contraception 2004;70:3–10.

31. Gerstman BB, Piper JM, Tomita DK, et al. Oral contraceptive estrogen dose and the risk of deep venous thromboembolic disease. Am J Epidemiol 1991;133:32–7.

32. Jick H, Jick SS, Gurewich V, et al. Risk of idiopathic cardiovascular death and nonfatal venous thromboembolism in women using oral contraceptives with differing progestagen components. Lancet 1995;346:1589–93.

33. Winkler UH, Schindler AE, Endrikat J, et al. A comparative study of the effects of the hemostatic system of two monophasic gestodene oral contraceptives containing 20 micrograms and 30 micrograms ethinylestradiol. Contraception 1996;53:75–84.

34. Endrikat J, Klipping C, Cronin M, et al. An open label, comparative study of the effects of a dose-reduced oral contraceptive containing 20 microg ethinyl estradiol and 100 microg levonorgestrel on hemostatic, lipids, and carbohydrate metabolism variables. Contraception 2002;65:215–21.

35. Skouby SO, Endrikat J, Dusterberg B, et al. A 1-year randomized study to evaluate the effects of a dose reduction in oral contraceptives on lipids and carbohydrate metabolism: 20 microg ethinyl estradiol combined with 100 microg levonorgestrel. Contraception 2005;71:111–7.

36. Klipping C, Marr J. Effects of two combined oral contraceptives containing ethinyl estradiol 20 microg combined with either drospirenone or desogestrel on lipids, hemostatic parameters and carbohydrate metabolism. Contraception 2005;71: 409–16.

37. Barkfeldt J, Virkkunen A, Dieben T. The effects of two progestogen-only pills containing either desogestrel (75 microg/day) or levonorgestrel (30 microg/day) on lipid metabolism. Contraception 2001;64:295–9.

38. Manson JE, Hsia J, Johnson KC, et al. Estrogen plus progestin and the risk of coronary heart disease. N Engl J Med 2003;349:523–34.

39. Bar J, Lahav J, Hod M, et al. Regulation of platelet aggregation and adenosine triphosphate release in vitro by 17beta-estradiol and medroxyprogesterone acetate in postmenopausal women. Thromb Haemost 2000;84:695–700.

40. Nakano Y, Oshima T, Matsuura H, et al. Effect of 17beta-estradiol on inhibition of platelet aggregation in vitro is mediated by an increase in NO synthesis. Arterioscler Thromb Vasc Biol 1998;18:961–7.

41. Zerr-Fouineau M, Jourdain M, Boesch C, et al. Certain progestins prevent the enhancing effect of 17beta-estradiol on NO-mediated inhibition of platelet aggregation by endothelial cells. Arterioscler Thromb Vasc Biol 2009;29:586–93.

42. Feuring M, Christ M, Roell A, et al. Alterations in platelet function during the ovarian cycle. Blood Coagul Fibrinolysis 2002;13:443–7.

43. Rosin C, Brunner M, Lehr S, et al. The formation of platelet-leukocyte aggregates varies during the menstrual cycle. Platelets 2006;17:61–6.

44. Roell A, Schueller P, Schultz A, et al. Effect of oral contraceptives and ovarian cycle on platelet function. Platelets 2007;18:165–70.
45. Nakano Y, Oshima T, Ozono R, et al. Estrogen replacement suppresses function of thrombin stimulated platelets by inhibiting Ca(2+) influx and raising cyclic adenosine monophosphate. Cardiovasc Res 2002;53:634–41.
46. Shifren JL, Schiff I. Role of hormone therapy in the management of menopause. Obstet Gynecol 2010;115:839–55.
47. Rossouw JE, Anderson GL, Prentice RL, et al. Risks and benefits of estrogen plus progestin in healthy postmenopausal women: principal results from the Women's Health Initiative randomized controlled trial. JAMA 2002;288:321–33.
48. Hulley S, Grady D, Bush T, et al. Randomized trial of estrogen plus progestin for secondary prevention of coronary heart disease in postmenopausal women. Heart and Estrogen/progestin Replacement Study (HERS) Research Group. JAMA 1998;280:605–13.
49. Maclennan AH, Broadbent JL, Lester S, et al. Oral oestrogen and combined oestrogen/progestogen therapy versus placebo for hot flushes. Cochrane Database Syst Rev 2004;4:CD002978.
50. Schiff I, Tulchinsky D, Cramer D, et al. Oral medroxyprogesterone in the treatment of postmenopausal symptoms. JAMA 1980;244:1443–5.
51. Burt VL, Whelton P, Roccella EJ, et al. Prevalence of hypertension in the US adult population. Results from the Third National Health and Nutrition Examination Survey, 1988-1991. Hypertension 1995;25:305–13.
52. Staessen JA, Ginocchio G, Thijs L, et al. Conventional and ambulatory blood pressure and menopause in a prospective population study. J Hum Hypertens 1997;11:507–14.
53. Hernandez Schulman I, Raij L. Salt sensitivity and hypertension after menopause: role of nitric oxide and angiotensin II. Am J Nephrol 2006;26:170–80.
54. Mallareddy M, Hanes V, White WB. Drospirenone, a new progestogen, for post-menopausal women with hypertension. Drugs Aging 2007;24:453–66.
55. Reckelhoff JF, Fortepiani LA. Novel mechanisms responsible for postmenopausal hypertension. Hypertension 2004;43:918–23.
56. Prelevic GM, Kwong P, Byrne DJ, et al. A cross-sectional study of the effects of hormone replacement therapy on the cardiovascular disease risk profile in healthy postmenopausal women. Fertil Steril 2002;77:945–51.
57. Anderson GL, Limacher M, Assaf AR, et al. Effects of conjugated equine estrogen in postmenopausal women with hysterectomy: the Women's Health Initiative randomized controlled trial. JAMA 2004;291:1701–12.
58. White WB, Pitt B, Preston RA, et al. Antihypertensive effects of drospirenone with 17beta-estradiol, a novel hormone treatment in postmenopausal women with stage 1 hypertension. Circulation 2005;112:1979–84.
59. White WB, Hanes V, Chauhan V, et al. Effects of a new hormone therapy, drospirenone and 17-beta-estradiol, in postmenopausal women with hypertension. Hypertension 2006;48:246–53.
60. Barrett-Connor E, Mosca L, Collins P, et al. Effects of raloxifene on cardiovascular events and breast cancer in postmenopausal women. N Engl J Med 2006;355:125–37.
61. Morgante G, Delia A, Musacchio MC, et al. Effects of raloxifene therapy on plasma renin and aldosterone levels and blood pressure in postmenopausal women. Gynecol Endocrinol 2006;22:376–80.
62. Sumino H, Ichikawa S, Kasama S, et al. Effects of raloxifene on brachial arterial endothelial function, carotid wall thickness, and arterial stiffness in osteoporotic postmenopausal women. Int Heart J 2010;51:60–7.

Ovarian Hypertension: Polycystic Ovary Syndrome

Rhonda Bentley-Lewis, MD, MBA, MMSc[a], Ellen Seely, MD[b],
Andrea Dunaif, MD[c],*

KEYWORDS

- Polycystic ovary syndrome • Hypertension
- Hyperandrogenism • Insulin • Obesity

Polycystic ovary syndrome (PCOS) was originally described by Stein and Leventhal in 1935 as a reproductive disorder characterized by oligo-amenorrhea, hirsutism, and polycystic ovary morphology.[1] Thirty years ago, it was first reported that women with PCOS had hyperinsulinemia.[2] Subsequent research indicated that PCOS was associated with a unique disorder of insulin action, as well as defects in insulin secretion, and together these abnormalities conferred a substantially increased risk of glucose intolerance.[3] Although the clinical manifestations of PCOS are heterogeneous, the hallmarks of the syndrome remain anovulation, androgen excess, and insulin resistance. Moreover, each of these features of the syndrome is responsible for the promotion of hypertension in this population. Therefore, therapy for hypertension should be targeted at treatment of these underlying abnormalities.

DIAGNOSTIC CRITERIA

The diagnostic criteria for PCOS have been a source of controversy. Outside the United States, the diagnosis has been based on the presence of polycystic ovary morphology (PCO) by ovarian ultrasound examination; affected women are then

---

This work was supported in part by Grant 5K23RR023333 from the National Institutes of Health and the Robert Wood Johnson Foundation Harold Amos Medical Faculty Development Program awarded to R.B.-L. and NIH grants P50 HD044405 and R01 DK073411 awarded to A.D. The authors have nothing to disclose.

[a] Diabetes Research Center and Diabetes Unit, Massachusetts General Hospital, 50 Staniford Street, Suite 301, Boston, MA 02114, USA
[b] Division of Endocrinology, Diabetes, and Hypertension, Brigham and Women's Hospital, 221 Longwood Avenue, Boston, MA 02115, USA
[c] Northwestern University, Feinberg School of Medicine, 303 East Chicago Avenue, Tarry Building 15-745, Chicago, IL 60611, USA
* Corresponding author.
E-mail address: a-dunaif@northwestern.edu

Endocrinol Metab Clin N Am 40 (2011) 433–449
doi:10.1016/j.ecl.2011.01.009
0889-8529/11/$ – see front matter © 2011 Elsevier Inc. All rights reserved.

further stratified based on ovulatory status. However, the finding that approximately 25% of normal women in many series can have PCO led investigators in the United States to focus on the biochemical features of the syndrome for diagnostic criteria.[4,5] The 1990 National Institutes of Health (NIH)/National Institute of Child Health and Human Development (NICHD) conference on PCOS proposed what have become known as the NIH diagnostic criteria: hyperandrogenism (clinical and/or biochemical) and chronic anovulation with the exclusion of specific disorders of the ovary, adrenal, and pituitary (**Table 1**).[4] PCO by ultrasound was not included as a criterion because of the lack of diagnostic specificity of this finding.[6] Ultrasonographically detected polycystic ovaries can be present in women with normal ovulation and sex hormone levels, whereas women with all the endocrine features of PCOS can have normal ovarian morphology by ultrasound examination.[6,7] The NIH criteria have been used to diagnose PCOS in the majority of studies on hypertension in affected women.

In 2003, an international conference in Rotterdam reassessed the diagnostic criteria for PCOS and proposed revised criteria that included PCO.[8] The Rotterdam criteria require 2 of 3 of the following findings: hyperandrogenism, chronic anovulation and PCO (see **Table 1**). Thus, these criteria would include all those women with PCOS by NIH criteria. However, the Rotterdam criteria also include women with hyperandrogenism and ovulatory cycles who would not be considered to have PCOS by NIH criteria. Because most ovulatory women with PCO have hyperandrogenism and increased luteinizing hormone (LH) levels, this additional group of women with PCOS according to Rotterdam criteria are analogous to the ovulatory PCO women identified by non–United States investigators on the basis of ovarian ultrasound morphology. There are studies to suggest that ovulatory women with PCO are not insulin resistant compared with anovulatory women with PCO,[9] although recent studies suggest they may have milder metabolic abnormalities.[10] Therefore, it is unclear whether these women should be grouped with those with the classic anovulatory form of the disorder. Recently, the Androgen Excess Society (AES) developed diagnostic criteria for PCOS based on the feature of androgen excess, endorsing the NIH criteria but also recommending that women with regular ovulation and polycystic ovaries on ultrasound be included as a PCOS phenotype.[11]

EPIDEMIOLOGY

PCOS is one of the most common endocrine disorders affecting women of reproductive age.[12] A recent Australian study examined the prevalence of PCOS in a retrospective birth cohort employing the NIH, Rotterdam, and AES diagnostic criteria.[13] These

Table 1 Diagnostic criteria for PCOS[a]	
NIH criteria[b]	Hyperandrogenism/hyperandrogenemia Chronic anovulation
Rotterdam criteria	Two of the following: hyperandrogenism/ hyperandrogenemia, chronic anovulation, polycystic ovaries
Androgen Excess Society criteria	Hyperandrogenism/hyperandrogenemia Infrequent or irregular ovulation OR regular ovulation and polycystic ovaries

[a] All criteria include the exclusion of other medical conditions, including thyroid or pituitary dysfunction, androgen-secreting tumors, Cushing syndrome, or congenital adrenal hyperplasia.
[b] NIH criteria developed with the National Institute of Child Health and Human Development.

data revealed prevalence based on NIH diagnostic criteria of 8.7% ± 2.0%, less than the 11.9% ± 2.4% and 10.2% ± 2.2% using Rotterdam and AES criteria, respectively. Prevalence estimates of PCOS among populations worldwide employing the NIH diagnostic criteria have been reported as approximately 6% in the Southeastern United States,[14] Spain,[15] the Mediterranean,[16] and Mexico.[17] Although studies have reported no statistically significant differences in the PCOS prevalence between black and white women,[14,18] there are data suggesting an increased prevalence of PCOS among Hispanic[19] and Mexican American[17] women compared with other racial and ethnic groups. Nonetheless, PCOS is likely underdiagnosed in clinical practice, so the use of chart-based data in prevalence estimate derivations is problematic.

PATHOPHYSIOLOGY

The biochemical reproductive phenotype in PCOS consists of increased LH relative to follicle-stimulating hormone (FSH) secretion and hyperandrogenism (**Fig. 1**).[4,5] There is increased frequency of LH pulsatile release, indicating that the frequency of gonadotropin-releasing hormone (GnRH) secretion is increased. There is also increased amplitude of LH pulses that is secondary, in part, to increased pituitary sensitivity to GnRH, which appears to be estrogen mediated. It is possible that there is also an increased amount of GnRH secreted per pulse. FSH release is relatively suppressed, and the late luteal and early follicular phase increases that are essential for normal follicular development are absent. One explanation for these FSH abnormalities is the increased frequency of GnRH secretion, which results in a selective suppression of FSH relative to LH release.[20] The elevated circulating androgens feedback on the hypothalamic-pituitary axis, both directly by decreasing sensitivity to the normal actions of estrogen and progesterone to slow the frequency of pulsatile GnRH release,[21] and by extragonadal aromatization to estrogen, to increase LH relative to FSH release, producing a self-sustaining syndrome.[4]

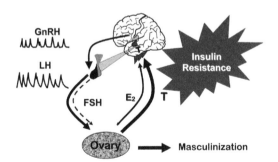

Fig. 1. Schema for the pathophysiology of PCOS. Increased gonadotropin-releasing hormone (GnRH) pulsatility leads to a selective increase in luteinizing hormone (LH) pulsatility while suppressing follicle-stimulating hormone (FSH) secretion. These gonadotropin secretory changes result in arrested follicular development and increased LH-dependent ovarian androgen production, increased theca cell androgen secretion, and decreased conversion of androgens to estrogens by the immature granulosa cells. These changes lead to increased ovarian androgen produc tion, which feedback on the hypothalamic-pituitary axis, both directly by decreasing sensitivity to the normal actions of estrogen and progesterone to slow the frequency of pulsatile GnRH release, and by extragonadal aromatization to estrogen, to increase LH relative to FSH release, producing a self-sustaining syndrome. E_2, estradiol; T, testosterone. (*Courtesy of* Andrea Dunaif, MD, Boston, MA; with permission.)

Under normal circumstances, the theca cells of the ovarian follicles produce androgens under the control of LH. These androgens are then aromatized into estrogens, primarily estradiol, by the adjacent granulosa cells.[22] FSH stimulates the granulosa cell growth and aromatase capacity. In PCOS, elevated LH levels stimulate enhanced theca cell androgen production. PCOS theca cells also have increased activity of multiple steroidogenic enzymes and produce increased amounts of androgens under basal circumstances as well as in response to LH.[22,23] Because of the acyclic FSH levels, there is arrested ovarian follicular development and decreased granulosa cell aromatase capacity, resulting in decreased conversion of androgens to estrogens. Increased adrenal androgen secretion is a common finding is PCOS, most likely caused by a shared defect in the steroid biosynthetic pathways common to the ovary and adrenals. The primary defect that initiates the reproductive features of PCOS remains unknown, because it has been shown experimentally that increasing either androgen levels[4] or GnRH release[24] can produce features of PCOS. However, the intrinsic abnormalities in thecal steroidogenesis taken together with recent family and genetic studies suggest that abnormalities in androgen biosynthesis may be a primary defect in many cases.[25]

An additional biochemical hallmark of PCOS is increased ovarian and, frequently, adrenal androgen production.[26] There is increased activity of multiple steroidogenic enzymes common to the ovaries and the adrenal glands. This abnormality is accounted for in part by increased transcription of genes encoding for steroidogenic enzymes, including 3-β-hydroxysteroid dehydrogenase (3β-HSD), cytochrome P450 enzyme 17α-hydroxylase (P450c17), and 20α-hydroxysteroid dehydrogenase (20α-HSD), as well as increased mRNA accumulation of cholesterol side-chain cleavage enzyme (P450scc), 3β-HSD, P450c17, and 20α-HSD.

Insulin Resistance and Pancreatic β-Cell Dysfunction

Although insulin resistance is a common feature of PCOS, not all women with PCOS are insulin resistant.[27] The insulin resistance in PCOS has been characterized in adipocytes by a post-binding defect in the insulin receptor-mediated signal transduction, which has also been confirmed in clinical studies of skeletal muscle action.[28] In addition, skin fibroblasts were used to demonstrate that defects in insulin signaling resulted from impaired insulin receptor tyrosine kinase activity.[27] This impairment has been determined to be secondary to increased receptor serine phosphorylation due to a serine kinase extrinsic to the receptor, which leads to selective resistance to the metabolic actions of insulin.[29]

In addition to insulin resistance, β-cell dysfunction is present in PCOS, and it is the combination of these two derangements that contributes to the development of type 2 diabetes mellitus (T2DM).[30] The β-cell dysfunction seen in women with PCOS has been evidenced by several methods demonstrating impaired insulin secretion response to glucose, and exists independently of impairment in glucose tolerance. Of note, the impaired insulin secretory response was observed most convincingly among the women who had first-degree family members with T2DM.

Impaired glucose tolerance (IGT) and T2DM are both increased in women with PCOS compared with women of similar body mass index (BMI; calculated as the weight in kilograms divided by height in meters squared, ie, kg/m^2) with regular menses.[31] In fact, in a large study of glucose intolerance among women with PCOS, 38.6% of the PCOS women had either IGT (31.1%) or diabetes (7.5%) by World Health Organization criteria. Of note, when examining the nonobese women with PCOS, 10.3% had IGT and 1.5% had diabetes.[31]

Obesity

Obesity is present in 30% to 70% of women with PCOS, depending on PCOS diagnostic criteria used and race/ethnicity of the population.[14,22] Conversely, one study showed that 30% of morbidly obese women met criteria for PCOS compared with 5% of the lean population.[32] The role of obesity in the development of PCOS has been supported by a prospective study revealing that abdominal obesity and weight gain after puberty were associated with the development of PCOS.[33] Obesity has also been shown to exacerbate the clinical complications of PCOS, including insulin resistance,[27] hirsutism,[34] and the prevalence of infertility.[35] Of note, bariatric surgery and correction of obesity have been shown to result in resolution of PCOS characteristics.[32]

Genetic Susceptibility

The etiology of PCOS is unknown; however, several possible mechanisms have been postulated. In addition to the abnormal gonadotropin secretion and androgen excess previously discussed, the high heritability of PCOS characteristics suggests a genetic susceptibility to the disorder.[25,36,37] Candidate gene studies were initiated, which examined genes associated with steroid hormone biosynthesis, gonadotropin, obesity, energy regulation, and insulin action.[38,39] However, the only susceptibility locus that has been replicated is a dinucleotide repeat polymorphism within an intron of the fibrillin-3 gene on chromosome 19.[40,41]

ASSOCIATED METABOLIC DISORDERS

PCOS is characterized by multiple metabolic derangements, which may contribute to the development of hypertension and cardiovascular disease seen in this condition. However, it must be noted that although women with PCOS manifest several cardiovascular disease risk factors, there have been no long-term prospective studies in women with PCOS that confirm the presence of increased cardiovascular disease events.[42] One study employed menstrual irregularity as a proxy for PCOS in a prospective cohort study of 82,439 female nurses aged 20 to 35 years.[43] During a 14-year follow-up, women with "usually irregular" or "very irregular" menstrual cycles had an increased risk for nonfatal or fatal coronary heart disease compared with women with "very regular" menstrual cycles (age-adjusted relative risks [RR], 1.25 and 1.67, respectively; 95% confidence intervals [CI], 1.07–1.47 and 1.35–2.06, respectively); a finding that was still significant after adjusting for BMI. There was also an insignificant increase in overall stroke risk (RR, 1.30; 95% CI, 0.97–1.74) and in ischemic stroke risk (RR, 1.40; 95% CI, 0.97–2.04) associated with "very irregular" menstrual cycles.

Metabolic Syndrome

Metabolic syndrome has been variably defined by several international organizations.[44-49] However, all of the definitions include measures of central obesity, glucose intolerance, dyslipidemia, and high blood pressure. The prevalence of the metabolic syndrome in PCOS has been reported to be 43% to 47%, which is twice as high as the prevalence in the general population of comparable age, even after adjusting for BMI.[50] The components of the metabolic syndrome most commonly present in PCOS are central obesity and low serum high-density lipoprotein cholesterol (HDL); however, elevated blood pressure, impaired fasting glucose, and glucose intolerance are commonly present.[50] There is also an increased prevalence of metabolic syndrome among the sisters of women with PCOS.[51]

Dyslipidemia

The dyslipidemia in PCOS is similar to that seen in metabolic syndrome,[52] character-ized by low levels of HDL, small particle size of low-density lipoprotein cholesterol (LDL), and high triglyceride cholesterol levels.[53] This pattern is more often seen in obese than in lean PCOS, likely secondary to the presence of greater insulin resistance in obesity.[4] The level of LDL cholesterol is also increased in women with PCOS and is less dependent on obesity than are HDL and triglyceride levels.[54] There is also evidence for heritability of dyslipidemia, so these lipid patterns can be seen not only in women with PCOS but also in their family members.[51]

Hypertension

Several studies suggest an increased prevalence of hypertension in women with PCOS compared with the general population.[55–62] However, a factor complicating the interpretation of the studies is that obesity, which is common in PCOS, is itself a significant risk factor for hypertension, and this variable was not consistently consid-ered in many studies. Moreover, in the studies that did adjust the analyses for BMI, either statistically or by study design involving matching control women by BMI, the association between hypertension and PCOS was not always clear.

Several studies demonstrated an association between PCOS and hypertension, but did not adjust for an elevated BMI. A Dutch study of PCOS women demonstrated a higher prevalence of hypertension among premenopausal women with PCOS compared with women without PCOS; however, the PCOS population was signifi-cantly more obese and the obesity could have been responsible for the greater prev-alence of hypertension in this population.[59] In addition, hypertension was examined in menopausal women with PCOS who had undergone ovarian wedge resection.[63] This surgical procedure was the first established treatment for women with PCOS[64] and was commonly performed prior to the 1970s; however, it was discontinued because of the ovarian adhesions that often followed this procedure.[65] This study revealed that menopausal women after ovarian wedge resection had a threefold increased like-lihood of being hypertensive compared with non-PCOS women.[63] These women with PCOS were also more obese than controls, and this comparison was not adjusted for BMI. Although this study examined a postmenopausal population, the full burden of hypertension in PCOS has not been assessed because women with PCOS have not been followed prospectively beyond their reproductive years. One study that attemp-ted to address this question was that of Wild and colleagues,[62] who conducted a retro-spective examination of women with PCOS diagnosed an average of 31 years previously and found an increased prevalence of hypertension compared with a cohort of control women. However, given the study design, BMI was not considered in the statistical analysis, and differences in BMI may explain the association with hypertension.

Additional studies demonstrated an association between PCOS and hypertension controlling for the influence of BMI. In one study, women with PCOS were 40% more likely to have elevated blood pressure than the non-PCOS women, independent of age, BMI, diabetes, or dyslipidemia (odds ratio [OR] 1.41, 95% CI 1.31–1.51).[19] Another population study from Brazil demonstrated similar findings in 69 women with PCOS when divided by BMI into normal, overweight, and obese categories, and revealed a hypertension prevalence of 20.3%; 78.6% of these were obese and 21.4% were overweight.[66] An examination of a Czech population of PCOS women in their early 30s compared with non-PCOS women revealed that, after adjusting for BMI, PCOS women had higher blood pressure.[58] In a population of Dutch women with PCOS aged 45 to 54 years, the prevalence of hypertension was 2.5 times greater than that of an age-matched Dutch female population.[59] Of note, the proportion of obese women with PCOS in this age group did not differ significantly from the control population.

In addition, an investigation of daytime ambulatory blood pressure monitoring (ABPM) among young (mean age approximately 26 years) overweight women (mean BMI approximately 26) revealed women with PCOS had higher blood pressures compared with regularly-menstruating control women. The women with PCOS compared with controls, although all normotensive, had systolic blood pressures in the prehypertensive range (mean ± SD, 126 ± 11 vs 119 ± 12 mm Hg, $P<.05$) and was independent of BMI.[60]

In addition to BMI, hypertension among women with PCOS may be affected by other background characteristics of the individual, such as race and ethnicity.[19] The investigation by Lo and colleagues[19] demonstrated that among women with PCOS, the prevalence of hypertension or elevated blood pressure was lowest among Asians and Hispanics and highest among Blacks. Even after adjusting for age, BMI, and diabetes status, Blacks had the highest (OR 1.32, 95% CI 1.19–1.38) and Hispanics had the lowest (OR 0.68, 95% CI 0.62–0.75) prevalence of blood pressure elevation when compared with the White population.

There are data to suggest that the nocturnal decrease in blood pressure characteristic of healthy vasculature is absent in women with PCOS, both in adolescent[67] and adult[68] women. In the study examining adolescent women with PCOS, there was no difference in BMI between the women who had normal glucose tolerance (NGT) and those with IGT. However, all of the women with NGT manifested normal systolic blood pressure nocturnal dipping, whereas only 40% of those PCOS women with IGT demonstrated this normal blood pressure response.[67] In adult women with PCOS, ABPM was found to be increased in 30% of women with PCOS, a finding largely explained by the increased prevalence of obesity in affected women.[68]

Other studies controlling for BMI have not revealed an association between PCOS and hypertension. A small study of 14 women with PCOS and 18 control obese women demonstrated no difference in blood pressures.[69] Another study of young lean PCOS women compared with age-matched control women did not reveal increased blood pressure among the PCOS women.[70] Conversely, a study of similarly overweight PCOS and control women did demonstrate a blood pressure discrepancy; however, the 50% prevalence of hypertension among PCOS women compared with 39% among control women did not reach statistical significance.[71] One study demonstrated that obese women with PCOS were hypertensive compared with lean PCOS and lean control women. However, the lean PCOS women were not hypertensive compared with the lean control women.[56] Similarly, in a study of 244 PCOS and an equal number of control women, BMI was a significant predictor of both systolic and diastolic blood pressure among women with PCOS.[57] In addition, there was no difference observed in ambulatory blood pressure in women with PCOS compared with control women with adjustment for BMI.[72]

Hypertension in Pregnancy

Pregnant women with PCOS have a greater risk of perinatal morbidity from pregnancy-induced hypertension (PIH) and preeclampsia (PE) than non-PCOS pregnancies, as demonstrated in a meta-analysis of pregnancy outcomes in women with PCOS compared with controls.[73] The studies included in the meta-analysis defined PIH as blood pressure 140/90 mm Hg or greater without proteinuria at a gestational age of more than 20 weeks, and defined PE as blood pressure 140/90 mm Hg or greater with proteinuria, either more than 0.3 g/24 h urine or 2+ or more on albustick at a gestational age of more than 20 weeks. The meta-analysis revealed an increased OR of nearly 3.5-fold for both PIH (OR 3.67, 95% CI 1.98–6.81), and PE (OR 3.47, 95% CI 1.95–6.17). All of the women with PCOS in the preeclampsia studies included in the meta-analysis had higher BMI than controls. However, of the 8 PIH studies included in the meta-analysis, 4 studies matched PCOS and control women on BMI, whereas in the other 4 studies PCOS women had significantly higher BMI than the control women. In addition, the control groups were mainly spontaneous conceptions as opposed to the variable assisted reproductive therapies used among the PCOS women, which may[74] or may not[75] also increase the risk of preeclampsia.

Cardiovascular Disease Risk Factors

In studies that have examined more nontraditional risk factors for coronary heart disease, including inflammatory biomarkers,[76,77] impaired vascular function,[78] and arterial stiffness,[79] derangements were not observed in the PCOS populations independent of obesity. Adiponectin, an adipokine inversely associated with atherosclerosis,[80] was also examined in PCOS and was found to be associated with insulin resistance and BMI, not with PCOS or testosterone levels.[81] An examination of plasminogen activator inhibitor 1 (PAI-1) activity and tissue plasminogen activator (tPA) mass concentration between patients with PCOS and control women demonstrated that obese women with PCOS had increased levels of PAI-1 and tPA compared with controls; however, the lean PCOS levels of these two factors did not differ from the levels seen among the control women.[82]

However, age-matched populations of women with PCOS have been found to have increased carotid intima-media thickness (cIMT) compared with control women, even after adjusting for BMI.[83–85] Another study observed that cIMT was increased and brachial artery flow-mediated dilation was decreased in women with PCOS compared with age- and BMI-matched control women.[86] Coronary artery calcification has also been observed to be greater among women with PCOS than in control women, even after adjusting for age and BMI.[87–89]

PATHOPHYSIOLOGY OF HYPERTENSION IN PCOS

Although the pathogenesis of PCOS has not yet been fully elucidated,[90] there are several mechanisms potentially responsible for the development of hypertension in PCOS (**Box 1**). Thus, the etiology of hypertension that occurs in the setting of PCOS is also multifactorial, including factors such as hyperandrogenemia, insulin resistance, obesity, and increased sympathetic nervous system activity.

Androgen Excess

There are data demonstrating that the hyperandrogenemia in PCOS women is associated with systolic and diastolic blood pressures in women with PCOS, independent

---

Box 1
Potential causes of hypertension in women with PCOS

- Hyperandrogenism
- Insulin resistance
- Obesity
- Increased sympathetic nervous system activity

of obesity or insulin resistance.[91] Androgen excess has also been associated with an increase in cIMT in women with PCOS.[85] Increased cIMT has been widely used as a reflection of preclinical atherosclerotic disease, a contributor to the development of hypertension.[92] A small study explored the relative impact of insulin resistance, another proposed cause of hypertension in this population, compared with hyperandrogenism by studying PCOS women treated with an oral contraceptive containing 35 μg of ethinyl estradiol and 2 mg of the antiandrogen cyproterone acetate (CPA-EE), to the insulin sensitizer, metformin, then measured ABPM and cIMT. The study revealed that CPA-EE use resulted in an increase in systolic, diastolic, and mean arterial blood pressures during the day whereas metformin decreased all of these measures. No differences were observed in the nighttime parameters in response to either of these therapies. In addition, there was no statistically significant change in cIMT, although there was a tendency toward reduction in PCOS women treated with either CPA-EE or metformin. This study suggests that insulin resistance is more responsible than androgen levels for the hypertension seen in women with PCOS. However, the increase in blood pressure seen with the CPA-EE relative to the metformin group may have been due to the estrogen component and may not reflect the antiandrogenic effect.

Insulin Resistance

Hypertension may be secondary to enhanced sodium retention occurring in the setting of hyperinsulinemia.[93] High insulin levels have been associated with a subsequent increase in intracellular sodium and calcium,[94] as well as an increased level of insulin-like growth factor-1 (IGF-1), which may be associated with vascular smooth muscle hypertrophy. In support of the role of insulin resistance in mediating hypertension in women with PCOS, the beneficial effects of metformin on blood pressure have been reported.[95] In addition, the insulin-sensitizing effects of metformin lead to a decrease in serum advanced glycated end products (AGEs),[96] molecules that permit the proliferation and migration of smooth muscles cells to the vascular intima.[97] Subsequently, the decrease in AGEs seen in the setting of insulin sensitizer therapy may lead to a decrease in cIMT. Moreover, other investigators have found an improvement in cIMT in response to metformin therapy in women with PCOS.[98]

Obesity

Obesity is a well-established risk factor for hypertension[99] and it has been considered the primary etiological factor implicated in the increased blood pressure in women with PCOS.[68] Current estimates internationally report that greater than 60% of women with PCOS are overweight or obese.[100-102] One population study demonstrated that women with PCOS were more than 4 times more likely to be obese (BMI $\geq$30) than non-PCOS women. In addition, blood pressure was more likely to be elevated among women who were obese than in those who were nonobese (43.1% vs 12.4%, $P<.001$).

Sympathetic Nervous System

The sympathetic nervous system has been implicated in the etiology of hypertension in this population. Greater sympathetic nerve activity was found in a study of 20 women with PCOS who were compared with 18 weight-matched and age-matched control women.[103] The sympathetic nerve activity to the muscle vascular bed among women with PCOS was increased and highly correlated with testosterone level and, to a lesser degree, the cholesterol level. In addition, androgen excess,[104] as well as insulin resistance[105] and obesity[106] have been implicated in stimulating the autonomic nervous system, each thereby serving as a potential mediator of the hypertension observed in PCOS.

Therapeutic Considerations

Therapy for PCOS is targeted toward ameliorating or eliminating the symptoms for each individual woman. Consequently, given the association of hypertension with all of the common PCOS manifestations, treating the manifestations of PCOS may treat concomitant hypertension or the risk for hypertension as well. In addition, one needs to assess hypertension in the context of assessing other cardiovascular risk factors.[107]

Treatment of hyperandrogenism revolves around the use of combination oral contraceptives (COC) or antiandrogens. However, the response to oral contraceptives has been inconsistent. The use of drospirenone, an antimineralocorticoid progestin, in combination with ethinyl estradiol, compared with use of the vaginal contraceptive ring was associated with a minimal but statistically significant increase of diurnal and 24-hour systolic blood pressure in women with PCOS (drospirenone, 5 mm Hg for both time periods, $P = .001$; and contraceptive ring, 6 mm Hg for both time periods).[108] Another study demonstrated a more convincing decrease in systolic blood pressure in response to a drospirenone containing COC of 1.9 mm Hg compared with a 1.7 mm Hg increase in systolic blood pressure in the desogestrel-containing COC group of women with PCOS.[109] However, other investigations in PCOS demonstrated no change in blood pressure with a drospirenone-containing COC.[110,111]

Another antiandrogenic therapy used in women with PCOS is spironolactone. This aldosterone antagonist has been used as a potassium-sparing diuretic in the setting of hypertension since the 1950s. It was serendipity that associated its use with improvement in hirsutism in a woman with PCOS undergoing treatment for hypertension,[112] and it has since become the most widely used antiandrogen for female pattern hair loss in the United States.[113] Studies have demonstrated the efficacy in the treatment of hirsutism in women with PCOS,[114] so its use for this indication exceeds that for hypertension among women with PCOS. In studies examining the effect of spironolactone on blood pressure, one Indian study of spironolactone versus metformin found no change in blood pressure evident with either drug.[115] In another investigation of PCOS women treated with spironolactone, 100 mg daily for 2 months, mean blood pressure decreased significantly from 118 ± 5/82 ± 4 mm Hg to 113 ± 4/72 ± 5 mm Hg ($P<.05$).[116]

Lifestyle modifications, including diet and physical activity, are critical in preventing hypertension for women with PCOS who are overweight or obese.[117] In addition, other methods of weight loss have shown promise for improving hypertension in the PCOS population. In a retrospective analysis of PCOS women who underwent a Roux-en-Y gastric bypass, normalization of blood pressure was observed in 78% of the previously hypertensive population.[118]

SUMMARY

Hypertension is a significant contributor to the risk of cardiovascular disease. The increased prevalence of hypertension in women with PCOS may contribute to the increased risk of cardiovascular disease in women with PCOS. Thus, the Androgen Excess and Polycystic Ovarian Societies recommend that blood pressure be obtained in women with PCOS at every visit and that prehypertension be detected and treated, given the potential benefit of lowering blood pressure for the prevention of CVD.[107]

Whether hypertension is associated with PCOS independent of obesity remains controversial. Nevertheless, detection and subsequent treatment of hypertension in this population should decrease the adverse sequelae from hypertensive cardiovascular disease. Moreover, treatment of the risk factors inherent to PCOS, such as hyperandrogenism, insulin resistance, and obesity, may minimize the risk not only for the development of hypertension but also for incident cardiovascular disease independent of hypertension.[107] Treatment of hypertension in the PCOS population may take the form of lifestyle modification or pharmacotherapy.

REFERENCES

1. Stein IF, Leventhal ML. Amenorrhea associated with bilateral polycystic ovaries. Am J Obstet Gynecol 1935;19:181–91.
2. Burghen GA, Givens JR, Kitabchi AE. Correlation of hyperandrogenism with hyperinsulinism in polycystic ovarian disease. J Clin Endocrinol Metab 1980; 50(1):113–6.
3. Dunaif A, Graf M, Mandeli J, et al. Characterization of groups of hyperandrogenic women with acanthosis nigricans, impaired glucose tolerance, and/or hyperinsulinemia. J Clin Endocrinol Metab 1987;65(3):499–507.
4. Dunaif A. Insulin resistance and the polycystic ovary syndrome: mechanism and implications for pathogenesis. Endocr Rev 1997;18(6):774–800.
5. Ehrmann DA. Polycystic ovary syndrome. N Engl J Med 2005;352(12):1223–36.
6. Polson DW, Adams J, Wadsworth J, et al. Polycystic ovaries—a common finding in normal women. Lancet 1988;1(8590):870–2.
7. Legro RS, Chiu P, Kunselman AR, et al. Polycystic ovaries are common in women with hyperandrogenic chronic anovulation but do not predict metabolic or reproductive phenotype. J Clin Endocrinol Metab 2005;90(5):2571–9.
8. Rotterdam ESHRE/ASRM-Sponsored PCOS Consensus Workshop Group. Revised 2003 consensus on diagnostic criteria and long-term health risks related to polycystic ovary syndrome. Fertil Steril 2004;81(1):19–25.
9. Robinson S, Kiddy D, Gelding SV, et al. The relationship of insulin insensitivity to menstrual pattern in women with hyperandrogenism and polycystic ovaries. Clin Endocrinol (Oxf) 1993;39(3):351–5.
10. Adams JM, Taylor AE, Crowley WF Jr, et al. Polycystic ovarian morphology with regular ovulatory cycles: insights into the pathophysiology of polycystic ovarian syndrome. J Clin Endocrinol Metab 2004;89(9):4343–50.
11. Azziz R, Carmina E, Dewailly D, et al. Criteria for defining polycystic ovary syndrome as a predominantly hyperandrogenic syndrome: an Androgen Excess Society guideline. J Clin Endocrinol Metab 2006;91(11):4237–45.
12. Carmina E, Lobo RA. Polycystic ovary syndrome (PCOS): arguably the most common endocrinopathy is associated with significant morbidity in women. J Clin Endocrinol Metab 1999;84:1897–9.
13. March WA, Moore VM, Willson KJ, et al. The prevalence of polycystic ovary syndrome in a community sample assessed under contrasting diagnostic criteria. Hum Reprod 2010;25(2):544–51.
14. Azziz R, Woods KS, Reyna R, et al. The prevalence and features of the polycystic ovary syndrome in an unselected population. J Clin Endocrinol Metab 2004;89(6):2745–9.
15. Asunción M, Calvo RM, San Millán JL, et al. A prospective study of the prevalence of the polycystic ovary syndrome in unselected Caucasian women from Spain. J Clin Endocrinol Metab 2000;85(7):2434–8.

16. Diamanti-Kandarakis E, Kouli CR, Bergiele AT, et al. A survey of the polycystic ovary syndrome in the Greek island of Lesbos: hormonal and metabolic profile. J Clin Endocrinol Metab 1999;84(11):4006–11.
17. Moran C, Tena G, Moran S, et al. Prevalence of polycystic ovary syndrome and related disorders in Mexican women. Gynecol Obstet Invest 2010; 69(4):274–80.
18. Knochenhauer ES, Key TJ, Kahsar-Miller M, et al. Prevalence of the polycystic ovary syndrome in unselected black and white women of the southeastern United States: a prospective study. J Clin Endocrinol Metab 1998;83(9): 3078–82.
19. Lo JC, Feigenbaum SL, Yang J, et al. Epidemiology and adverse cardiovascular risk profile of diagnosed polycystic ovary syndrome. J Clin Endocrinol Metab 2006;91(4):1357–63.
20. Marshall JC, Eagleson CA. Neuroendocrine aspects of polycystic ovary syndrome. Endocrinol Metab Clin North Am 1999;28:295–324.
21. Eagleson CA, Gingrich MB, Pastor CL, et al. Polycystic ovarian syndrome: evidence that flutamide restores sensitivity of the gonadotropin-releasing hormone pulse generator to inhibition by estradiol and progesterone. J Clin Endocrinol Metab 2000;85(11):4047–52.
22. Franks S. Polycystic ovary syndrome. Trends Endocrinol Metab 1989;1(2):60–3.
23. Nelson VL, Qin KN, Rosenfield RL, et al. The biochemical basis for increased testosterone production in theca cells propagated from patients with polycystic ovary syndrome. J Clin Endocrinol Metab 2001;86(12):5925–33.
24. Reid RL, Leopold GR, Yen SS. Induction of ovulation and pregnancy with pulsatile luteinizing hormone releasing factor: dosage and mode of delivery. Fertil Steril 1981;36(5):553–9.
25. Legro RS, Driscoll D, Strauss JF 3rd, et al. Evidence for a genetic basis for hyperandrogenemia in polycystic ovary syndrome. Proc Natl Acad Sci U S A 1998;95(25):14956–60.
26. Wickenheisser JK, Quinn PG, Nelson VL, et al. Differential activity of the cytochrome P450 17alpha-hydroxylase and steroidogenic acute regulatory protein gene promoters in normal and polycystic ovary syndrome theca cells. J Clin Endocrinol Metab 2000;85(6):2304–11.
27. Dunaif A. Insulin action in the polycystic ovary syndrome. Endocrinol Metab Clin North Am 1999;28:341–59.
28. Dunaif A, Wu X, Lee A, et al. Defects in insulin receptor signaling in vivo in the polycystic ovary syndrome (PCOS). Am J Physiol Endocrinol Metab 2001; 281(2):E392–9.
29. Book CB, Dunaif A. Selective insulin resistance in the polycystic ovary syndrome. J Clin Endocrinol Metab 1999;84(9):3110–6.
30. Ehrmann DA, Sturis J, Byrne MM, et al. Insulin secretory defects in polycystic ovary syndrome. Relationship to insulin sensitivity and family history of non-insulin-dependent diabetes mellitus. J Clin Invest 1995;96:520–7.
31. Legro RS, Kunselman AR, Dodson WC, et al. Prevalence and predictors of risk for type 2 diabetes mellitus and impaired glucose tolerance in polycystic ovary syndrome: a prospective, controlled study in 254 affected women. J Clin Endocrinol Metab 1999;84(1):165–9.
32. Escobar-Morreale HF, Botella-Carretero JI, Alvarez-Blasco F, et al. The polycystic ovary syndrome associated with morbid obesity may resolve after weight loss induced by bariatric surgery. J Clin Endocrinol Metab 2005; 90(12):6364–9.

33. Laitinen J, Taponen S, Martikainen H, et al. Body size from birth to adulthood as a predictor of self-reported polycystic ovary syndrome symptoms. Int J Obes Relat Metab Disord 2003;27(6):710–5.
34. Hoeger KM. Obesity and lifestyle management in polycystic ovary syndrome. Clin Obstet Gynecol 2007;50(1):277–94.
35. Grodstein F, Goldman MB, Cramer DW. Body mass index and ovulatory infertility. Epidemiology 1994;5(2):247–50.
36. Legro RS, Kunselman AR, Demers L, et al. Elevated dehydroepiandrosterone sulfate levels as the reproductive phenotype in the brothers of women with polycystic ovary syndrome. J Clin Endocrinol Metab 2002;87(5):2134–8.
37. Legro RS, Bentley-Lewis R, Driscoll D, et al. Insulin resistance in the sisters of women with polycystic ovary syndrome: association with hyperandrogenemia rather than menstrual irregularity. J Clin Endocrinol Metab 2002;87(5):2128–33.
38. Urbanek M, Legro RS, Driscoll DA, et al. Thirty-seven candidate genes for polycystic ovary syndrome: strongest evidence for linkage is with follistatin. Proc Natl Acad Sci U S A 1999;96(15):8573–8.
39. Urbanek M, Wu X, Vickery KR, et al. Allelic variants of the follistatin gene in polycystic ovary syndrome. J Clin Endocrinol Metab 2000;85(12):4455–61.
40. Urbanek M, Sam S, Legro RS, et al. Identification of a polycystic ovary syndrome susceptibility variant in fibrillin-3 and association with a metabolic phenotype. J Clin Endocrinol Metab 2007;92(11):4191–8.
41. Ewens KG, Stewart DR, Ankener W, et al. Family-based analysis of candidate genes for polycystic ovary syndrome. J Clin Endocrinol Metab 2010;95(5):2306–15.
42. Legro RS. Polycystic ovary syndrome and cardiovascular disease: a premature association? Endocr Rev 2003;24(3):302–12.
43. Solomon CG, Hu FB, Dunaif A, et al. Menstrual cycle irregularity and risk for future cardiovascular disease. J Clin Endocrinol Metab 2002;87(5):2013–7.
44. National Cholesterol Education Program (NCEP) Expert Panel on Detection E and Treatment of High Blood Cholesterol in Adults (Adult Treatment Panel III). Third Report of the National Cholesterol Education Program (NCEP) expert panel on detection, evaluation, and treatment of high blood cholesterol in adults (Adult Treatment Panel III) final report. Circulation 2002;106:3143–421.
45. Grundy SM, Cleeman JI, Daniels SR, et al. Diagnosis and management of the metabolic syndrome: an American Heart Association/National Heart, Lung, and Blood Institute scientific statement. Circulation 2005;112(17):2735–52.
46. Einhorn D, Reaven GM, Cobin RH, et al. American College of Endocrinology position statement on the insulin resistance syndrome. Endocr Pract 2003;9(3):237–52.
47. International Diabetes Federation. Worldwide definition of the metabolic syndrome. 2006. Available at: http://www.idf.org/webdata/docs/MetS_def_update2006.pdf. Accessed March 7, 2011.
48. Balkau B, Charles MA. Comment on the provisional report from the WHO consultation. European Group for the Study of Insulin Resistance (EGIR). Diabet Med 1999;16:442–3.
49. Alberti KG, Zimmet PZ. Definition, diagnosis and classification of diabetes mellitus and its complications. Part 1: diagnosis and classification of diabetes mellitus provisional report of a WHO consultation. Diabet Med 1998;15:539–53.
50. Essah PA, Nestler JE. Metabolic syndrome in women with polycystic ovary syndrome. Fertil Steril 2006;86:S18–9.

51. Sam S, Legro RS, Bentley-Lewis R, et al. Dyslipidemia and metabolic syndrome in the sisters of women with polycystic ovary syndrome. J Clin Endocrinol Metab 2005;90(8):4797–802.
52. Bentley-Lewis R, Koruda K, Seely EW. The metabolic syndrome in women. Nat Clin Pract Endocrinol Metab 2007;3(10):696–704.
53. Legato MJ. Dyslipidemia, gender, and the role of high-density lipoprotein cholesterol: implications for therapy. Am J Cardiol 2000;86(12A):15L–8L.
54. Valkenburg O, Steegers-Theunissen RP, Smedts HP, et al. A more atherogenic serum lipoprotein profile is present in women with polycystic ovary syndrome: a case-control study. J Clin Endocrinol Metab 2008;93(2):470–6.
55. Carmina E. Cardiovascular risk and events in polycystic ovary syndrome. Climacteric 2009;12(Suppl 1):22–5.
56. Conway GS, Agrawal R, Betteridge DJ, et al. Risk factors for coronary artery disease in lean and obese women with the polycystic ovary syndrome. Clin Endocrinol (Oxf) 1992;37(2):119–25.
57. Talbott E, Clerici A, Berga SL, et al. Adverse lipid and coronary heart disease risk profiles in young women with polycystic ovary syndrome: results of a case-control study. J Clin Epidemiol 1998;51(5):415–22.
58. Vrbíková J, Cífková R, Jirkovská A, et al. Cardiovascular risk factors in young Czech females with polycystic ovary syndrome. Hum Reprod 2003;18(5): 980–4.
59. Elting MW, Korsen TJ, Bezemer PD, et al. Prevalence of diabetes mellitus, hypertension and cardiac complaints in a follow-up study of a Dutch PCOS population. Hum Reprod 2001;16(3):556–60.
60. Holte J, Gennarelli G, Berne C, et al. Elevated ambulatory day-time blood pressure in women with polycystic ovary syndrome: a sign of a pre-hypertensive state? Hum Reprod 1996;11(1):23–8.
61. Orbetzova MM, Shigarminova RG, Genchev GG, et al. Role of 24-hour monitoring in assessing blood pressure changes in polycystic ovary syndrome. Folia Med (Plovdiv) 2003;45(3):21–5.
62. Wild S, Pierpoint T, Jacobs H, et al. Long-term consequences of polycystic ovary syndrome: results of a 31 year follow-up study. Hum Fertil (Camb) 2000;3(2):101–5.
63. Dahlgren E, Johansson S, Lindstedt G, et al. Women with polycystic ovary syndrome wedge resected in 1956 to 1965: a long-term follow-up focusing on natural history and circulating hormones. Fertil Steril 1992;57(3):505–13.
64. Farquhar C, Lilford RJ, Marjoribanks J, et al. Laparoscopic 'drilling' by diathermy or laser for ovulation induction in anovulatory polycystic ovary syndrome. Cochrane Database Syst Rev 2007;3:CD001122.
65. Buttram VC, Vaquero C. Post-ovarian wedge resection adhesive disease. Fertil Steril 1975;26:874–6.
66. Barcellos CR, Rocha MP, Hayashida SA, et al. Impact of body mass index on blood pressure levels in patients with polycystic ovary syndrome. Arq Bras Endocrinol Metabol 2007;51(7):1104–9.
67. Arslanian SA, Lewy VD, Danadian K. Glucose intolerance in obese adolescents with polycystic ovary syndrome: roles of insulin resistance and beta-cell dysfunction and risk of cardiovascular disease. J Clin Endocrinol Metab 2001; 86(1):66–71.
68. Luque-Ramírez M, Alvarez-Blasco F, Mendieta-Azcona C, et al. Obesity is the major determinant of the abnormalities in blood pressure found in young women with the polycystic ovary syndrome. J Clin Endocrinol Metab 2007;92(6):2141–8.

69. Zimmermann S, Phillips RA, Dunaif A, et al. Polycystic ovary syndrome: lack of hypertension despite profound insulin resistance. J Clin Endocrinol Metab 1992; 75(2):508–13.

70. Sampson M, Kong C, Patel A, et al. Ambulatory blood pressure profiles and plasminogen activator inhibitor (PAI-1) activity in lean women with and without the polycystic ovary syndrome. Clin Endocrinol (Oxf) 1996;45(5):623–9.

71. Cibula D, Cífková R, Fanta M, et al. Increased risk of non-insulin dependent diabetes mellitus, arterial hypertension and coronary artery disease in perimenopausal women with a history of the polycystic ovary syndrome. Hum Reprod 2000;15(4):785–9.

72. Meyer C, McGrath BP, Teede HJ. Overweight women with polycystic ovary syndrome have evidence of subclinical cardiovascular disease. J Clin Endocrinol Metab 2005;90(10):5711–6.

73. Boomsma CM, Fauser BC, Macklon NS. Pregnancy complications in women with polycystic ovary syndrome. Semin Reprod Med 2008;26(1):72–84.

74. Ludwig M. Risk during pregnancy and birth after assisted reproductive technologies: an integral view of the problem. Semin Reprod Med 2005;23(4): 363–70.

75. Sun LM, Walker MC, Cao HL, et al. Assisted reproductive technology and placenta-mediated adverse pregnancy outcomes. Obstet Gynecol 2009; 114(4):818–24.

76. Möhlig M, Spranger J, Osterhoff M, et al. The polycystic ovary syndrome per se is not associated with increased chronic inflammation. Eur J Endocrinol 2004; 150(4):525–32.

77. Escobar-Morreale HF, Villuendas G, Botella-Carretero JI, et al. Obesity, and not insulin resistance, is the major determinant of serum inflammatory cardiovascular risk markers in pre-menopausal women. Diabetologia 2003;46(5):625–33.

78. Ketel IJ, Stehouwer CD, Serné EH, et al. Obese but not normal-weight women with polycystic ovary syndrome are characterized by metabolic and microvascular insulin resistance. J Clin Endocrinol Metab 2008;93(9):3365–72.

79. Ketel IJ, Stehouwer CD, Henry RM, et al. Greater arterial stiffness in polycystic ovary syndrome (PCOS) is an obesity—but not a PCOS-associated phenomenon. J Clin Endocrinol Metab 2010;95(10):4566–75.

80. Libby P, Okamoto Y, Rocha VZ, et al. Inflammation in atherosclerosis: transition from theory to practice. Circ J 2010;74(2):213–20.

81. Spranger J, Möhlig M, Wegewitz U, et al. Adiponectin is independently associated with insulin sensitivity in women with polycystic ovary syndrome. Clin Endocrinol (Oxf) 2004;61(6):738–46.

82. Lindholm A, Bixo M, Eliasson M, et al. Tissue plasminogen activator and plasminogen activator inhibitor 1 in obese and lean patients with polycystic ovary syndrome. Gynecol Endocrinol 2010;26(10):743–8.

83. Guzick DS, Talbott EO, Sutton-Tyrrell K, et al. Carotid atherosclerosis in women with polycystic ovary syndrome: initial results from a case-control study. Am J Obstet Gynecol 1996;174:1224–32.

84. Talbott EO, Guzick DS, Sutton-Tyrrell K, et al. Evidence for association between polycystic ovary syndrome and premature carotid atherosclerosis in middle-aged women. Arterioscler Thromb Vasc Biol 2000;20:2414–21.

85. Luque-Ramírez M, Mendieta-Azcona C, Alvarez-Blasco F, et al. Androgen excess is associated with the increased carotid intima-media thickness observed in young women with polycystic ovary syndrome. Hum Reprod 2007;22(12): 3197–203.

86. Carmina E, Orio F, Palomba S, et al. Endothelial dysfunction in PCOS: role of obesity and adipose hormones. Am J Med 2006;119(4):356.e1–6.
87. Christian RC, Dumesic DA, Behrenbeck T, et al. Prevalence and predictors of coronary artery calcification in women with polycystic ovary syndrome. J Clin Endocrinol Metab 2003;88:2562–8.
88. Talbott EO, Zborowski JV, Rager JR, et al. Evidence for an association between metabolic cardiovascular syndrome and coronary and aortic calcification among women with polycystic ovary syndrome. J Clin Endocrinol Metab 2004;89:5454–61.
89. Talbott EO, Zborowski J, Rager J, et al. Is there an independent effect of polycystic ovary syndrome (PCOS) and menopause on the prevalence of subclinical atherosclerosis in middle aged women? Vasc Health Risk Manag 2008;4(2):453–62.
90. Norman RJ, Dewailly D, Legro RS, et al. Polycystic ovary syndrome. Lancet 2007;370(9588):685–97.
91. Chen MJ, Yang WS, Yang JH, et al. Relationship between androgen levels and blood pressure in young women with polycystic ovary syndrome. Hypertension 2007;49(6):1442–7.
92. Riccioni G. The effect of antihypertensive drugs on carotid intima media thickness: an up-to-date review. Curr Med Chem 2009;16(8):988–96.
93. Zavaroni I, Coruzzi P, Bonini L, et al. Association between salt sensitivity and insulin concentrations in patients with hypertension. Am J Hypertens 1995;8(8):855–8.
94. Resnick LM. Cellular ions in hypertension, insulin resistance, obesity, and diabetes: a unifying theme. J Am Soc Nephrol 1992;3(Suppl 4):S78–85.
95. Lord JM, Flight IH, Norman RJ. Insulin-sensitising drugs (metformin, troglitazone, rosiglitazone, pioglitazone, D-chiro-inositol) for polycystic ovary syndrome. Cochrane Database Syst Rev 2003;3:CD003053.
96. Diamanti-Kandarakis E, Alexandraki K, Piperi C, et al. Effect of metformin administration on plasma advanced glycation end product levels in women with polycystic ovary syndrome. Metabolism 2007;56(1):129–34.
97. Hattori Y, Suzuki M, Hattori S, et al. Vascular smooth muscle cell activation by glycated albumin (Amadori adducts). Hypertension 2002;39(1):22–8.
98. Orio F Jr, Palomba S, Cascella T, et al. Improvement in endothelial structure and function after metformin treatment in young normal-weight women with polycystic ovary syndrome: results of a 6-month study. J Clin Endocrinol Metab 2005;90(11):6072–6.
99. Kannel WB. Fifty years of Framingham study contributions to understanding hypertension. J Hum Hypertens 2000;14(2):83–90.
100. Cupisti S, Kajaia N, Dittrich R, et al. Body mass index and ovarian function are associated with endocrine and metabolic abnormalities in women with hyperandrogenic syndrome. Eur J Endocrinol 2008;158(5):711–9.
101. Glintborg D, Henriksen JE, Andersen M, et al. Prevalence of endocrine diseases and abnormal glucose tolerance tests in 340 Caucasian premenopausal women with hirsutism as the referral diagnosis. Fertil Steril 2004;82(6):1570–9.
102. Azziz R, Sanchez LA, Knochenhauer ES, et al. Androgen excess in women: experience with over 1000 consecutive patients. J Clin Endocrinol Metab 2004;89(2):453–62.
103. Sverrisdottir YB, Mogren T, Kataoka J, et al. Is polycystic ovary syndrome associated with high sympathetic nerve activity and size at birth? Am J Physiol Endocrinol Metab 2008;294:E576–81.

104. Yildirir A, Aybar F, Kabakci G, et al. Heart rate variability in young women with polycystic ovary syndrome. Ann Noninvasive Electrocardiol 2006;11(4):306–12.
105. Muniyappa R, Montagnani M, Koh KK, et al. Cardiovascular actions of insulin. Endocr Rev 2007;28(5):463–91.
106. Müller-Wieland D, Kotzka J, Knebel B, et al. Metabolic syndrome and hypertension: pathophysiology and molecular basis of insulin resistance. Basic Res Cardiol 1998;93(Suppl 2):131–4.
107. Wild RA, Carmina E, Diamanti-Kandarakis E, et al. Assessment of cardiovascular risk and prevention of cardiovascular disease in women with the polycystic ovary syndrome: a consensus statement by the Androgen Excess and Polycystic Ovary Syndrome (AE-PCOS) Society. J Clin Endocrinol Metab 2010; 95(5):2038–49.
108. Battaglia C, Mancini F, Fabbri R, et al. Polycystic ovary syndrome and cardiovascular risk in young patients treated with drospirenone-ethinylestradiol or contraceptive vaginal ring. A prospective, randomized, pilot study. Fertil Steril 2010;94(4):1417–25.
109. Kriplani A, Periyasamy AJ, Agarwal N, et al. Effect of oral contraceptive containing ethinyl estradiol combined with drospirenone vs. desogestrel on clinical and biochemical parameters in patients with polycystic ovary syndrome. Contraception 2010;82(2):139–46.
110. Fruzzetti F, Perini D, Lazzarini V, et al. Comparison of effects of 3 mg drospirenone plus 20 µg ethinyl estradiol alone or combined with metformin or cyproterone acetate on classic metabolic cardiovascular risk factors in nonobese women with polycystic ovary syndrome. Fertil Steril 2010;94(5):1793–8.
111. Guido M, Romualdi D, Giuliani M, et al. Drospirenone for the treatment of hirsute women with polycystic ovary syndrome: a clinical, endocrinological, metabolic pilot study. J Clin Endocrinol Metab 2004;89(6):2817–23.
112. Ober KP, Hennessy JF. Spironolactone therapy for hirsutism in a hyperandrogenic woman. Ann Intern Med 1978;89:643–4.
113. Rathnayake D, Sinclair R. Innovative use of spironolactone as an antiandrogen in the treatment of female pattern hair loss. Dermatol Clin 2010;28(3):611–8.
114. Christy NA, Franks AS, Cross LB. Spironolactone for hirsutism in polycystic ovary syndrome. Ann Pharmacother 2005;39(9):1517–21.
115. Ganie MA, Khurana ML, Eunice M, et al. Comparison of efficacy of spironolactone with metformin in the management of polycystic ovary syndrome: an open-labeled study. J Clin Endocrinol Metab 2004;89(6):2756–62.
116. Armanini D, Castello R, Scaroni C, et al. Treatment of polycystic ovary syndrome with spironolactone plus licorice. Eur J Obstet Gynecol Reprod Biol 2007; 131(1):61–7.
117. Norman RJ, Davies MJ, Lord J, et al. The role of lifestyle modification in polycystic ovary syndrome. Trends Endocrinol Metab 2002;13(6):251–7.
118. Eid GM, Cottam DR, Velcu LM, et al. Effective treatment of polycystic ovarian syndrome with Roux-en-Y gastric bypass. Surg Obes Relat Dis 2005;1(2): 77–80.

Index

Note: Page numbers of article titles are in **boldface** type.

A

ACTH. See *Adrenocorticotropic hormone (ACTH)*.
Adrenal synthetic defects, in low-renin hypertension of childhood, 369–372
Adrenal vein sampling, in primary aldosteronism evaluation, 322–324
Adrenal-endocrine hypertension, screening for, **279–294**. See also *Hypertension, adrenal-endocrine, screening for.*
Adrenocorticotropic hormone (ACTH), Cushing syndrome due to, 393–394
Aldosterone/renin ratio (ARR), in primary aldosteronism evaluation, 286, 319–320
   diagnostic accuracy of, 286–288
Aldosteronism
   glucocorticoid-remediable, **333–341**. See also *Glucocorticoid-remediable aldosteronism (GRA).*
   primary, **343–354**. See also *Primary aldosteronism.*
AME. See *Apparent mineralocorticoid excess (AME).*
Androgen excess, hypertension in PCOS and, 440–441
Apparent mineralocorticoid excess (AME)
   genetics of, 374
   in low-renin hypertension of childhood, 373–376
   mild forms of, 376
   pathophysiology of, 373
   treatment of, 374–375
L-Arginine, availability and delivery of, in nitric oxide synthesis, 397–398
ARR. See *Aldosterone/renin ratio (ARR).*

B

Blood pressure
   in Cushing's syndrome, physiology of, 381–382
   oral contraceptives effects on, **419–432**. See also *Hypertension, OCP-induced.*

C

Cardiovascular disease, PCOS and, 440
Cardiovascular system
   glucocorticoid effects on, **409–417**
   hypercatecholamine effects on, 301–303
   OCP effects on, 423–426
      raloxifene, 428–429
Catecholamine(s)
   action of, 296–298

Endocrinol Metab Clin N Am 40 (2011) 451–458
doi:10.1016/S0889-8529(11)00044-2
0889-8529/11/$ – see front matter © 2011 Elsevier Inc. All rights reserved.

endo.theclinics.com

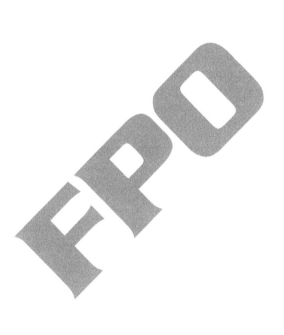

Moving?

Make sure your subscription moves with you!

To notify us of your new address, find your **Clinics Account Number** (located on your mailing label above your name), and contact customer service at:

Email: journalscustomerservice-usa@elsevier.com

800-654-2452 (subscribers in the U.S. & Canada)
314-447-8871 (subscribers outside of the U.S. & Canada)

Fax number: 314-447-8029

Elsevier Health Sciences Division
Subscription Customer Service
3251 Riverport Lane
Maryland Heights, MO 63043

*To ensure uninterrupted delivery of your subscription, please notify us at least 4 weeks in advance of move.

Printed and bound by CPI Group (UK) Ltd, Croydon, CR0 4YY

03/10/2024

01040446-0001